Med-Math

*Dosage Calculation,
Preparation and Administration*

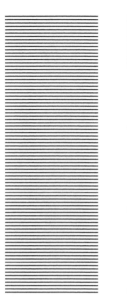

Med-Math

*Dosage
Calculation,
Preparation
and
Administration*

Grace Henke, S.C., R.N., M.S.N., Ed.D.

*Instructor
St. Vincent's Hospital School of Nursing
New York, New York
Adjunct Professor
College of Mount St. Vincent
Riverdale, New York*

J. B. LIPPINCOTT COMPANY
Philadelphia

New York   St. Louis   London   Sydney   Tokyo

Acquisitions Editor: Ellen M. Campbell
Coordinating Editorial Assistant: Amy Stonehouse
Project Editor: Tom Gibbons
Indexer: Mary Rose Muccie
Art Director: Ellen C. Dawson
Cover Designer: Miriam Recio
Interior Designer: Ellen C. Dawson
Production Manager: Helen Ewan
Production Coordinator: Sharon McCarthy
Compositor: TAPSCO
Printer/Binder: Murray Printing Company

1 3 5 6 4 2

Library of Congress Cataloging-in-Publication Data

Henke, Grace.
  Med-math : dosage calculation, preparation and administration /
Grace Henke.
    p.   cm.
  Includes index.
  ISBN 0-397-54792-7 (paper)
  1. Pharmaceutical arithmetic.   I. Title.
  [DNLM: 1. Drugs—administration & dosage—nurses' instruction.
2. Drugs—administration & dosage—programmed instruction.
3. Mathematics—nurses' instruction.   4. Mathematics—programmed
instruction.   QV   18 H512m]
  RS57.H46   1990
  615.5'8'01513—dc20
  DNLM/DLC
  for Library of Congress   90-6484
                                                              CIP

Any procedure or practice described in this book should be applied by the health-care practitioner under appropriate supervision in accordance with professional standards of care used with regard to the unique circumstances that apply in each practice situation. Care has been taken to confirm the accuracy of information presented and to describe generally accepted practices. However, the authors, editors, and publisher cannot accept any responsibility for errors or omissions or for any consequences from application of the information in this book and make no warranty, express or implied, with respect to the contents of the book.

Every effort has been made to ensure drug selections and dosages are in accordance with current recommendations and practice. Because of ongoing research, changes in government regulations and the constant flow of information on drug therapy, reactions and interactions, the reader is cautioned to check the package insert for each drug for indications, dosages, warnings and precautions, particularly if the drug is new or infrequently used.

For my students past and present
and
for my mother
You all light up my life

Preface

Med-Math: Dosage Calculation, Preparation and Administration is a clinically oriented, self-instructional learning tool that provides practical information about the proper dosage and administration of medications. Designed to meet the needs of students in every type of nursing program, it is suitable for any health care professional who administers drugs, including practicing nurses in need of review and nurses returning to practice after some time.

The workbook takes a step-by-step approach to dosage calculation, preparation, and administration in order to improve the reader's understanding of the basic knowledge and specific skills needed. Students in introductory courses should complete the chapters in order. Practicing nurses using the workbook as a refresher may wish to do the dosage competency tests in Chapter 11 and then return to beginning chapters as needed to drill in identified areas of weakness.

Chapter 1 explains the language of prescriptions and demonstrates how to interpret medication orders. Chapter 2 describes how to read and interpret drug labels. Chapter 3 reviews mathematical operations needed to solve dosage problems. Multiplication and division tables are provided, along with exercises designed to test the reader's knowledge of basic math. These are important and necessary drills for students who experience difficulty in calculation and even for those who do not, since, regardless of how proficient one is in mathematics, careless medication errors still can occur. Therefore, students should not skip this arithmetic review; those who believe their skills are satisfactory should at least complete the practice exercises.

The reader is encouraged to practice solving dosage problems mentally or, if necessary, using paper and pencil rather than a calculator. Doing so makes one think logically about the dosage problem and then evaluate the answer in relation to the physician's order; it will increase speed and efficiency in preparing medications.

In Chapter 4 the reader studies the differences between measurement systems and learns how to convert measures from one system to another. Chapter 5 describes types of drug preparations and the equipment used to measure doses.

Chapters 6 through 9 present dosage problems by route of administration: oral solids and oral liquids in Chapter 6, injections from liquids in Chapter 7, injections from powders in Chapter 8, and intravenous and "piggyback" drips in Chapter 9. Directions found on actual drug labels and package inserts are included for problems involving the dilution of powders, and drawings of syringes and oral liquid measurement cups are also included to help the student visualize the correct answer as an actual dose.

In Chapter 10, the student practices solving dosage problems for infants and children and determines the safety of each dose based on body weight and body surface area. Chapter 11 offers a series of dosage competency tests for review or further drill.

Chapter 12 provides the student with important drug information essential to the safe administration of medications, including legal considerations concerning medications, how to handle errors in medication, and how malpractice claims can be avoided. Ethical principles are also addressed. The chapter concludes with a listing of practical points.

Chapter 13 discusses the Universal Safeguards recommended by the Centers for Disease Control (CDC) as they apply to the administration of medications. These procedural guidelines are advocated by the CDC in order to protect health care workers from hepatitis B virus and the human immunodeficiency virus (HIV); those presented here concern the administration of oral, injectable, and topical drugs. The use of tickets, unit dose packaging, stock containers, and the mobile cart is also discussed.

Throughout the workbook, dosage problems, presented as physicians' orders, range from simple to complex. Easy-to-learn formulas and a step-by-step approach aid the reader in solving the problems; abundant examples and practice problems allow the reader to test his or her new knowledge and skills before proceeding to the next chapter. Answers to all problems are provided at the end of each chapter.

Med-Math: Dosage Calculation, Preparation and Administration offers a down-to-earth approach to the calculation and administration of drug dosages. It is my hope that this knowledge will instill a sense of confidence in the reader, ensuring that the right drug in the right dose is given to the right patient at the right time by the right route!

Sister Grace Henke

Acknowledgments

I am grateful to many colleagues and friends for their support and encouragement, especially Sister Mary Robert, R.N., M.S., M.Ed., Director, School of Nursing; Sister Miriam Kevin, R.N., M.S., M.Ed., Associate Director; and Virginia Sweeny, R.N., M.S., C.N.A.A., Vice President for Nursing at St. Vincent's Hospital and Medical Center.

I wish to extend sincere appreciation to the following persons who reviewed and validated content and made pertinent suggestions: Curtis Kellner, M.S., R.Ph.—drug forms and preparations; Mary Ann Going, R.N.C., M.A., and Mary Ann Dono, R.N., M.A.—pediatric dosage; Anne Marie O'Brien, R.N., B.S.N., C.I.C., Infection Control Coordinator—guidelines for universal safeguards in administering drugs; and Christopher Clones, Director of Central Supply—intravenous fluids and equipment. Thanks, too, to Gary Margolis, who did the initial line drawings, and to Sheila Maroney, who typed the manuscript.

I am indebted to Ellen Campbell and Tom Gibbons, editors at Lippincott, for their support and help in planning, writing, and producing the text.

Finally, I wish to acknowledge the following pharmaceutical companies that provided drug labels and package inserts: Abbott Laboratories; Beecham Laboratories; Bristol-Myers, U. S. Pharmaceuticals; Burroughs Wellcome Laboratories; Hoechst-Roussel Pharmaceuticals; Eli Lilly & Company; Merck, Sharp & Dohme; Roerig Pfizer Pharmaceuticals; Ross Laboratories; Smith Kline & French Laboratories; E. R. Squibb and Sons, Inc.; and Wyeth-Ayerst Laboratories.

Contents

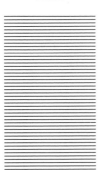

Interpreting the Language of Prescriptions

Every medication order contains the name and dosage of the drug and the route and time of administration. The dosage, route, and time are written in shorthand using abbreviations. Learn this shorthand to become proficient in reading and interpreting prescriptions.

In writing orders, some physicians use capital letters, whereas others use lower-case letters; some use periods after abbreviations, others do not. These variations reflect individual writing style and are not important. Concentrate on understanding the meaning of the abbreviation in the context of the order.

Here are three medication orders that will make sense to you after studying the material in this chapter:

Morphine sulfate 15 mg SC stat and 10 mg q4h prn

Neomycin ophthalmic oint OS bid

Ampicillin 1 g IVPB q6h

TIME OF ADMINISTRATION OF DRUGS

The abbreviations for times of drug administration are based on Latin words. They are included here under *Learning Aid* for your information, but it is not necessary for you to study or learn the Latin words. Learn the abbreviations, their meanings, and the sample times that indicate how the abbreviations are interpreted.

Time Abbreviation	Meaning	Learning Aid
ac	Before meals	Latin, *ante cibum* ‖ *Sample time:* 7:30 AM, 11:30 AM, 4:30 PM
pc	After meals	Latin, *post cibum* ‖ *Sample time:* 10 AM, 2 PM, 6 PM
qd	Every day, daily	Latin, *quaque die* ‖ *Sample time:* 10 AM
bid	Twice a day	Latin, *bis in die* ‖ *Sample time:* 10 AM, 6 PM

(continued)

Time Abbreviation	Meaning	Learning Aid
tid	Three times a day	Latin, *ter in die* ‖ **Sample time:** 10 AM, 2 PM, 6 PM
qid	Four times a day	Latin, *quater in die* ‖ **Sample time:** 10 AM, 2 PM, 6 PM, 10 PM
qh	Every hour	Latin, *quaque hora* Because the drug is given every hour, it will be given 24 times in one day.
hs	At bedtime, hour of sleep	Latin, *hora somni* ‖ **Sample time:** 10 PM
qn	Every night	Latin, *quaque nocte* ‖ **Sample time:** 10 PM
stat	Immediately	Latin, *statim* ‖ **Sample time:** now!

The following time abbreviations are based on a 24-hour day. To determine the number of times a medication will be given in a day, divide 24 by the number given in the abbreviation.

Time Abbreviation	Meaning	Learning Aid
q2h or q2°	Every 2 hours	The drug will be given 12 times in a 24-hour period (24 ÷ 2). ‖ **Sample times:** even hours at 2 AM, 4 AM, 6 AM, 8 AM, 10 AM, 12 noon, 2 PM, 4 PM, 6 PM, 8 PM, 10 PM, 12 midnight
q4h or q4°	Every 4 hours	The drug will be given six times in a 24-hour period (24 ÷ 4). ‖ **Sample times:** 2 AM, 6 AM, 10 AM, 2 PM, 6 PM, 10 PM
q6h or q6°	Every 6 hours	The drug will be given four times in a 24-hour period (24 ÷ 6). ‖ **Sample times:** 6 AM, 12 noon, 6 PM, 12 midnight
q8h or q8°	Every 8 hours	The drug will be given three times in a 24-hour period (24 ÷ 8). ‖ **Sample times:** 6 AM, 2 PM, 10 PM
q12 h or q12°	Every 12 hours	The drug will be given twice in a 24-hour period (24 ÷ 12). ‖ **Sample times:** 6 AM, 6 PM

There are four additional time abbreviations that require explanation. They are as follows:

Time Abbreviation	Meaning	Learning Aid

qod	Every other day	Latin, *quaque otra die*
		 This abbreviation is interpreted by the days of the **month**: the nurse writes on the medication record:
		       qod odd days of the month
		 ‖ **Sample time:** 10 AM on the first, third, fifth day, and so on
		 The nurse might write:
		       qod even days of the month
		 ‖ **Sample time:** 10 AM on the second, fourth, sixth day, and so on

prn	As needed	Latin, *pro re nata* This abbreviation is usually combined with a time abbreviation.

Time Abbreviation	Meaning	Learning Aid
		Example: q4h prn (every 4 hours as needed).
		This permits the nurse to assess the patient and make a nursing judgment about whether or not to administer the medication.
		Sample: acetaminophen 650 mg po q4h prn (650 milligrams of acetaminophen by mouth, every 4 hours as needed for pain)
		The nurse assesses the patient for pain every 4 hours; if the patient has pain, the nurse may administer the drug. This abbreviation has three administration implications:
		1. The nurse **must wait** 4 hours before giving the next dose.
		2. Once 4 hours has elapsed, the dose may be given at any time thereafter.
		3. Sample times are not given because the nurse does not know when the patient will need the drug.
tiw	Three times per week	Latin, *ter in vicis* Time relates to days of the **week.**
		Sample time: 10 AM on Monday, Wednesday, Friday
		Do not confuse with tid (three times per **day**).
biw	Twice per week	Latin, *bis in vicis* Time relates to days of the **week.**
		Sample time: 10 AM on Monday, Thursday
		Do not confuse with bid (twice per **day**).

SELF-TEST 1

After studying the abbreviations for times of administration, give the meaning of the following terms. Include sample times. Answers are given at the end of the chapter.

1. tid _____   9. q4h _____

2. qn _____   10. ac _____

3. pc _____   11. qd _____

4. qod _____   12. q8h _____

5. bid _____   13. qh _____

6. hs _____   14. prn _____

7. stat _____   15. q4h prn _____

8. qid _____

ROUTES OF ADMINISTRATION

Some of these abbreviations are based on Latin words, whereas others are not. Again, the Latin words are included for your information, but it is not necessary to study them. Alternative abbreviations are given in parentheses.

Route Abbreviation	Meaning	Learning Aid
IM	Intramuscularly	The injection is given at a 90° angle into a muscle.
IV	Intravenously	The injection is given into a vein.
IVPB	Intravenous piggyback	Medication prepared in a small volume of fluid is attached to an IV (which is already infusing fluid into a patient's vein) at specified times (Fig. 1-1).
NGT (ng)	Nasogastric tube	Medication is placed in the stomach through a tube in the nose.
OD	In the right eye	Latin, *oculus dextra*
OS	In the left eye	Latin, *oculus sinister*
OU	In both eyes	Latin, *oculi utrique*
po (PO)	By mouth	Latin, *per os*
pr (PR)	In the rectum	Latin, *per rectum*
SC (SQ)	Subcutaneously	The injection is usually given at a 45° angle into subcutaneous tissue.
SL	Sublingual, under the tongue	Latin, *sub lingua*
S & S	Swish and swallow	By using tongue and cheek muscles, the patient coats his mouth with a liquid medication.

═══ SELF-TEST 2 ═══

After studying the abbreviations for route of administration, give the meaning of the following terms. Answers are given at the end of the chapter.

1. SL _____

2. OU _____

3. NGT _____

4. IV _____

5. po _____

6. OD _____

7. IVPB _____

8. OS _____

9. IM _____

10. pr _____

11. S & S _____

12. SC _____

METRIC ABBREVIATIONS

Metric abbreviations relate to the measure of a drug's weight or volume. Although several systems and abbreviations of measure are in use, these are gradually being replaced by the International System of Units (Systèm International d'Unités; SI). This system provides unambiguous symbols that are standard in all languages. The preferred SI metric abbreviations will be

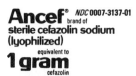

Ancef® *NDC* 0007-3137-01
brand of
sterile cefazolin sodium
(lyophilized)
equivalent to
1 gram
cefazolin
"Piggyback" Vial For
Intravenous Admixture
Smith Kline & French Laboratories
Division of SmithKline Beckman Corporation
Philadelphia, Pa. 19101

Figure 1-1.   Label states the route of administration. (Courtesy of Smith Kline & French Laboratories.)

used throughout this workbook. However, because these abbreviations are still not universally used, you should be aware of the alternative forms (given in parentheses) that may be used by physicians when writing orders or by pharmaceutical companies on their package labels and inserts.

Weight measures are used for solid forms of drugs, whereas volume measures are used for the liquid forms. Study the meanings of the metric abbreviations listed in the following table. Under *Learning Aid,* one equivalent is given for each abbreviation to give you an understanding of what kinds of quantities are involved; it is not yet necessary for you to study the equivalents.

Metric Abbreviation	Meaning	Learning Aid
cc	Cubic centimeter	This is a measure of volume. It is now usually reserved for measuring gases; however you may still find it used as a liquid measure. (One cubic centimeter is approximately equal to 16 drops from a medicine dropper.)
g (gm, Gm)	Gram	This is a solid measure of weight. (One gram is approximately equal to the weight of two paper clips.)
kg (Kg)	Kilogram	This is a weight measure. (One kilogram equals 2.2 pounds.)
L	Liter	This is a liquid measure. (One liter is a little more than a quart.)
μg (mcg)	Microgram	This is a measure of weight. (One thousand micrograms make up 1 milligram: 1000 μg = 1 mg)
mEq	Milliequivalent	No equivalent necessary. Drugs are prepared and ordered in this weight measure.
mg	Milligram	This is a measure of weight. (One thousand milligrams make up 1 gram: 1000 mg = 1 g)
ml (mL)	Milliliter	This is a liquid measure. The terms *cubic centimeter* (cc) and *milliliter* (ml) are interchangeable in dosage (1 cc = 1 ml).
unit (U)	Unit	This is a measure of biologic activity. Nurses do not calculate this measure.
		Example: penicillin potassium 300,000 units
		Important: It is considered safer to write the word *unit* rather than use the abbreviation, because the *U* could be read as a zero and a medication error might result.

SELF-TEST 3

After studying metric abbreviations, write the meaning of the following terms. Answers can be found at the end of the chapter.

1. 0.3 g _____

2. 150 mcg _____

3. 80 U _____

4. 0.5 ml _____

5. 1.7 cc _____

_____

6. 0.25 mg _____

_____

7. 14 kg _____

8. 20 mEq _____

9. 1.5 L _____

10. 50 μg _____

APOTHECARY ABBREVIATIONS

The archaic apothecary system of measures has been largely replaced by the more precise metric system. However, because some physicians still order in apothecary terms, several of these abbreviations are listed in the following table. The meanings given are commonly accepted interpretations used in nursing practice. The system requires notation in Roman numerals and fractions.

Apothecary Abbreviation	Meaning	Learning Aid
ʒ	Dram	This is a liquid measure. It is slightly less than a household teaspoon. (One dram equals 4 milliliters: ʒi = 4 ml)
℥	Ounce	This is a liquid measure. It is slightly more than a household ounce. (One ounce equals 30 milliliters: ℥i = 30 ml)
gr	Grain	Latin, *granum.* This solid measure was based on the weight of a grain of wheat in ancient times. There is no commonly used equivalent to the grain in the metric system.
gtt	Drop	Latin, *guttae.* This liquid measure was based on a drop of water. (One drop equals 1 milliliter: 1 gtt = 1 ml)
m (M,Mₓ)	Minim	Latin, *minim.* (One minim equals one drop: 1 m = 1 gtt) (Fig. 1-2)
ss	One-half	Latin, *semis.*
i	One	*Example:* gr i = grains 1
i ss	One-and-a-half	*Example:* gr i ss = grains 1$\frac{1}{2}$
ii	Two	*Example:* gr ii = grains 2
iii	Three	*Example:* gr iii = grains 3
iv	Four	*Example:* gr iv = grains 4
		ʒ iv = drams 4
v	Five	*Example:* gr v = grains 5
		m v = minims 5
vii	Seven	*Example:* gr vii = grains 7
vii ss	Seven-and-a-half	*Example:* gr vii ss = grains 7$\frac{1}{2}$
x	Ten	*Example:* gr x = grains 10
		m x = minims 10
xv	Fifteen	*Example:* gr xv = grains 15
		m xv = minims 15

SELF-TEST 4

After studying the apothecary abbreviations, write the meaning of the following terms. Answers can be found at the end of the chapter.

1. m x _____   5. ℥ i _____   8. gr x _____

2. ʒ ii _____   6. ʒ viii _____   9. m v _____

3. gr v _____   7. ℥ ss _____   10. gr i ss _____

4. gtt x _____

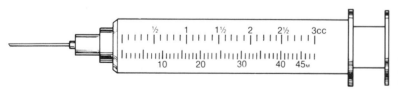

Figure 1-2. A 3-ml (cc) syringe calibrated in tenths of a milliliter and in minims.

HOUSEHOLD ABBREVIATIONS

Physicians may use these common household measures to order drugs. Metric equivalents are included in the *Learning Aid* column for your information.

Household Abbreviation	Meaning	Learning Aid
pt	Pint	One pint is approximately equal to 500 milliliters (1 pt ≅ 500 ml).
qt	Quart	One quart is approximately equal to 1 liter, which is equal to 1000 milliliters (1 qt ≅ 1 L = 1000 ml). One-half a quart is approximately equal to 1 pint $\left(\dfrac{1}{2}\ qt \cong 1\ pt = 500\ ml\right)$.
tbsp	Tablespoon	One tablespoon equals 15 milliliters (1 tbsp = 15 ml).
tsp	Teaspoon	One teaspoon equals 5 milliliters (1 tsp = 5 ml).
oz	Ounce	One ounce equals 30 milliliters (1 oz = 30 ml). 6 tsp = 1 oz = 30 ml $3\ tsp = \dfrac{1}{2}\ oz = 15\ ml$ 2 tbsp = 1 oz = 30 ml = 6 tsp (Fig. 1-3)

SELF-TEST 5

After studying household measures, write the meaning of the following terms. Answers can be found at the end of the chapter.

1. 3 tsp _____

2. 1 oz _____

3. $\dfrac{1}{2}$ qt _____

4. 1 tsp _____

5. 1 pt _____

6. 2 tbsp_____

TERMS AND ABBREVIATIONS FOR DRUG PREPARATIONS

The following abbreviations and terms are used to describe selected drug preparations.

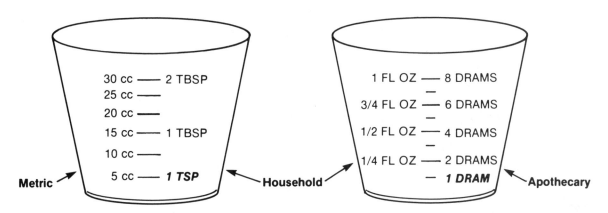

Figure 1-3. *A medicine cup with metric, household, and apothecary equivalents. Two sides of the cup are shown.*

Term Abbreviation	Meaning	Learning Aid
cap, caps	Capsule	Medication is encased in a gelatin shell.
CR	Controlled-release	These abbreviations indicate that the drug has been prepared in a form that allows extended action. Therefore, the drug is given less frequently.
LA	Long-acting	
SA	Sustained-action	
SR	Slow-release	
DS	Double-strength	
EC	Enteric-coated	The tablet is coated with a substance that will not dissolve in the acid secretions of the stomach, but, instead, it dissolves in the more alkaline secretions of the intestines.
el, elix	Elixir	A drug is dissolved in a hydroalcoholic sweetened base.
sol	Solution	The drug is contained in a clear liquid preparation.
sp	Spirit	An alcoholic solution of a volatile substance (e.g., spirit of ammonia).
sup, supp	Suppository	A solid, cylindrically shaped drug that can be inserted into a body opening (e.g., the rectum or vagina).
susp	Suspension	Small particles of drug are dispersed in a liquid base and must be shaken before pouring. Gels and magmas are also suspensions.
syr	Syrup	A sugar is dissolved in a liquid medication and flavored to disguise the taste.
tab, tabs	Tablet	Medication is compressed or molded into a solid form; additional ingredients are used to shape and color the tablet.
tr, tinct.	Tincture	This is a liquid alcoholic or hydroalcoholic solution of a drug.
ung, oint.	Ointment	This is a semisolid drug preparation that is applied to the skin (for external use only).
KVO	Keep vein open	*Example order:* 1000 ml dextrose 5% in water IVKVO. The nurse is to continue infusing this fluid.
D/C	Discontinue	*Example order:* D/C ampicillin
NKA	No known allergies	This is an important assessment that is noted on the medication record of a patient.

SELF-TEST 6

After studying the abbreviations for drug forms, write out the meaning of the following terms. Answers can be found at the end of the chapter.

1. elix _____
2. DS _____
3. NKA _____
4. caps _____
5. susp _____

6. tab _____
7. SR _____
8. D/C _____
9. supp _____
10. tr _____

EXERCISE IN READING PRESCRIPTIONS

Now that you have studied the language of prescriptions, you are ready to interpret medication orders! Write the following orders in longhand. Give sample times. Answers are given at the end of this chapter.

1. Nembutal 100 mg hs prn po _____

2. Propranolol hydrochloride 40 mg po bid _____

3. Ampicillin 1 g IVPB q6h _____

4. Demerol 50 mg IM q4h prn for pain _____

5. Tylenol 325 mg tabs ii po stat _____

6. Pilocarpine gtt ii OU q3h _____

7. Scopolamine 0.8 mg SC stat _____

8. El Digoxin 0.25 mg po qd _____

9. Kaochlor 30 mEq po bid _____

10. Liquaemin sodium 6000 units SC q4h _____

11. Tobramycin 70 mg IM q8h _____

12. Maalox ℥ i po AC and hs _____

13. Humulin insulin units 15 SC qd 7:30 AM _____

14. Vitamin B_{12} 1000 μg IM tiw _____

15. Tr belladonna gtt xv and Amphojel ℥ ss̈ qid po _____

16. Aspirin gr x po q4h prn for temperature over 101° _____

17. Neomycin ophthalmic oint 1% OS tid _____

18. Prednisone 10 mg po qod _____

19. Milk of magnesia 1 tbsp po hs qn _____

(continued)

======= EXERCISE IN READING PRESCRIPTIONS (*Continued*) =======

20. Septra DS tab i qd po _____

_____

21. Morphine sulfate 15 mg SC stat and 10 mg q4h prn _____

_____

_____

ANSWERS

SELF-TEST 1

1. Three times a day. (*Sample times:* 10 AM, 2 PM, 6 PM)

2. Every night. (*Sample time:* 10 PM)

3. After meals. (*Sample times:* 10 AM, 2 PM, 6 PM)

4. Every other day. (*Sample times:* odd days of month at 10 AM)

5. Twice a day. (*Sample times:* 10 AM, 6 PM)

6. Hour of sleep. (*Sample time:* 10 PM)

7. Immediately. (*Sample time:* whatever the time is now)

8. Four times a day. (*Sample times:* 10 AM, 2 PM, 6 PM, 10 PM)

9. Every 4 hours. (*Sample times:* 2 AM, 6 AM, 10 AM, 2 PM, 6 PM, 10 PM)

10. Before meals. (*Sample times:* 7:30 AM, 11:30 AM, 4:30 PM)

11. Every day. (*Sample time:* 10 AM)

12. Every 8 hours. (*Sample times:* 6 AM, 2 PM, 10 PM)

13. Every hour.

14. Whenever necessary. (*Sample times:* No time routine can be written.)

15. Every 4 hours as needed. (*Sample times:* No time routine is written because we do not know when the drug will be needed.)

SELF-TEST 2

1. Sublingual; under the tongue
2. Both eyes
3. Nasogastric tube
4. Intravenously
5. By mouth
6. Right eye
7. Intravenous piggyback
8. Left eye
9. Intramuscularly
10. Rectally
11. Swish and swallow
12. Subcutaneously

SELF-TEST 3

1. Three-tenths of a gram
2. One hundred fifty micrograms
3. Eighty units
4. Five-tenths of a milliliter
5. One and seven-tenths of a cubic centimeter
6. Twenty-five hundredths of a milligram
7. Fourteen kilograms
8. Twenty milliequivalents
9. One and five-tenths liters
10. Fifty micrograms

SELF-TEST 4

1. Minims 10
2. Drams 2
3. Grains 5
4. Drops 10
5. Ounces 1
6. Drams 8
7. Ounces $\frac{1}{2}$ (0.5)
8. Grains 10
9. Minims 5
10. Grains $1\frac{1}{2}$ (1.5)

SELF-TEST 5

1. Three teaspoons
2. One ounce
3. One-half quart
4. One teaspoon
5. One pint
6. Two tablespoons

SELF-TEST 6

1. Elixir
2. Double-strength
3. No known allergies
4. Capsules
5. Suspension
6. Tablet
7. Slow-release
8. Discontinue
9. Suppository
10. Tincture

EXERCISE IN READING PRESCRIPTIONS

1. Nembutal one hundred milligrams at the hour of sleep, as needed, by mouth (e.g., 10 PM)
2. Propranolol hydrochloride forty milligrams by mouth twice a day (e.g., 10 AM, 6 PM)
3. Ampicillin one gram intravenous piggyback every 6 hours (e.g., 6 AM, 12 noon, 6 PM, 12 midnight)
4. Demerol fifty milligrams intramuscularly every 4 hours as needed for pain
5. Tylenol three hundred twenty-five milligrams, two tablets by mouth immediately. (Give two tablets of Tylenol. Each tablet is 325 mg.)
6. Pilocarpine drops two in both eyes every 3 hours (e.g., 3 AM, 6 AM, 9 AM, 12 noon, 3 PM, 6 PM, 9 PM, 12 midnight)
7. Scopolamine eight-tenths milligram subcutaneously immediately
8. Elixir of digoxin twenty-five hundredths of a milligram by mouth every day (e.g., 10 AM)
9. Kaochlor thirty milliequivalents by mouth twice a day (e.g., 10 AM and 6 PM)
10. Liquaemin sodium six thousand units subcutaneously every 4 hours (e.g., 2 AM, 6 AM, 10 AM, 2 PM, 6 PM, 10 PM)
11. Tobramycin seventy milligrams intramuscularly every 8 hours (e.g., 6 AM, 2 PM, 10 PM)
12. Maalox one ounce by mouth before meals and at the hour of sleep (e.g., 7:30 AM, 11:30 AM, 4:30 PM, 10 PM)
13. Humulin insulin fifteen units subcutaneously every day at seven-thirty in the morning
14. Vitamin B_{12} one thousand micrograms intramuscularly three times a week (e.g., Monday, Wednesday, Friday at 10 AM)
15. Tincture of belladonna drops fifteen and Amphojel ounces one-half four times a day by mouth (e.g., 10 AM, 2 PM, 6 PM, 10 PM)
16. Aspirin grains ten by mouth every 4 hours as needed for temperature over one hundred one degrees
17. Neomycin ophthalmic ointment one percent left eye three times a day (e.g., 10 AM, 2 PM, 6 PM)
18. Prednisone ten milligrams by mouth every other day (e.g., even days of the month at 10 AM). You might substitute qod, "odd days of the month".
19. Milk of magnesia one tablespoon by mouth at the hour of sleep every night (e.g., 10 PM)
20. Septra one double-strength tablet every day by mouth (e.g., 10 AM)
21. Morphine sulfate fifteen milligrams subcutaneously immediately and ten milligrams every 4 hours as needed. The stat time given determines when the next dose can be administered. (Next dose must be *at least 4 hours later.*)

2

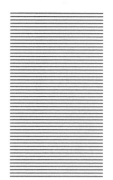

Drug Labels and Packaging

Nurses must read and interpret label information to be able to prepare, administer, and store drugs safely. When needed information is not on the label, the nurse should consult the professional literature accompanying the drug, check reliable references, or consult the pharmacist.

In general, there are two types of drug labels, those that contain detailed information, and those that are limited to specific facts.

LABELS THAT CONTAIN DETAILED INFORMATION

In the institutional setting, this type of label is found on drugs that are dispensed in a dry (powder) form and must be reconstituted, or dissolved, by the nurse before they are administered to a patient. The following information is common on this type of label:

NDC Number.   The National Drug Code (NDC) is a number used by the pharmacist to identify the drug and the method of packaging.

|| ***EXAMPLE:***   NDC 71-771-52

Total Amount of Drug in the Container.   This information is usually found at the top of the label to the left.

|| ***EXAMPLE:***   200 tablets; 1000 ml

Trade Name.   The term *trade name,* which is also referred to as a brand name or a proprietary name, may be identified by the symbol ® that follows the name. Several companies may manufacture the same drug under different trade names. Trade names may be capitalized on the labels, or they may have an initial capital only. They are always written with the first letter capitalized.

|| ***EXAMPLE:***

   Monocid® is the trade name of a drug manufactured by Smith Kline & French Laboratories.

Generic Name.   The generic name is the official accepted name of a drug, as listed in the United States Pharmacopeia (USP) and the National Formulary (NF). A drug may have several trade names but only one official generic name. The generic name is not capitalized.

|| ***EXAMPLE:***

   ampicillin sodium is distributed as Omnipen-N; Polycillin-N; SK Ampicillin-N; Totacillin-N.

Strength of the Drug. Solid drugs are given in metric weights; liquids are stated as a solution of drug in solvent.

| | *EXAMPLE:* cefonicid 5 g; dicloxacillin 100 mg/5 ml

Form of the Drug. The label specifies the type of preparation in the container.

| | *EXAMPLE:* tablet, capsule, oral suspension, aqueous solution

Usual Dosage. This states how much drug is given at a single time, or over a 24-hour period, and also identifies who should receive the drug.

| | *EXAMPLE:* Adults 1–2 teaspoons every 4 hours

Route of Administration. The label specifies how the drug is to be given: orally, parenterally (an injection of some type), or topically (applied to skin or mucous membranes). *When the label does not specify the route, the drug is in an oral form.*

Storage. This information describes the conditions necessary to protect the drug from losing its potency (effectiveness). Some drugs come in a dry form and must be dissolved, that is, reconstituted. The drug may be stored one way when dry and another way after reconstitution.

> *EXAMPLE:*
>
> Before reconstitution protect from light and store at controlled room temperature (59°–86°). After reconstitution, stable at room temperature for 18 hours or 7 days if refrigerated.

Directions for Preparation. The drug comes as a powder and must be dissolved. The amount and type of liquid to be used in reconstituting the drug and the resulting solution will be stated by the manufacturer.

| | *EXAMPLE:* Dilute powder with 2 ml sterile water for injection to make 50 mg/ml.

Expiration Date. The drug cannot be used after the last day of the month indicated.

Precautions. These are specific instructions related to safety, effectiveness, or administration that must be noted and followed.

Manufacturer's Name. Any questions about the drug should be directed to this company.

Lot Number. This number indicates the batch of drug from which this stock came.

Additives. The manufacturer may have used substances to bind the drug, to aid in dissolving the drug, to produce a specific pH, and so on. This information may be found on the label or in the literature accompanying the drug.

EXERCISE 1

Read the label in Figure 2–1 and give the information requested. Answers may be found at the end of the chapter.

1. What is the trade name? _____

2. What is the generic or official name? _____

Pharmacist: do not remove this panel

TO PATIENT
Shake well before using. (Oversize bottle permits shaking space.)
Keep tightly closed.
When stored at room temperature, discard unused portion after 7 days; when stored in refrigerator, discard unused portion after 14 days.
Date prepared: _____

H.

(detach here)

100 ml.   *NDC* 0007-3174-72

Anspor® 125 mg./5ml.
brand of   (when reconstituted as directed)
cephradine
for oral suspension

CAUTION—Federal law prohibits dispensing without prescription.
Bottle contains 2.5 grams cephradine in a dry, pleasantly flavored mixture. When prepared as directed, each 5 ml. teaspoonful provides 125 mg. cephradine.
Usual dosage: Adults—2 teaspoonfuls every 6 hours or 4 teaspoonfuls every 12 hours. Children—25 to 50 mg./kg./day total, in equally divided doses every 6 or 12 hours. See accompanying folder for complete prescribing information.
Do not store above 86°F. in dry form.
DIRECTIONS FOR PREPARATION: Use 61 ml. of water to prepare 100 ml. oral suspension. (1) Shake to loosen powder. (2) Add 61 ml. of water and shake vigorously.   U.S. Pat. 3,485,819
DISPENSE IN THIS CONTAINER

Mfd. for **Smith Kline &French Laboratories**
Div. of SmithKline Beckman Corp., Phila., Pa. 19101
by Squibb Manufacturing, Inc., Humacao, P.R. 00661
Subsidiary of E.R. Squibb & Sons, Inc.   **SK&F**

Figure 2-1. *Label of a drug that must be reconstituted for po use. (Courtesy of Smith Kline & French Laboratories.)*

3. What is the total amount of drug in the container as dispensed by the manufacturer? _____
   _____

4. In what form is the drug prepared by the manufacturer? _____

5. When reconstituted, what will be the strength of the drug? _____

6. When reconstituted, how much liquid will be in the container? _____

7. What is the usual dosage for a child? _____
   _____

8. What is the route of administration? _____

9. What are the directions for preparation? _____
   _____
   _____

10. List two ways the drug can be stored. For each way give the expiration time. _____
    _____
    _____

11. Name the manufacturer. _____

12. Give six precautions listed on the label. _____
    _____
    _____
    _____

EXERCISE 2

Read the label in Figure 2-2 and give the information requested. Answers may be found at the end of the chapter.

1. What is the trade name? _____

2. What is the generic or official name? _____

(continued)

NDC 0007-3130-01

Ancef® brand of
sterile cefazolin
sodium
(lyophilized)

equivalent to
1 gram
cefazolin

Expires:
T.Lot:

CAUTION— Federal law prohibits
dispensing without prescription
U.S. Pat. 3,516,997

Smith Kline &French Labs., Div. of SmithKline Beckman Corp., Phila., Pa. 19101

For I.V. or I.M. use
Usual Adult Dose—250 mg. to
1 gram every six to eight hours.
See literature.
For I.M. use, add 2.5 ml. Sterile
Water for Injection and shake.
Provides an approximate volume
of 3.0 ml. (330 mg./ml.) For I.V.
use see accompanying literature.
Reconstituted "Ancef" is stable
24 hours at room temperature
or 96 hours if refrigerated.

Patient _____
Date prepared _____ Time _____

Figure 2-2. Label of a drug that must be reconstituted for IM or IV use. (Courtesy of Smith Kline & French Laboratories.)

EXERCISE 2 (*Continued*)

3. What is the total amount of drug in the container? _____

4. In what form is the drug dispensed by the manufacturer? _____

5. By what route(s) may the drug be given? _____

6. What is the usual dose for an adult? _____

7. Can the drug be given to a child? Explain. _____
_____
_____

8. How should the drug be prepared for IM use? _____
_____

9. What is the amount and strength of the solution when prepared as directed for IM use? _____
_____

10. What must be done to prepare the drug for IV use? _____
_____
_____

11. List two ways the drug can be stored. For each way give the expiration time. _____
_____
_____

LABELS LIMITED TO SPECIFIC FACTS

Drugs with these types of labels are designed to be administered in the form in which they are packaged. The form may be solid or liquid. The following information is typical of this type of label:

- NDC number
- Total amount of drug in the container
- Trade and generic names
- Strength and form of the drug
- Manufacturer's name
- Expiration date and lot number

Some information, including route of administration, usual dose, and storage may not be on the label, usually because the container is too small. When the nurse needs further information, professional references should be consulted.

Labels for some combination drugs may not list any strength. Instead they give the ingredients in the combination. These drugs are ordered by the number to give if they are solid forms. Liquids are ordered in metric or household measures.

|| **EXAMPLE:** Multivitamin tabs 1 po qd; Robitussin DM cough mixture 1 tsp po q4h prn

EXERCISE 3

Read the label in Figure 2–3 and give the information requested. Answers may be found at the end of the chapter.

1. What is the trade name? _____

2. What is the generic name? _____

3. By what route(s) may this drug be given? _____

4. In what form is the drug dispensed? _____

5. What is the strength of the drug? _____

6. What is the total amount of drug in the container? _____

7. How should the drug be stored? _____
    _____

8. What information will the package insert contain? _____
    _____

EXERCISE 4

Read the label in Figure 2–4 and give the information requested. Answers may be found at the end of the chapter.

1. In what form does the drug come? _____

2. What is the trade name? _____

3. What is the generic name? _____

4. What is the strength of each drug unit? _____

5. Name the usual dosage. _____
    _____

(continued)

100 Tablets   NDC-0081-0168-55

For indications, dosage, precautions, etc., see accompanying package insert.

CARDILATE®
(ERYTHRITYL TETRANITRATE)
FOR ORAL OR SUBLINGUAL USE
Each scored tablet contains
10 mg
CAUTION: Federal law prohibits
dispensing without prescription.

BURROUGHS WELLCOME CO.
Research Triangle Park, NC 27709

Store at 15°–25°C (59°–77°F) in a dry place. Dispense in glass, tight container as defined in the U.S.P.

Made in U.S.A.

444721

Figure 2-3. Label of a drug that does not require reconstitution for po or SL use. (Courtesy of Burroughs Wellcome Co.) (Note: Cardilate is no longer manufactured.)

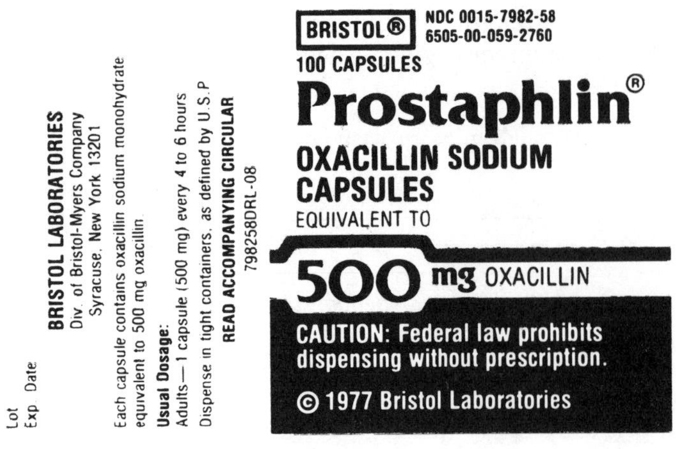

BRISTOL LABORATORIES
Div. of Bristol-Myers Company
Syracuse, New York 13201

Each capsule contains oxacillin sodium monohydrate
equivalent to 500 mg oxacillin

Usual Dosage:
Adults— 1 capsule (500 mg) every 4 to 6 hours
Dispense in tight containers, as defined by U.S.P.
READ ACCOMPANYING CIRCULAR
79825BDRL-08

Lot
Exp Date

BRISTOL®   NDC 0015-7982-58
            6505-00-059-2760
100 CAPSULES

Prostaphlin®

**OXACILLIN SODIUM
CAPSULES**
EQUIVALENT TO

500 mg OXACILLIN

CAUTION: Federal law prohibits
dispensing without prescription.

© 1977 Bristol Laboratories

*Figure 2-4. Label of a solid drug that does
not require reconstitution for po use. (Courtesy of Bristol Laboratories.)*

═══ EXERCISE 4 (Continued) ═══

6. Is there literature with the drug? _____

7. Are storage directions on the label? _____

8. Is the route of administration specified on the label? _____

_____

_____

═══ EXERCISE 5 ═══

*Read the label in Figure 2-5 and give the information requested. Answers may be found at the end of the
chapter.*

1. Give the drug name. _____

2. What is the generic name? _____

3. By what route(s) may this drug be administered? _____

4. What is the strength of the drug? _____

5. In what form is the drug dispensed and how do you know this? _____

_____

_____

6. In what type of container is the drug? _____

7. Give the additives. _____

_____

_____

8. List three cautions in storing the drug. _____

_____

_____

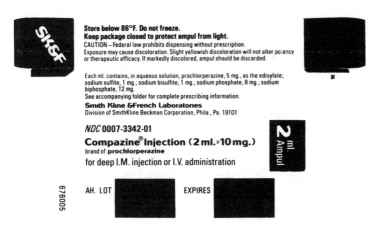

Store below 86°F. Do not freeze.
Keep package closed to protect ampul from light.
CAUTION—Federal law prohibits dispensing without prescription.
Exposure may cause discoloration. Slight yellowish discoloration will not alter potency or therapeutic efficacy. If markedly discolored, ampul should be discarded.

Each ml. contains, in aqueous solution, prochlorperazine, 5 mg., as the edisylate; sodium sulfite, 1 mg.; sodium bisulfite, 1 mg.; sodium phosphate, 8 mg.; sodium biphosphate, 12 mg.
See accompanying folder for complete prescribing information.
Smith Kline &French Laboratories
Division of SmithKline Beckman Corporation, Phila., Pa. 19101

NDC 0007-3342-01
Compazine®Injection (2 ml.=10 mg.)
brand of **prochlorperazine**
for deep I.M. injection or I.V. administration

2 ml.
Ampul

676005

AH. LOT   EXPIRES

Figure 2-5. Label of a liquid drug that does not require reconstitution for IM or IV use. (Courtesy of Smith Kline & French Laboratories.)

9. What precaution is given about the color of the drug? _____

_____

_____

_____

_____

DRUG PACKAGING

In the future, innovative delivery systems will revolutionize the ways in which drugs are administered. In this chapter, however, we focus on the common types of containers that nurses handle as they prepare medications.

There are two types of packaging: *unit-dose* and *multidose.* Each type may contain a solid or liquid form of the drug for oral, parenteral, or topical use. Most institutions use a combination of unit-dose and multidose.

Unit-Dose Packaging

Each dose is individually wrapped and labeled, and a 24-hour supply is prepared by the pharmacy and dispensed. A major value of unit-dose packaging is that two professionals check the drug and the dose—the pharmacist and the nurse—thereby decreasing the possibility of error.

It should be stressed that unit-dose packaging does not relieve the nurse of the responsibility to *check the label three times* and to calculate the amount of drug needed. Unit-dose drugs come in different strengths, and there is always a chance of error when trade names are ordered instead of generic names. Fractions of doses are also possible.

> **EXAMPLE:**
> A nurse has a unit-dose 100-mg tablet. If an order calls for 50 mg, only half the tablet would be administered.

For the Oral Route. For oral administration, unit-dose packaging may consist of

1. Plastic bubble, foil, or paper wrappers containing tablets or capsules (Fig. 2–6A).
2. Plastic or glass containers that hold a single dose of a liquid or powder. The powder is reconstituted to a liquid form by following the directions given on the label (see Fig. 2–6B).

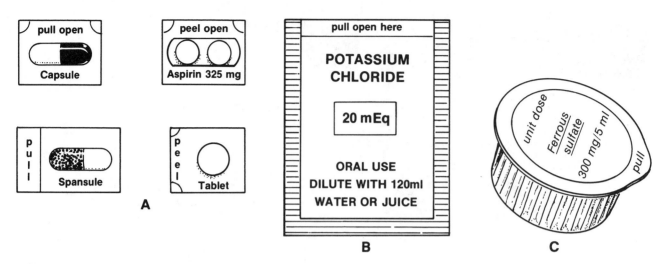

Figure 2-6. (**A**) *Unit-dose tablets and capsules in foil wrappers.* (**B**) *Unit-dose powder, in a sealed packet, that is diluted before giving.* (**C**) *Sealed cup containing one dose of a liquid medication ready to administer.*

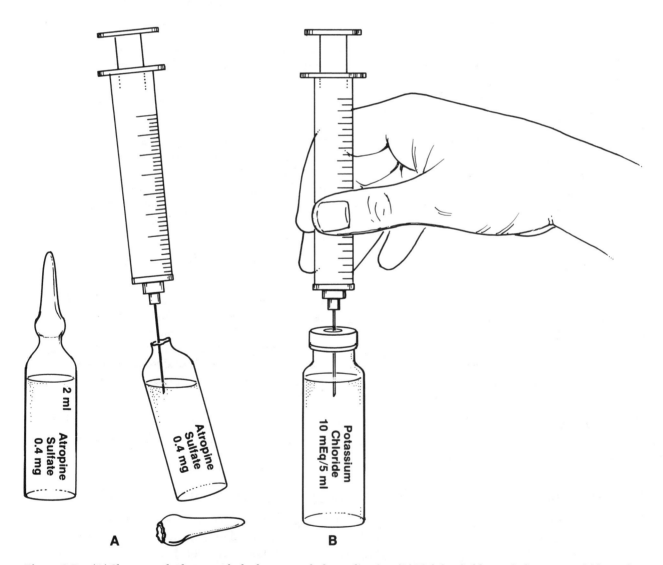

Figure 2-7. (**A**) *Glass ampule that must be broken to reach the medication.* (**B**) *Vial that holds a unit dose or a multidose. The rubber top seals to keep the medication sterile.*

3. A sealed medication cup containing one dose of a liquid. The nurse removes the cover and the dose is ready to administer (see Fig. 2–6C).

For the Parenteral Route. These drugs are given by injection. The route must be specified in the order (e.g., IM, SC, IVPB). Drugs in such containers are sterile, and sterile technique is used for their preparation and administration. The drugs may come in a solid or liquid form.

1. An *ampule* (ampoule) is a glass container that holds a single sterile dose of drug. The container has a narrow neck that must be broken to reach the drug. A sterile syringe is used to withdraw the medication (Fig. 2–7A). The drug in the ampule may come as a liquid, a powder, or a crystal. Directions must be followed to reconstitute the solid forms. Once the glass is broken, any portion of drug not used must be discarded because the drug cannot be kept sterile.
2. A *vial* is a glass container with a sealed rubber top. It may contain a sterile liquid or a sterile powder that must be reconstituted with a sterile diluent and syringe. Single-dose vials do not contain a preservative or a bacteriostatic agent. Therefore, any medication remaining after the dose is prepared should be discarded (see Fig. 2–7B).
3. Flexible *plastic bags* or *glass vials* may hold sterile medication for intravenous use. The fluid is administered with use of IV tubing which is connected to a needle or catheter placed in the patient's blood vessel (Fig. 2–8).
4. Prefilled syringes contain liquid, sterile medication that is ready to administer without further preparation. This type of unit-dose packaging is expensive but lifesaving in an emergency in which speed is essential (Fig. 2–9A).
5. *Prefilled cartridges* are actually small vials, with a needle attached, that fit into a metal or plastic holder and eject one unit-dose of a sterile drug in liquid form (see Fig. 2–9B).

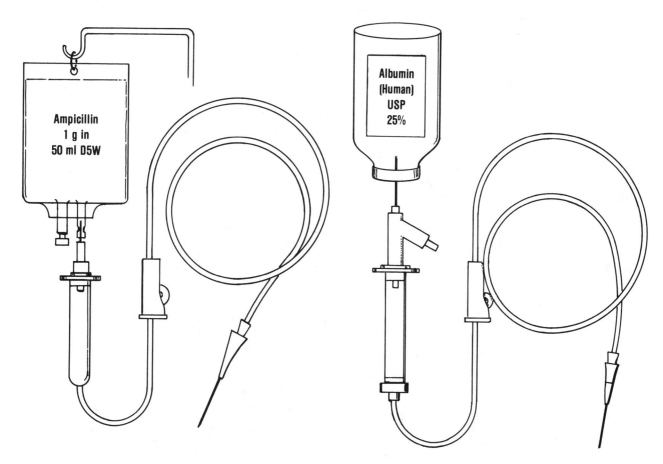

Ampicillin
1 g in
50 ml D5W

Albumin
(Human)
USP
25%

Figure 2-8. *Plastic or glass containers hold medication for IV use.*

For Topical Administration.   Drugs are applied to the skin or mucous membranes to achieve a local effect or to act systemically throughout the body.

1. *Transdermal patches or pads* are adhesive bandages placed on the skin. They hold a drug form that is slowly absorbed into the circulation over a period, ranging from hours to several days (Fig. 2–10).
2. *Lozenges and pastilles* are disklike solids that are slowly dissolved in the mouth (e.g., cough drops).
3. *Suppositories,* in foil or plastic wrappers are molded forms that can be inserted into the rectum, vagina, or urethra. They hold medication in a substance, such as cocoa butter, that melts at body temperature and releases the drug (Fig. 2–11).
4. Plastic, disposable, squeezable containers hold prepared solutions for the vagina (douches) or enema solutions that are administered rectally. The containers for enemas have a lubricated nozzle for ease in insertion. As the container is squeezed, the solution is forced out (Fig. 2–12).

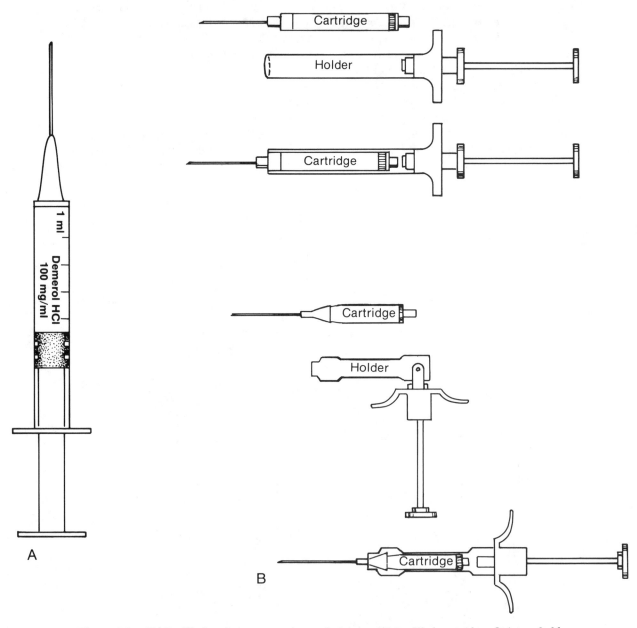

Figure 2-9. (**A**) *Prefilled syringes are ready to administer.* (**B**) *Prefilled cartridges fit into a holder.*

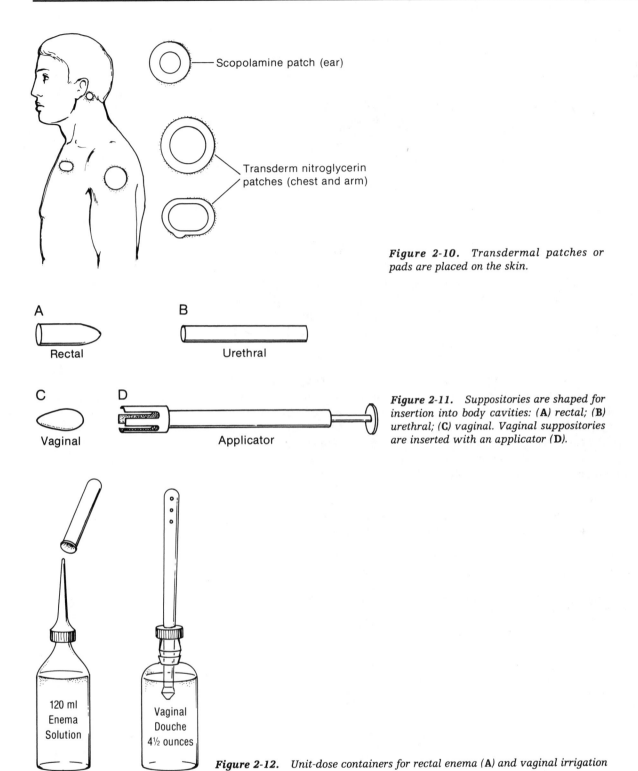

Figure 2-10. *Transdermal patches or pads are placed on the skin.*

Figure 2-11. *Suppositories are shaped for insertion into body cavities: (**A**) rectal; (**B**) urethral; (**C**) vaginal. Vaginal suppositories are inserted with an applicator (**D**).*

Figure 2-12. *Unit-dose containers for rectal enema (**A**) and vaginal irrigation (**B**).*

Multidose Packaging

Each patient unit receives large, stock containers of medications commonly used in that area. The nurse identifies the drug, checks the strength, and calculates and prepares the dose. This type of packaging reduces the pharmacy's workload, but it requires more nursing time. The possibility of error is increased.

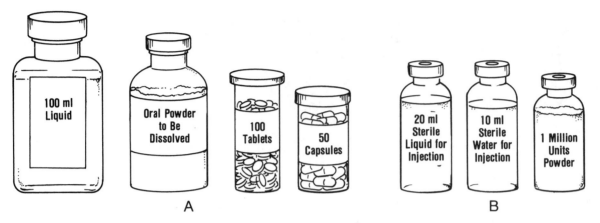

Figure 2-13. *Multidose containers: (A) for the oral route; (B) for the parenteral route.*

For the Oral Route.   Stock bottles contain a liquid or a solid form, such as tablets, capsules, powders. When powders are reconstituted, the date and time of preparation must be written on the label and storage directions and expiration carefully noted. Large stock bottles hold medication that is dispensed over a period of days (Fig. 2–13A).

For the Parenteral Route.   Large-volume vials contain a sterile liquid or powder to be reconstituted, using sterile technique. As with powders for oral use, the nurse must write the date and time of preparation on the powder label and note storage directions and expiration (see Fig. 2–13B).

For Topical Administration.   Care must be exercised to avoid contaminating these containers because they will be used over an extended period. Whenever possible, label the container with the patient's name and reserve its use for that one patient. The following types of containers may be used:

1. *Metal or plastic tubes* that contain ointments or creams to be applied to the skin or mucous membranes are squeezed to release the medication (Fig. 2–14A).

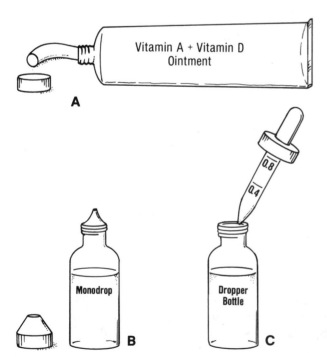

Figure 2-14. *Topical multidose containers: (A) tubes for creams or ointments; (B) monodrop containers—the dropper is attached; (C) removable dropper is sometimes calibrated for liquid measures.*

2. Medication is removed from *jars for creams, ointments, pastes* by using a sterile tongue blade or sterile glove to avoid contamination.

3. To prevent cross-contamination, *dropper bottles* for eye, ear, or nose medications should be labeled with one patient's name. The nurse must be careful to avoid touching mucous membranes with the dropper, because contamination of the dropper could result in the growth of pathogens.

   There are two kinds of droppers: monodrop containers that are squeezed to release the medication and those in which the dropper can be removed from the bottle. Separate, packaged droppers are available to administer medications. These are calibrated, that is, marked in milliliters (see Figs. 2–14*B,C*).

   Eye medications are labeled "ophthalmic" or "for the eye." Ear drugs are labeled "otic" or "auric" or "for the ear." Drugs for nasal administration are labeled "nose drops." Routes must *never* be interchanged.

4. *Lozenges and pastilles* may be packaged in multidose as well as unit-dose containers.

5. *Metered-dose inhalers (MDI)* are aerosol devices that consist of two parts: a canister under pressure and a mouthpiece. The canister contains multiple drug doses in a liquid form or as a microfine powder or crystal. The mouthpiece fits on the canister. Finger pressure on the mouthpiece opens a valve on the canister that discharges one dose. The physician's order will state the number of inhalations or "puffs" to be taken (Fig. 2–15).

   Medications for inhalation may also be packaged as liquids in vials or bottles to be used with a hand-held nebulizer, or with an intermittent positive-pressure breathing apparatus (IPPB).

EXERCISE 6

Match Column A with the letters in Column B to identify the meaning of terms used in drug packaging. Answers may be found at the end of the chapter.

Column A

1. _____ Unit dose
2. _____ Ampule
3. _____ Parenteral
4. _____ Prefilled cartridge
5. _____ Reconstitution
6. _____ Topical

Column B

a. Dissolving a powder into a solution

b. Glass container with a sealed rubber top

c. Route of administration to skin or mucous membranes

d. Individually wrapped and labeled drugs

e. Disklike solid that dissolves in the mouth

f. Suppository ingredient that melts at body temperature

(continued)

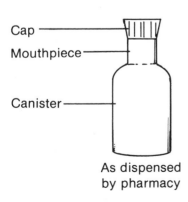

Cap —
Mouthpiece —
Canister —

As dispensed
by pharmacy

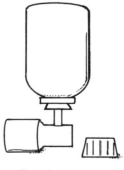

Ready to use

Figure 2-15. *Metered-dose inhaler as dispensed by the pharmacy (**left**), and prepared for use (**right**).*

EXERCISE 6 (Continued)

7. _____ Transdermal patch   g. General term for an injection route

8. _____ Vial   h. Adhesive bandage applied to the skin that gradually releases a drug

9. _____ Lozenge   i. Small vial, with a needle attached, that fits into a syringe holder

10. _____ Cocoa butter   j. Glass container that must be broken to obtain the drug

EXERCISE 7

Complete these statements related to drug packaging. Answers may be found at the end of the chapter.

1. Date and time of reconstitution must be written _____
_____
_____ .

2. The best way to avoid cross-contamination of a multidose tube of ointment is to _____
_____ .

3. To remove medication from a jar of paste the nurse should use _____
_____ .

4. Dropper bottles for eye medications will be labeled _____
_____ .

5. Doses of medication that require use of a metered-dose inhaler are ordered in _____
_____ .

6. Medications for the ear will be labeled _____ .

7. The term "multidose" refers to _____
_____ .

8. The type of drug packaging that decreases the possibility of error is termed _____
_____ .

9. Drugs administered topically for a local effect may be absorbed and produce another effect that is
called a _____
_____
_____ .

10. The word "lozenge" describes _____
_____
_____ .

=========== **ANSWERS** ===========

EXERCISE 1

1. Anspor
2. cephradine
3. Contains 2.5 g cephradine in a dry form
4. Dry mixture
5. 125 mg/5 ml
6. 100 ml
7. 25 to 50 mg/kg per day total, in equally divided doses every 6 or 12 hours
8. Oral
9. Use 61 ml of water to prepare 100 ml oral suspension. (1) Shake to loosen powder. (2) Add 61 ml of water and shake vigorously.
10. Store at room temperature—discard unused portion after 7 days; store in refrigerator—discard unused portion after 14 days.
11. Smith Kline & French Laboratories
12. Federal law prohibits dispensing without prescription; see accompanying folder for complete prescribing information; do not store above 86°F in dry form; dispense in this container; shake well before using; keep tightly closed

EXERCISE 2

1. Ancef
2. cefazolin sodium
3. 1 g cefazolin
4. Lyophilized (freeze-dried)
5. IV or IM
6. 250 mg to 1 g every 6 to 8 hours
7. You cannot tell from the label and must read the literature accompanying the drug.
8. Add 2.5 ml of sterile water for injection and shake
9. Volume is now 3 ml, 330 mg/ml.
10. You must read the accompanying literature to find out how to prepare the drug for IV use.
11. Can be stored at room temperature—discard after 24 hours; stored in the refrigerator the drug is potent for 96 hours.

EXERCISE 3

1. Cardilate
2. erythrityl tetranitrate
3. Oral or sublingual (po or SL)
4. Scored tablet
5. 10 mg
6. 100 tablets
7. Store at 15°–25°C (59°–77°F) in a dry place.
8. Package insert will give indications, dosage, precautions, etc.

EXERCISE 4

1. Capsules
2. Prostaphlin
3. oxacillin sodium
4. 500 mg/capsule
5. For adults—1 capsule (500 mg) every 4 to 6 hours
6. Yes, there is a circular (another name for package insert).
7. No
8. No. Capsules are administered po unless specified otherwise. Check the circular.

EXERCISE 5

1. Compazine Injection
2. prochlorperazine
3. Deep IM or IV administration
4. 2 ml = 10 mg
5. As a liquid. (This is implied because of the way the drug strength is given. The actual drug would appear liquid if you could see it.) Also note that the information on the additives states this is an aqueous solution.
6. A 2-ml ampule—a sealed glass vessel
7. Sodium sulfite, 1 mg; sodium bisulfite, 1 mg; sodium phosphate, 8 mg; sodium biphosphate, 12 mg
8. Store below 86°F; do not freeze; keep package closed to protect ampule from light.
9. Exposure to light may cause discoloration. Slight yellowish discoloration will not alter potency or therapeutic efficacy. If markedly discolored, ampule should be discarded.

EXERCISE 6

1.	d	6.	c
2.	j	7.	h
3.	g	8.	b
4.	i	9.	e
5.	a	10.	f

EXERCISE 7

1. On the label of any powder that the nurse dissolves. Powders begin to lose their potency as soon as they are placed in solution. By writing the date and time on the label, the nurse will be able to check for expiration time.
2. Label the tube with one patient's name and restrict its use to that one patient.
3. A sterile tongue blade or sterile gloves to prevent contamination of the jar contents.
4. "Ophthalmic" or "for the eye"
5. Number of inhalations or puffs
6. "Otic" or "auric"
7. Large stock containers that hold many doses of a drug
8. Unit-dose
9. A systemic effect; the drug reaches the circulation and is carried to other parts of the body.
10. A disklike solid that is slowly dissolved in the mouth (e.g., a cough drop)

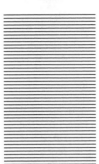

Arithmetic Needed for Dosage

Drugs come in fixed amounts; for example, adult aspirin tablets contain 325 mg, whereas those for children contain 65 mg. When a physician's order differs from the fixed amount at which the drug is supplied, the nurse must calculate the dose needed. Calculation requires knowledge of the systems of measurement and the ability to solve arithmetic. This chapter covers those common arithmetic functions that the nurse needs for the safe administration of drugs.

Students ask why this information must be learned when calculators are so readily available. The reason is that solving the arithmetic forces nurses to think logically about the dose ordered and evaluate their answer (the dose calculated) in relation to the order. Solving dosage problems also mentally increases speed and efficiency in preparing medications. There may be occasions when a problem that will require a calculator arises in the clinical area; however, all arithmetic problems in this chapter can be completed without a calculator.

The arithmetic operations needed for dosage calculations are multiplying whole numbers and fractions; dividing whole numbers, fractions, and decimals; reducing fractions; and reading decimals and using percentage.

MULTIPLYING WHOLE NUMBERS

The multiplication table (Fig. 3-1) is provided for review. Study the table for the numbers 1 through 12. You should achieve 100% accuracy without referring to the table.

> *EXAMPLE:*
>
> Multiply 8 by 7 (8 × 7)
>
> 1. Find column number 8.
> 2. Find row number 7.
> 3. Read across row 7 until you intersect column number 8. The answer is 56.

═══════════════════ **SELF-TEST 1** ═══════════════════

After studying the multiplication table, write the answers to these problems. Answers are given at the end of the chapter; if you do not achieve 100%, you need more study time.

1. 2 × 6 = _____   3. 4 × 8 = _____   5. 12 × 9 = _____

2. 9 × 7 = _____   4. 5 × 9 = _____   6. 8 × 3 = _____

(continued)

1	2	3	4	5	6	⑦	8	9	10	11	12
2	4	6	8	10	12	14	16	18	20	22	24
3	6	9	12	15	18	21	24	27	30	33	36
4	8	12	16	20	24	28	32	36	40	44	48
5	10	15	20	25	30	35	40	45	50	55	60
6	12	18	24	30	36	42	48	54	60	66	72
7	14	21	28	35	42	49	56	63	70	77	84
⑧	16	24	32	40	48	㊼	64	72	80	88	96
9	18	27	36	45	54	63	72	81	90	99	108
10	20	30	40	50	60	70	80	90	100	110	120
11	22	33	44	55	66	77	88	99	110	121	132
12	24	36	48	60	72	84	96	108	120	132	144

Figure 3-1. The multiplication table. The numbers going down the left side (from 1 to 12) are the column numbers. The numbers going across the top (from 1 to 12) are the row numbers. To multiply any two numbers from 1 to 12, find the column for one number, find the row for the other number, and read across the row until you intersect the column.

SELF-TEST 1 (Continued)

7. $11 \times 10 =$ _____

8. $2 \times 7 =$ _____

9. $8 \times 6 =$ _____

10. $8 \times 9 =$ _____

11. $3 \times 5 =$ _____

12. $6 \times 7 =$ _____

13. $4 \times 6 =$ _____

14. $9 \times 6 =$ _____

15. $8 \times 8 =$ _____

16. $7 \times 8 =$ _____

17. $2 \times 9 =$ _____

18. $8 \times 11 =$ _____

19. $4 \times 9 =$ _____

20. $3 \times 8 =$ _____

21. $12 \times 11 =$ _____

22. $9 \times 5 =$ _____

23. $9 \times 9 =$ _____

24. $7 \times 5 =$ _____

DIVIDING WHOLE NUMBERS

The multiplication table is also helpful in dividing large numbers by smaller ones. Study the table for the division of numbers 2 through 12 (Fig. 3–2). Again, you should be able to achieve 100% accuracy without referring to the table; if not, study it again.

EXAMPLE:

Divide 108 by 12 ($108 \div 12$)

1. Find 12 (the smaller number) in the left column.
2. Read across that row until you find 108 (the larger number).
3. The number at the top of that column is the answer, 9.

Remember, because $9 \times 12 = 108$, then $108 \div 12 = 9$ (see Fig. 3–2).

SELF-TEST 2

After studying the division of larger numbers by smaller numbers, write the answers to the following problems. Answers can be found at the end of the chapter.

1. $63 \div 7 =$ _____

2. $24 \div 6 =$ _____

3. $36 \div 12 =$ _____

4. $42 \div 6 =$ _____

5. $35 \div 5 =$ _____

6. $96 \div 12 =$ _____

1	2	3	4	5	6	7	8	⑨	10	11	12
2	4	6	8	10	12	14	16	18	20	22	24
3	6	9	12	15	18	21	24	27	30	33	36
4	8	12	16	20	24	28	32	36	40	44	48
5	10	15	20	25	30	35	40	45	50	55	60
6	12	18	24	30	36	42	48	54	60	66	72
7	14	21	28	35	42	49	56	63	70	77	84
8	16	24	32	40	48	56	64	72	80	88	96
9	18	27	36	45	54	63	72	81	90	99	108
10	20	30	40	50	60	70	80	90	100	110	120
11	22	33	44	55	66	77	88	99	110	121	132
⑫	24	36	48	60	72	84	96	⑩⑧	120	132	144

Figure 3-2. Division table.

7. 12 ÷ 3 = _____

8. 27 ÷ 9 = _____

9. 49 ÷ 7 = _____

10. 18 ÷ 3 = _____

11. 72 ÷ 8 = _____

12. 48 ÷ 8 = _____

13. 28 ÷ 7 = _____

14. 21 ÷ 7 = _____

15. 24 ÷ 8 = _____

16. 84 ÷ 12 = _____

17. 81 ÷ 9 = _____

18. 32 ÷ 8 = _____

19. 36 ÷ 6 = _____

20. 18 ÷ 9 = _____

21. 21 ÷ 3 = _____

22. 48 ÷ 4 = _____

23. 144 ÷ 12 = _____

24. 56 ÷ 8 = _____

FRACTIONS

A *fraction* is a portion of a whole number. The top number is called the *numerator*. The bottom number is called the *denominator*.

EXAMPLE:

$\dfrac{1}{4}$ → numerator
→ denominator

LEARNING AID

The line between the numerator and the denominator is a division sign. Therefore, the fraction can be read as one divided by four.

Types of Fractions

In a *proper* fraction, the numerator is smaller than the denominator.

EXAMPLE: $\dfrac{2}{5}$ (Read as two-fifths.)

In an *improper* fraction, the numerator is larger than the denominator.

EXAMPLE: $\dfrac{5}{2}$ (Read as five halves.)

A *mixed number* has a whole number plus a fraction.

EXAMPLE: $1\frac{2}{3}$ (Read as one and two-thirds.)

In a *complex* fraction, both the numerator and the denominator are already fractions.

EXAMPLE: $\dfrac{\frac{1}{2}}{\frac{1}{4}}$ (Read as one-half divided by one-fourth.)

Reducing Fractions

Find the largest number that can be divided evenly into the numerator *and* the denominator.

EXAMPLE:

Reduce $\dfrac{4}{12}$

$$\dfrac{\overset{1}{\cancel{4}}}{\underset{3}{\cancel{12}}} = \dfrac{1}{3}$$

EXAMPLE:

Reduce $\dfrac{7}{49}$

$$\dfrac{\overset{1}{\cancel{7}}}{\underset{7}{\cancel{49}}} = \dfrac{1}{7}$$

> **LEARNING AID**
> Check to see if the denominator is evenly divisible by the numerator. The number 7 can be evenly divided into 49.

Sometimes fractions are more difficult to reduce because the answer is not obvious.

EXAMPLE:

Reduce $\dfrac{56}{96}$

$$\dfrac{56}{96} = \dfrac{\overset{1}{\cancel{8}} \times 7}{\underset{1}{\cancel{8}} \times 12} = \dfrac{7}{12}$$

EXAMPLE:

Reduce $\dfrac{54}{99}$

$$\dfrac{54}{99} = \dfrac{\overset{1}{\cancel{9}} \times 6}{\underset{1}{\cancel{9}} \times 11} = \dfrac{6}{11}$$

> **LEARNING AID**
> Your knowledge of the multiplication table can help you. Change the numbers to their multiples.

Patience is required to reduce a very large fraction. It may be difficult to find the largest number that will divide evenly into the numerator and the denominator, and you may have to reduce several times.

EXAMPLE:

Reduce $\dfrac{189}{216}$

Try to divide both by 3
$$\dfrac{\overset{63}{\cancel{189}}}{\underset{72}{\cancel{216}}} = \dfrac{63}{72}$$

Then use multiples
$$\dfrac{63}{72} = \dfrac{\overset{1}{\cancel{9}} \times 7}{\underset{1}{\cancel{9}} \times 8} = \dfrac{7}{8}$$

> **LEARNING AID**
> Certain numbers are called prime numbers because they cannot be reduced further. Examples are 2, 3, 5, 7, and 11.
>   In reducing, if the last number is even or a zero, try 2.
>   If the last number is a zero or 5, try 5.
>   If the last number is odd, try 3, 7, or 11.

EXAMPLE:

Reduce $\dfrac{27}{135}$

Try to divide both by 3

$$\dfrac{\overset{9}{\cancel{27}}}{\underset{45}{\cancel{135}}} = \dfrac{\overset{1}{\cancel{9}}}{\underset{5}{\cancel{45}}} = \dfrac{1}{5}$$

SELF-TEST 3

Reduce these fractions to their lowest terms. Answers may be found at the end of the chapter. Be patient!

1. $\dfrac{16}{24}$

2. $\dfrac{36}{216}$

3. $\dfrac{18}{96}$

4. $\dfrac{70}{490}$

5. $\dfrac{18}{81}$

6. $\dfrac{8}{48}$

7. $\dfrac{12}{30}$

8. $\dfrac{68}{136}$

9. $\dfrac{55}{121}$

10. $\dfrac{15}{60}$

Multiplying Fractions

There are two ways to multiply fractions.

FIRST WAY

Multiply the numerators across. Multiply denominators across.
Reduce the answer to its lowest terms.

EXAMPLE:

$$\dfrac{2}{7} \times \dfrac{3}{4} = \dfrac{6}{28}$$

$$\dfrac{6}{28} = \dfrac{3 \times \overset{1}{\cancel{2}}}{14 \times \underset{1}{\cancel{2}}} = \dfrac{3}{14}$$

> **LEARNING AID**
> In multiplying fractions, sometimes one way will be easier. Use whichever method is more comfortable for you.

SECOND WAY (WHEN THERE ARE SEVERAL FRACTIONS)

Reduce by dividing numerators into denominators evenly. Multiply remaining numerators across. Multiply remaining denominators across. Check to see if further reductions can be made.

EXAMPLE:

$$\frac{3}{14} \times \frac{7}{10} \times \frac{5}{12} =$$

$$\frac{\overset{1}{\cancel{3}}}{\underset{2}{\cancel{14}}} \times \frac{\overset{1}{\cancel{7}}}{\underset{2}{\cancel{10}}} \times \frac{\overset{1}{\cancel{5}}}{\underset{4}{\cancel{12}}} = \frac{1}{16}$$

LEARNING AID
$12 \div 3 = 4$
$14 \div 7 = 2$
$10 \div 5 = 2$

EXAMPLE:

$$1\frac{1}{2} \times \frac{4}{6} =$$

$$\frac{\overset{1}{\cancel{3}}}{\underset{1}{\cancel{2}}} \times \frac{\overset{2}{\cancel{4}}}{\underset{2}{\cancel{6}}} = \frac{\overset{}{\cancel{2}}}{\underset{}{\cancel{2}}} = 1$$

LEARNING AID
Mixed numbers must be changed to improper fractions.
$1\frac{1}{2} = 1 \times 2 + 1 = \frac{3}{2}$

EXAMPLE:

$$\frac{4}{5} \times 6\frac{2}{3} =$$

$$\frac{4}{\underset{1}{\cancel{5}}} \times \frac{\overset{4}{\cancel{20}}}{3} = \frac{16}{3}$$

LEARNING AID
$6 \times 3 = 18 + 2 = \frac{20}{3}$

SELF-TEST 4

Multiply these fractions. Answers may be found at the end of the chapter.

1. $\dfrac{1}{6} \times \dfrac{4}{5} \times \dfrac{5}{2} =$

2. $\dfrac{4}{15} \times \dfrac{3}{2} =$

3. $1\dfrac{1}{2} \times 4\dfrac{2}{3} =$

4. $\dfrac{1}{5} \times \dfrac{15}{45} =$

5. $3\dfrac{3}{4} \times 10\dfrac{2}{3} =$

6. $\dfrac{7}{20} \times \dfrac{2}{14} =$

7. $\dfrac{9}{2} \times \dfrac{3}{2} =$

8. $6\dfrac{1}{4} \times 7\dfrac{1}{9} \times \dfrac{9}{5} =$

Dividing Fractions

Fractions can be divided by inverting the number after the division sign and then changing the division sign to a multiplication sign.

EXAMPLE: $\dfrac{1}{75} \div \dfrac{1}{150} = \dfrac{1}{\underset{1}{\cancel{75}}} \times \dfrac{\overset{2}{\cancel{150}}}{1} = 2$

EXAMPLE:

$$\frac{\dfrac{1}{4}}{\dfrac{3}{8}} = \frac{1}{4} \div \frac{3}{8} = \frac{1}{\cancel{4}} \times \frac{\cancel{8}}{3} = \frac{2}{3}$$

EXAMPLE:

$$\frac{1\dfrac{1}{5}}{\dfrac{2}{3}} = \frac{6}{5} \div \frac{2}{3} =$$

$$\frac{\cancel{6}}{5} \times \frac{3}{\cancel{2}} = \frac{9}{5}$$

LEARNING AID

Complex fractions such as

$$\frac{\dfrac{1}{4}}{\dfrac{3}{8}} \text{ may be read as } \frac{1}{4} \div \frac{3}{8}.$$

Remember, the long line represents a division sign.

SELF-TEST 5

Divide these fractions. This operation is important in calculating dosage correctly. Answers may be found at the end of the chapter.

1. $\dfrac{1}{75} \div \dfrac{1}{150} =$

2. $\dfrac{1}{8} \div \dfrac{1}{4} =$

3. $2\dfrac{2}{3} \div \dfrac{1}{2} =$

4. $75 \div 12\dfrac{1}{2} =$

5. $\dfrac{7}{25} \div \dfrac{7}{75} =$

6. $\dfrac{1}{2} \div \dfrac{1}{4} =$

7. $\dfrac{3}{4} \div \dfrac{8}{3} =$

8. $\dfrac{1}{60} \div \dfrac{7}{10} =$

Changing Fractions to Decimals

This can be accomplished by dividing the numerator by the denominator. Remember the line between the numerator and the denominator is a division sign; hence, $\dfrac{1}{4}$ can be read as $1 \div 4$.

In division, the number being divided is called the *dividend;* the number that does the dividing is called the *divisor;* the answer is called the *quotient.*

$$\begin{array}{r} 40. \leftarrow \text{quotient} \\ \text{Divisor} \rightarrow 16\overline{)640.} \leftarrow \text{dividend} \\ \underline{64} \\ 0 \end{array}$$

1. Look at the fraction $\dfrac{1}{4}$

> $\underline{1}$ ← numerator = dividend
> 4 ← denominator = divisor

2. Write

> $4\overline{)1}$

3. If you have difficulty setting this up, you can continue the line for the fraction and place the number above the line into the box.

> $\dfrac{1}{4} = 4\overline{)1}$

4. Once the division problem is set up, place a decimal point immediately after the dividend and also bring the decimal point up to the quotient.

> ⟍_____. ← quotient
> $4\,)\,1.$ ← dividend

Important! Failure to place decimal points carefully can lead to serious dosage errors.

5. Carry out the division.

> $\dfrac{1}{4}\ \dfrac{.25}{)1.00} = 0.25$
> $\underline{8}$
> 20
> $\underline{20}$
> 0

LEARNING AID

If the answer does not have a whole number, place a zero before the decimal. This prevents misreading the answer: .25 is incorrect; 0.25 is correct.

The number of places to report your answer will vary depending upon the way the stock drug comes and the equipment you use. For these exercises, carry answers to three places.

EXAMPLE:

> $\dfrac{5}{16} = 16\dfrac{0.312}{)5.000} = 0.312$
> $\underline{4\,8}$
> 20
> $\underline{16}$
> 40
> $\underline{32}$
> 8

EXAMPLE:

> $\dfrac{1}{75} = 75\dfrac{.013}{)1.000} = 0.013$
> $\underline{75}$
> 250
> $\underline{225}$
> 25

LEARNING AID

Note that there is a space between the 8 and the decimal point in the answer. When this occurs, place a zero in the space to complete the answer.

EXAMPLE:

> $\dfrac{640}{8} = \dfrac{640}{8}\ \dfrac{80.}{)640.} = 80$

SELF-TEST 6

Divide these fractions to produce decimals. Answers will be found at the end of the chapter. Carry decimal places to three if necessary.

1. $\dfrac{1}{6}$

4. $\dfrac{9}{40}$

2. $\dfrac{6}{8}$

5. $\dfrac{1}{8}$

3. $\dfrac{4}{5}$

6. $\dfrac{1}{7}$

DECIMALS

Most medication orders are written in the metric system, which uses decimals.

Reading Decimals

Count the number of places after the decimal point. As you read the decimal, you also create a fraction.

0.1 is read as one tenth $\left(\dfrac{1}{10}\right)$

0.01 is read as one hundredth $\left(\dfrac{1}{100}\right)$

0.001 is read as one thousandth $\left(\dfrac{1}{1000}\right)$

> **LEARNING AID**
> The first number after a decimal point is the tenth place.
>   The second number after the decimal point is the 100th place.
>   The third number after the decimal point is the 1000th place.

EXAMPLES:

0.56 = fifty-six hundredths $\left(\dfrac{56}{100}\right)$

0.2 = two tenths $\left(\dfrac{2}{10}\right)$

0.194 = one hundred and ninety-four thousandths $\left(\dfrac{194}{1000}\right)$

0.31 = thirty-one hundredths $\left(\dfrac{31}{100}\right)$

> **LEARNING AID**
> In reading decimals, read the number first, then count off the decimal places.
>   Whole numbers preceding decimals are read in the usual way.

$$1.6 = \text{one and six tenths} \left(1\frac{6}{10}\right)$$

$$17.354 = \text{seventeen and three hundred and fifty-four thousandths} \left(17\frac{354}{1000}\right)$$

SELF-TEST 7

Write these decimals in longhand and as fractions. Answers may be found at the end of the chapter.

1. 0.25 _____

2. 0.004 _____

3. 1.7 _____

4. 0.5 _____

5. 0.334 _____

6. 136.75 _____

7. 0.1 _____

8. 0.150 _____

Dividing Decimals

Again, in division the number that is being divided is called the dividend; the number that does the dividing is called the divisor and the answer is called the quotient.

$$\text{divisor} \rightarrow 16\overline{)5.000} \rightarrow \text{dividend}$$
$$0.312 \rightarrow \text{quotient}$$

Note that a decimal point is placed immediately after the dividend is written, and is also moved up to the quotient.

EXAMPLE: $\dfrac{13}{16}$ $16\overline{)13.}$

Division is then completed.

EXAMPLE:

```
        0.812
  16)13.000
     12 8
        20
        16
        40
        32
         8
```

Clearing the Divisor of Decimal Points

Before dividing one decimal by another, the divisor must be cleared of decimal points. To do this, move the decimal point to the far right. Move the decimal point in the dividend *the same number of places* and bring the decimal point up to the quotient in the same place.

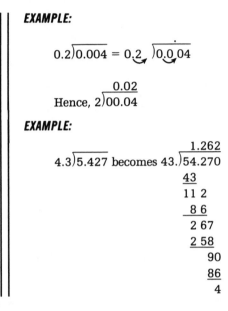

EXAMPLE:

$$0.2\overline{)0.004} = 0.2\overline{)0.0\,04}$$

Hence, $2\overline{)00.04}$ with quotient 0.02

EXAMPLE:

$4.3\overline{)5.427}$ becomes
$$
\begin{array}{r}
1.262 \\
43\overline{)54.270} \\
\underline{43} \\
11\,2 \\
\underline{8\,6} \\
2\,67 \\
\underline{2\,58} \\
90 \\
\underline{86} \\
4
\end{array}
$$

=== **SELF-TEST 8** ===

Do these problems in division of decimals. The answers may be found at the end of this chapter. If necessary, carry answer to three places.

1. $24\overline{)0.0048}$

2. $0.004\overline{)0.1}$

3. $0.02\overline{)0.2}$

4. $7.8\overline{)140}$

5. $6\overline{)140}$

6. $0.025\overline{)10}$

Rounding off Decimals

How do you determine how many places to carry your division? For the nurse, the answer must relate to the materials being used. Some syringes are marked to the tenth place; some to the hundredth place. Some tablets can be broken into halves or fourths; some liquids come in units of measurement in the tenths, hundredths, or thousandths. As you become familiar with dosage you will learn how far you need to round out your answer. At this point let us review the general rule for rounding off decimals.

The rule is: When the number to be dropped is 5 or more, drop the number and add 1 to the previous number. When the last number is 4 or less, drop the number.

EXAMPLE:

0.864 becomes 0.86   4.562 becomes 4.56

1.55 becomes 1.6   2.38 becomes 2.4

0.33 becomes 0.3

Suppose you wanted answers to the nearest tenth. Look at the number in the hundredth place and follow the rules for rounding off.

EXAMPLE:

0.12 becomes 0.1

0.667 becomes 0.7

1.46 becomes 1.5

Suppose you wanted answers to the nearest hundredth. Look at the number in the thousandth place and follow the rules for rounding off.

EXAMPLE:

0.664 becomes 0.66

0.148 becomes 0.15

2.375 becomes 2.38

Suppose you wanted answers to the nearest thousandth. Look at the number in the ten-thousandth place and follow the rules for rounding off.

EXAMPLE:

1.3758 becomes 1.376

0.0024 becomes 0.002

4.5555 becomes 4.556

SELF-TEST 9

Round off these decimals as indicated. Answers may be found at the end of the chapter.

Nearest Tenth	Nearest Hundredth	Nearest Thousandth
1. 0.25 = _____	6. 1.268 = _____	11. 1.3254 = _____
2. 1.84 = _____	7. 0.750 = _____	12. 0.0025 = _____
3. 3.27 = _____	8. 0.677 = _____	13. 0.4520 = _____
4. 0.05 = _____	9. 4.539 = _____	14. 0.7259 = _____
5. 0.63 = _____	10. 1.222 = _____	15. 0.3482 = _____

Comparing the Value of Decimals

Understanding which decimal is larger or smaller is often a help in solving dosage problems. For example, will I need more than one tablet, or less than one tablet?

The rule is: The decimal with the higher number in the tenth place has the greater value.

> *EXAMPLE:*
>
> Compare 0.25 with 0.5
> It is clear that 0.5 is greater because the number 5 is higher than the number 2.

SELF-TEST 10

In each pair, underline the decimal with the greater value. Answers may be found at the end of the chapter.

1. 0.125 and 0.25   **4.** 0.1 and 0.2   **7.** 0.25 and 0.4

2. 0.04 and 0.1   **5.** 0.825 and 0.44   **8.** 0.7 and 0.350

3. 0.5 and 0.125   **6.** 0.9 and 0.5

PERCENT

Percent means parts per hundred. Percent is a fraction with the number becoming the numerator and 100 becoming the denominator. Whole numbers, fractions, and decimals may be written as percent. Percents may be changed to decimals or to fractions.

> *EXAMPLE:*
>
> Whole number: 4% (four percent)
>
> Decimal: 0.2% (two-tenths percent)
>
> Fraction: $\frac{1}{4}$ % (one-fourth percent)

Percents That Are Whole Numbers

> *EXAMPLE:*
>
> Change to a fraction
>
> $4\% = \frac{4}{100} = \frac{1}{25}$
>
> *EXAMPLE:*
>
> Change to a decimal
>
> $4\% = \frac{4}{100} \begin{array}{r} .04 \\ \overline{)4.00} \end{array} = 0.04$

LEARNING AID

Note that 4% means four parts per 100. The 100th place has two decimal points. A quick rule to change a percent to a decimal is to move the decimal point two places to the left.
4% = 0.04
25% = 0.25

Percents That Are Decimals

These may be changed in three ways:

1. By using the quick rule (see Learning Aid)

$$0.2\% = 00.2 = 0.002$$

2. By keeping the decimal

$$0.2\% = \frac{0.2}{100} = 100\overline{)0.200}\ 0.002 = 0.002$$

3. By changing to a complex fraction

$$0.2\% = \frac{\frac{2}{10}}{100} =$$

$$\frac{2}{10} \div 100 =$$

$$\frac{2}{10} \times \frac{1}{100} = \frac{2}{1000}$$

$$\frac{\overset{1}{\cancel{2}}}{\underset{500}{\cancel{1000}}} = \frac{1}{500}$$

> **LEARNING AID**
> Quick rule: To remove a % sign, move the decimal point two places to the left.

> **LEARNING AID**
> Remember that the number after a division sign is inverted. The sign is changed to a multiplication sign.
> Every whole number is understood to have a denominator of 1.
>
> $$\frac{2}{10} \div 100 = \frac{2}{10} \times \frac{1}{100}$$

Percents That Are Fractions

EXAMPLE:

$$\frac{1}{4}\% = \frac{\frac{1}{4}}{100} = \frac{1}{4} \div 100$$

$$\frac{1}{4} \div 100 = \frac{1}{4} \times \frac{1}{100} = \frac{1}{400}$$

EXAMPLE:

$$\frac{1}{2}\% = \frac{\frac{1}{2}}{100} = \frac{1}{2} \div \frac{100}{1}$$

$$\frac{1}{2} \times \frac{1}{100} = \frac{1}{200}$$

Alternative Way. Because $\frac{1}{2} = 0.5$, the percent could also be written as 0.5%. By using the quick rule of moving the decimal point two places to the left to clear a percent, you have 00.5% = 0.005.

Note that 0.005 is $\frac{5}{1000} = \frac{1}{200}$

═══════ SELF-TEST 11 ═══════

*Change these percents to both a **fraction** and a **decimal**. Answers may be found at the end of the chapter.*

1. 10% _____ _____

2. 0.9% _____ _____

3. $\frac{1}{5}$ % _____ _____

RATIO

Medication labels may be stated as a ratio to indicate the relationship of one quantity to another in solution. Ratios are actually fractions. The first number is the numerator. The number after the colon (:) is the denominator.

EXAMPLE: **EXAMPLE:**

$$1:10 = \frac{1}{10} \qquad 1:500 = \frac{1}{500}$$

Proportion shows the relationship between two ratios. Proportions can be written as follows:

$$1:5 :: 25:125$$

This is read as: one is to five as twenty-five is to one hundred twenty-five.

In dosage, a nurse often has the physician's order and an equivalent measure such as 1 g = 1000 mg. To calculate the dose needed, a proportion is set up using x as the unknown, the amount to give the patient. This concept will be discussed in succeeding chapters.

ANSWERS

SELF-TEST 1

1.	12	**7.**	110	**13.**	24	**19.**	36
2.	63	**8.**	14	**14.**	54	**20.**	24
3.	32	**9.**	48	**15.**	64	**21.**	132
4.	45	**10.**	72	**16.**	56	**22.**	45
5.	108	**11.**	15	**17.**	18	**23.**	81
6.	24	**12.**	42	**18.**	88	**24.**	35

SELF-TEST 2

1.	9	**7.**	4	**13.**	4	**19.**	6
2.	4	**8.**	3	**14.**	3	**20.**	2
3.	3	**9.**	7	**15.**	3	**21.**	7
4.	7	**10.**	6	**16.**	7	**22.**	12
5.	7	**11.**	9	**17.**	9	**23.**	12
6.	8	**12.**	6	**18.**	4	**24.**	7

SELF-TEST 3

1. $\dfrac{16}{24} = \dfrac{4}{6} = \dfrac{2}{3}$ (divide by 4, then 2)

Alternatively: $\dfrac{16}{24} = \dfrac{2}{3}$ (divide by 8)

2. $\dfrac{36}{216} = \dfrac{6}{36} = \dfrac{1}{6}$ (divide by 6, then 6)

3. $\dfrac{18}{96} = \dfrac{9}{48} = \dfrac{3}{16}$ (divide by 2, then 3)

4. $\dfrac{70}{490} = \dfrac{7}{49} = \dfrac{1}{7}$ (divide by 10, then 7)

5. $\dfrac{18}{81} = \dfrac{2}{9}$ (divide by 9)

6. $\dfrac{8}{48} = \dfrac{1}{6}$ (divide by 8)

7. $\dfrac{12}{30} = \dfrac{6}{15} = \dfrac{2}{5}$ (divide by 2, then 3)

Alternatively: $\dfrac{12}{30} = \dfrac{2}{5}$ (divide by 6)

8. $\dfrac{68}{136} = \dfrac{34}{68} = \dfrac{1}{2}$ (divide by 2, then 34)

9. $\dfrac{55}{121} = \dfrac{5}{11}$ (divide by 11)

10. $\dfrac{15}{60} = \dfrac{1}{4}$ (divide by 15)

Alternatively: $\dfrac{15}{60} = \dfrac{3}{12} = \dfrac{1}{4}$ (divide by 5, then 3)

SELF-TEST 4

First Way

1. $\dfrac{1}{6} \times \dfrac{4}{5} \times \dfrac{5}{2} = \dfrac{20}{60} = \dfrac{1}{3}$

2. $\dfrac{4}{15} \times \dfrac{3}{2} = \dfrac{\overset{2}{\cancel{12}}}{\cancel{30}} = \dfrac{2}{5}$
               5
(Divide by 6)

3. $1\dfrac{1}{2} \times 4\dfrac{2}{3} = \dfrac{3}{2} \times \dfrac{14}{3} = \dfrac{42}{6} = 7$

4. $\dfrac{1}{5} \times \dfrac{15}{45} = \dfrac{\overset{3}{\cancel{15}}}{\cancel{225}} = \dfrac{3}{45} = \dfrac{1}{15}$
             45
(Divide by 5)

5. $3\dfrac{3}{4} \times 10\dfrac{2}{3} = \dfrac{15}{4} \times \dfrac{32}{3}$
   (Too confusing! Use the second way.)

6. $\dfrac{7}{20} \times \dfrac{2}{14}$
   (Too difficult. Use the second way.)

7. $\dfrac{9}{2} \times \dfrac{3}{2} = \dfrac{27}{4}$
   (Cannot reduce)

8. $6\dfrac{1}{4} \times 7\dfrac{1}{9} \times \dfrac{9}{5} = \dfrac{25}{4} \times \dfrac{64}{9} \times \dfrac{9}{5}$
   (Too difficult. Use the second way.)

Second Way

1. $\dfrac{1}{6} \times \dfrac{4}{5} \times \dfrac{5}{2} = \dfrac{2}{6} = \dfrac{1}{3}$

2. $\dfrac{4}{15} \times \dfrac{3}{2} = \dfrac{2}{5}$

3. $1\dfrac{1}{2} \times 4\dfrac{2}{3} = \dfrac{3}{2} \times \dfrac{14}{3} = 7$

4. $\dfrac{1}{5} \times \dfrac{15}{45} = \dfrac{1}{15}$

5. $\dfrac{15}{4} \times \dfrac{32}{3} = 40$

6. $\dfrac{7}{20} \times \dfrac{2}{14} = \dfrac{1}{20}$

8. $\dfrac{25}{4} \times \dfrac{64}{9} \times \dfrac{9}{5} = 80$

SELF-TEST 5

1. $\dfrac{1}{75} \div \dfrac{1}{150} = \dfrac{1}{75} \times \dfrac{150}{1} = 2$

2. $\dfrac{1}{8} \div \dfrac{1}{4} = \dfrac{1}{8} \times \dfrac{4}{1} = \dfrac{1}{2}$

3. $2\dfrac{2}{3} \div \dfrac{1}{2} = \dfrac{8}{3} \times \dfrac{2}{1} = \dfrac{16}{3}$

6. $\dfrac{1}{2} \div \dfrac{1}{4} = \dfrac{1}{\cancel{2}} \times \dfrac{\overset{2}{\cancel{4}}}{1} = 2$

4. $75 \div 12\dfrac{1}{2} = 75 \div \dfrac{25}{2} = \cancel{75} \times \dfrac{2}{\underset{1}{\cancel{25}}} = \overset{3}{} \cdot 6 = 6$

7. $\dfrac{3}{4} \div \dfrac{8}{3} = \dfrac{3}{4} \times \dfrac{3}{8} = \dfrac{9}{32}$

5. $\dfrac{7}{25} \div \dfrac{7}{75} = \dfrac{\overset{1}{\cancel{7}}}{\underset{1}{\cancel{25}}} \times \dfrac{\overset{3}{\cancel{75}}}{\underset{1}{\cancel{7}}} = 3$

8. $\dfrac{1}{60} \div \dfrac{7}{10} = \dfrac{1}{\underset{6}{\cancel{60}}} \times \dfrac{\overset{1}{\cancel{10}}}{7} = \dfrac{1}{42}$

SELF-TEST 6

1. $\dfrac{1}{6}$ $6\,\overline{)\,1.000}^{\,.166}$ $= 0.166$

$\quad\underline{6}$
$\quad40$
$\quad\underline{36}$
$\quad40$
$\quad\underline{36}$
$\quad4$

4. $\dfrac{9}{40}$ $40\,\overline{)\,9.000}^{\,.225}$ $= 0.225$

$\quad\underline{8\,0}$
$\quad1\,00$
$\quad\underline{80}$
$\quad200$
$\quad\underline{200}$
$\quad0$

2. $\dfrac{\cancel{6}}{\cancel{8}} = \dfrac{3}{4}$ $4\,\overline{)\,3.00}^{\,.75}$ $= 0.75$

$\overset{3}{}\quad4\quad\underline{2\,8}$
$\qquad\quad20$
$\qquad\quad\underline{20}$
$\qquad\quad0$

5. $\dfrac{1}{8}$ $8\,\overline{)\,1.000}^{\,.125}$ $= 0.125$

$\quad\underline{8}$
$\quad20$
$\quad\underline{16}$
$\quad40$
$\quad\underline{40}$
$\quad0$

3. $\dfrac{4}{5}$ $5\,\overline{)\,4.0}^{\,.8}$ $= 0.8$

$\quad\underline{4\,0}$
$\quad0$

6. $\dfrac{1}{7}$ $7\,\overline{)\,1.000}^{\,.142}$ $= 0.142$

$\quad\underline{7}$
$\quad30$
$\quad\underline{28}$
$\quad20$
$\quad\underline{14}$
$\quad6$

SELF-TEST 7

1. Twenty-five hundredths $\left(\dfrac{25}{100}\right)$

2. Four thousandths $\left(\dfrac{4}{1000}\right)$

3. One and seven tenths $\left(1\dfrac{7}{10}\right)$

4. Five tenths $\left(\dfrac{5}{10}\right)$

5. Three hundred thirty-four thousandths $\left(\dfrac{334}{1000}\right)$

6. One hundred thirty-six and seventy-five hundredths $\left(136\dfrac{75}{100}\right)$

7. One tenth $\left(\dfrac{1}{10}\right)$

8. One hundred fifty thousandths $\left(\dfrac{150}{1000}\right)$. The zero at the end of 0.150 is not necessary. The number could be read as fifteen hundredths $\left(\dfrac{15}{100}\right)$.

SELF-TEST 8

1. $24\overline{)0.0048}$ 0.0002   No decimals in the divisor, so no need to move the decimal in the dividend.

2. $0.004\overline{)0.100}$ Now it is $4\overline{)100.}$ 25.

3. $0.02\overline{)0.20}$ Now it is $2\overline{)20}$ 10.

4. $7.8\overline{)140.0}$ Now it is $78\overline{)1400.000}$ 17.948

```
   17.948
78)1400.000
   78
   620
   546
    74 0
    70 2
     3 80
     3 12
       680
       624
        56
```

5.
```
   23.333
6)140.000
  12
  20
  18
   20
   18
    20
    18
    20
    18
     2
```

6. $0.025\overline{)10.000}$ Now it is $25\overline{)10000.}$ 400.

Note that because there are two places between the 4 and the decimal, you had to add 2 zeros.

SELF-TEST 9

Nearest Tenth		Nearest Hundredth		Nearest Thousandth
1. 0.3	**6.**	1.27	**11.**	1.325
2. 1.8	**7.**	0.75	**12.**	0.003
3. 3.3	**8.**	0.68	**13.**	0.452
4. 0.1	**9.**	4.54	**14.**	0.726
5. 0.6	**10.**	1.22	**15.**	0.348

SELF-TEST 10

1. 0.25   **5.** 0.825
2. 0.1   **6.** 0.9
3. 0.5   **7.** 0.4
4. 0.2   **8.** 0.7

SELF-TEST 11

1. Fraction $10\% = \dfrac{\overset{1}{\cancel{10}}}{\underset{10}{\cancel{100}}} = \dfrac{1}{10}$

   Decimal $10\% = \dfrac{10}{100}$ $100\overline{)10.0}\,^{.1} = 0.1$

   Quick rule decimal $10.\% = 0.1$

2. Fraction $0.9\% = \dfrac{\frac{9}{10}}{100} = \dfrac{9}{10} \div 100 = \dfrac{9}{10} \times \dfrac{1}{100} = \dfrac{9}{1000}$

   Decimal $0.9\% = \dfrac{0.9}{100}$ $100\overline{)0.900}\,^{.009} = 0.009$

   Quick rule decimal $00.9 = 0.009$

3. Fraction $\dfrac{1}{5}\% = \dfrac{\frac{1}{5}}{100} = \dfrac{1}{5} \div 100 = \dfrac{1}{5} \times \dfrac{1}{100} = \dfrac{1}{500}$

   Decimal $\dfrac{1}{5}\% = \dfrac{1}{5} \div 100 = \dfrac{1}{500}$ $500\overline{)1.000}\,^{.002} = 0.002$

   Quick rule decimal $\dfrac{1}{5}\% = \dfrac{1}{5}$ $5\overline{)1.0}\,^{.2} = 0.2\%$

   $00.2 = 0.002$

4

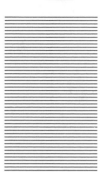

Dosage Measurement Systems

Most medication orders are written in the metric system. However, some physicians do order drugs in the apothecary and household systems. Therefore, nurses must be familiar with all three systems and be able to convert doses from one system to another.

METRIC SYSTEM

The metric system is a decimal system based on tens; it has three basic units of measurement: gram (weight), liter (volume), and meter (length). Measures of length will not be discussed because medication orders are written for weight and volume.

The metric system uses arabic numbers (e.g., 1, 2, 3) and decimals (e.g., 0.4, 0.008).

Measures of Weight

Solid measures in the metric system are

Gram: abbreviated g or Gm or gm (g is preferred)

Milligram: abbreviated mg or mgm (mg is preferred)

Microgram: abbreviated μg or mcg (μg, which uses the Greek letter *mu* (μ), is printed; mcg is written)

Kilogram: abbreviated kg or Kg (kg is preferred)

Weight Equivalents

The basic weight equivalents in the metric system are:

1 g = 1000 mg

1 mg = 1000 μg (mcg)

Note that the gram is larger than a milligram. It takes 1000 mg to equal the weight of 1 g. A milligram is itself larger than a microgram; it takes 1000 μg to equal the weight of 1 mg. These relationships can be indicated using the symbol >, which means "is greater than":

g > mg > μg

Read: A gram is greater than a milligram, which is greater than a microgram.

Converting Solid Equivalents

The nurse will have to calculate how much of a drug to give if the supply on hand is not in the same weight measure as the medication order.

> **EXAMPLE:**
>
> Order: 0.25 g
> Supply: tablets labeled 125 mg

We know the equivalent 1 g = 1000 mg. Therefore, we could change 0.25 g to milligrams by multiplying the number of grams by 1000.

$$
\begin{array}{r}
0.25 \\
\times 1000 \\
\hline
250.00
\end{array}
$$

The answer, then, is that 0.25 g = 250 mg.

There is a shortcut. In decimals, the thousandth place is three numbers after the decimal point. We can change grams to milligrams by moving the decimal point three places to the right, which produces the same answer as multiplying by 1000. We can also change milligrams to grams by moving the decimal point three places to the left, which is the same as dividing by 1000. This is the method we will learn.

TO CHANGE GRAMS TO MILLIGRAMS

Rule: Move the decimal point three places to the right. This means to multiply by 1000.

> **EXAMPLE:**   0.25 g = _____ mg
> 0.250 = 250
> 0.25 g = 250 mg

> **EXAMPLE:**   0.1 g = _____ mg
> 0.100 = 100
> 0.1 g = 100 mg

Grams to Milligrams Quick Rule: Some students have difficulty deciding whether to move decimal points to the left or the right. Here is a method that might be helpful.

1. Write the order first.
2. Write the equivalent measure needed.
3. Use an arrow to show which way the decimal point should move.
4. The open part of the arrow always faces the *larger* measure.
5. In the equivalent 1 g = 1000 mg, the gram is the larger measure. It takes 1000 mg to make 1 g.

> **EXAMPLE:**
>
> Order: 0.25 g
> Supply: 125 mg
> You want to convert grams to milligrams
> 0.25 g > _____ mg
> The arrow is telling you to move the decimal point three places to the right.
> 0.250 = 250
> Hence, 0.25 g = 250 mg

(*continued*)

> **EXAMPLE:**
>
> Order: 1.5 g
> Supply: 500 mg
> You want to convert grams to milligrams
> 1.5 g > _____ mg
> 1.500 = 1500
> Hence, 1.5 g = 1500 mg

EXERCISE 1

Try these conversions from grams to milligrams. Answers may be found at the end of the chapter.

1. 0.3 g = _____ mg   **5.** 5 g = _____ mg

2. 0.001 g = _____ mg   **6.** 0.4 g = _____ mg

3. 0.02 g = _____ mg   **7.** 0.08 g = _____ mg

4. 1.2 g = _____ mg   **8.** 0.275 g = _____ mg

TO CHANGE MILLIGRAMS TO GRAMS

> Rule: Move the decimal point three places to the left. This means to divide by 1000.
>
> **EXAMPLE:**   **EXAMPLE:**
>
> 100 mg = _____ g   8 mg = _____ g
> 100. = 0.1   008. = 0.008
> 100 mg = 0.1 g   8 mg = 0.008 g
>
> *Milligrams to Grams Quick Rule:* The arrow method also works to convert milligrams to grams. Remember the steps:
>
> 1. Write the order first.
> 2. Write the equivalent measure needed.
> 3. Use an arrow to show which way the decimal point should move.
> 4. The open part of the arrow always faces the *larger* measure.
> 5. In the equivalent 1 g = 1000 mg, the gram is the larger measure.
>
> **EXAMPLE:**
>
> Order: 15 mg
> Supply: 0.03 g
> You want to convert milligrams to grams
> 15 mg < g
> The arrow tells you to move the decimal point three places to the left.
> 015. = 0.015
> 15 mg = 0.015 g

(*continued*)

(continued)

> **EXAMPLE:**
>
> Order: 500 mg
> Supply: 1 g
> You want to convert mg to g
> 500 mg = _____ g
> 500 < g
> The arrow tells you to move the decimal point three places to the left.
> $\overset{\curvearrowleft}{500.}$ = 0.5
> 500 mg = 0.5 g

=== **EXERCISE 2** ===

Try these conversions from milligrams to grams. Answers may be found at the end of the chapter.

1. 4 mg = _____ g   5. 250 mg = _____ g

2. 120 mg = _____ g   6. 1 mg = _____ g

3. 40 mg = _____ g   7. 50 mg = _____ g

4. 75 mg = _____ g   8. 600 mg = _____ g

The second major weight equivalent in the metric system is

$$1 \text{ mg} = 1000 \text{ } \mu g$$

Some medications are so powerful that minute microgram doses are sufficient to produce a therapeutic effect. It is easier to write orders in micrograms as whole numbers than to use milligrams written as decimals.

TO CHANGE MILLIGRAMS TO MICROGRAMS

> Rule: Move the decimal point three places to the right. This means to multiply by 1000.
>
> > **EXAMPLE:**
> >
> > 0.1 mg = _____ μg
> > $0.\underset{\curvearrowright}{100}$ = 100
> > 0.1 mg = 100 μg
> >
> > **EXAMPLE:**
> >
> > 0.25 mg = _____ μg
> > $0.\underset{\curvearrowright}{250}$ = 250
> > 0.25 mg = 250 μg

(*continued*)

Milligrams to Micrograms Quick Rule: Some students have difficulty deciding whether to move decimal points to the left or the right.

1. Write the order first.
2. Write the equivalent measure needed.
3. Use an arrow to show which way the decimal point should move.
4. The open part of the arrow always faces the *larger* measure.
5. In the equivalent 1 mg = 1000 μg, the milligram is the larger measure. It takes 1000 μg to make 1 mg.

EXAMPLE:

Order: 0.1 mg
Supply: 200 μg
You want to convert milligrams to micrograms.
0.1 mg > _____ μg
The arrow is telling you to move the decimal point three places to the right.
0.100 = 100
Hence: 0.1 mg = 100 μg

EXAMPLE:

Order: 0.3 mg
Supply: 600 μg
You want to convert milligrams to micrograms.
0.3 mg > _____ μg
0.300 = 300
Hence, 0.3 mg = 300 μg

EXERCISE 3

Try these conversions from milligrams to micrograms. Use either method. Answers may be found at the end of the chapter.

1. 0.3 mg = _____ μg
2. 0.001 mg = _____ μg
3. 0.02 mg = _____ μg
4. 0.08 mg = _____ μg
5. 1.2 mg = _____ μg
6. 0.4 mg = _____ μg
7. 5 mg = _____ μg
8. 0.7 mg = _____ μg

TO CHANGE MICROGRAMS TO MILLIGRAMS

Rule: Move the decimal point three places to the left. This means to divide by 1000.

EXAMPLE:

300 μg = _____ mg
300. = 0.3
300 μg = 0.3 mg

EXAMPLE:

50 μg = _____ mg
050. = 0.05
50 μg = 0.05 mg

(*continued*)

(continued)

Micrograms to Milligrams Quick Rule: The arrow method also works to convert micrograms to milligrams. Remember the steps.

1. Write the order first.
2. Write the equivalent measure needed.
3. Use an arrow to show which way the decimal point should move.
4. The open part of the arrow always faces the *larger* measure.
5. In the equivalent 1 mg = 1000 μg, the milligram is the larger measure.

EXAMPLE:

Order: 100 μg
Supply: 0.1 mg
You want to convert micrograms to milligrams.
100 μg < mg
The arrow tells you to move the decimal point three places to the left.
100. = 0.1
100 μg = 0.1 mg

EXAMPLE:

Order: 50 μg
Supply: 0.1 mg
You want to convert micrograms to milligrams.
50 μg = _____ mg
μg < mg
The arrow tells you to move the decimal point three places to the left.
050. = 0.05
50 μg = 0.05 mg

EXERCISE 4

Try these conversions from micrograms to milligrams. Answers may be found at the end of the chapter.

1. 800 μg = _____ mg   5. 1 μg   = _____ mg

2. 4 μg   = _____ mg   6. 200 μg = _____ mg

3. 14 μg = _____ mg   7. 50 μg = _____ mg

4. 25 μg = _____ mg   8. 750 μg = _____ mg

EXERCISE 5

Now try mixed conversions in metric weight measures. Be careful when reading and take the time to think and apply the rules you have learned. Answers may be found at the end of the chapter.

1. 0.3 mg = _____ g   3. 15 μg = _____ mg

2. 0.03 g = _____ mg   4. 0.1 g   = _____ mg

=========== **EXERCISE 5** (*Continued*) ===========

5. 100 μg = _____ mg   8. 200 mg = _____ g

6. 50 mg = _____ g   9. 0.2 mg = _____ μg

7. 0.014 g = _____ mg   10. 0.65 mg = _____ μg

Table of Common Metric Solid Equivalents

Most practicing nurses know certain common equivalents in the metric system. Study Table 4–1 to familiarize yourself with them.

Metric Liquid Measures

Liquid measures in the metric system are

    Liter: abbreviated L

    Milliliter: abbreviated ml or mL

    Cubic centimeter: abbreviated cc

Metric Liquid Equivalents

The basic liquid equivalents in the metric system are

    1 ml = 1 cc

    1 L = 1000 ml or 1000 cc

Table 4-1.   Common Metric Weight Equivalents

Weight	Equivalent
1000 mg	1 g
600 mg	0.6 g
500 mg	0.5 g
300 mg	0.3 g
200 mg	0.2 g
100 mg	0.1 g
60 mg	0.06 g
30 mg	0.03 g
15 mg	0.15 g
10 mg	0.01 g
1 mg	1000 μg
0.6 mg	600 μg
0.4 mg	400 μg
0.3 mg	300 μg
0.1 mg	100 μg

It is not necessary to study liquid conversions within the metric system, because orders are given and supplies are in the same measure.

APOTHECARY SYSTEM

The apothecary system of measurement was brought to the United States from England during the colonial era. Some physicians still order medications this way, and some pharmacists label drugs in the apothecary system as well as the metric system. Therefore, nurses should be familiar with the basic apothecary measures.

Overview

The system is expressed in fractions (e.g., $\frac{1}{4}, \frac{1}{2}$) and in Roman numerals. The Roman numerals are made up of letters of the alphabet.

    M = 1000   x = 10

    D = 500   v = 5

    C = 100   i = 1

    L = 50

(x, v, and i may or may not be capitalized)

When a smaller numeral precedes a larger numeral, the smaller numeral is **subtracted** from the larger.

XL = 40 (10 from 50)

IX = 9 (1 from 10)

When the smaller numeral follows a larger numeral, the smaller numeral is **added** to the larger.

MX = 1010 (1000 plus 10)

LII = 52 (50 plus 1 plus 1)

XI = 11 (10 plus 1)

Roman numerals never use more than three of the same digit in a row.
The year 1991 would be written by analyzing its component parts.

```
1000 = M  (1000)
 900 = CM (100 from 1000)
  90 = XC (10 from 100)
   1 = I   (one)
```
1991 = MCMXCI

Roman Numerals Used in Apothecary Dosage

Arabic Number	Roman Number	Arabic Number	Roman Number
$\frac{1}{2}$	ss	6	vi
1	i	7	vii
$1\frac{1}{2}$	iss	$7\frac{1}{2}$	viiss
2	ii	8	viii
3	iii	9	ix
4	iv	10	x
5	v	20	xx
		30	xxx

Grain

The solid measure in the apothecary system is the grain (abbreviated gr). An example of an order is gr v. Note that the Roman numeral follows the measure. Some physicians write this order using Arabic numbers, so you might see 5 gr or 10 gr.

Liquid Measures

In the apothecary system, the liquid measures are

Minim: abbreviated M or M̡

Dram: abbreviated ʒ or dr

Ounce: abbreviated ʒ

Drop: abbreviated gtt

Remember that an ounce is larger than a dram; hence, the symbol for an ounce has two loops.

Common Liquid Equivalents

In the apothecary system, the common liquid equivalents are

Spoken	Written
1 minim = 1 drop	m i = gtt i
60 minims = 1 dram	m LX = ʒi = 1 dr
1 dram = 4 ml	ʒi = 1 dr = 4 ml
8 drams = 1 ounce	ʒviii = 8 dr = ℥i

HOUSEHOLD MEASURES

Although used in the home, these measures are acceptable in preparing medications in the medical setting when a standard medication receptacle is used. Household measures are

Teaspoon: abbreviated tsp

Tablespoon: abbreviated tbsp or T

Ounce: abbreviated oz

Pint: abbreviated pt

Quart: abbreviated qt

Common Equivalents in the Household System

Spoken	Written
One teaspoon = 5 milliliters	1 tsp = 5 ml
One tablespoon = 15 milliliters	1 tbsp = 15 ml
One ounce = 30 milliliters	1 oz = 30 ml
One pint = 500 milliliters	1 pt = 500 ml
One quart = 1 liter = 1000 milliliters	1 qt = 1 L = 1000 ml
2.2 pounds = 1 kilogram	2.2 lb = 1 kg

CONVERSIONS AMONG METRIC, APOTHECARY, AND HOUSEHOLD SYSTEMS

Solid Equivalents

The physician's drug order may not be written in the same system as the supply. The nurse must convert either the order *or* the supply amount to calculate the dose needed. In changing from one system to another, conversions are not exact. Table 4-2 lists common equivalents the nurse should know.

Three equivalents require explanation:

gr x = 0.6 g = 600 mg or 650 mg

gr v = 0.3 g = 300 mg or 325 mg

gr i = 0.06 g = 60 mg or 65 mg

Look at the table. Note that gr xv = 1 g = 1000 mg. Also, note that gr i = 60 mg. If you multiply 15 gr by 60 mg, the answer is 900 mg. According to the table, 15 gr is equivalent to 1000 mg, not 900 mg. A discrepancy exists. To remedy this problem, some drug companies have manufactured the grain to contain 65 mg; 5 gr to contain 325 mg; 10 gr to contain 650 mg.

**Table 4-2.   Common Solid Metric
and Apothecary Equivalents**

Milligram	Gram*	Grain	Microgram
1000 mg	1 g	gr xv	
(650)† 600 mg	0.6 g	gr x	
500 mg	0.5 g	gr vii s̈s	
(325)† 300 mg	0.3 g	gr v	
200 mg	0.2 g	gr iii	
100 mg	0.1 g	gr i s̈s	
(65)† 60 mg	0.06 g	gr i	
30 mg	0.03 g	gr s̈s or gr $\frac{1}{2}$	
15 mg	0.015 g	gr $\frac{1}{4}$	
10 mg	0.01 g	gr $\frac{1}{6}$	
0.6 mg		gr $\frac{1}{100}$	600 μg
0.4 mg		gr $\frac{1}{150}$	400 μg
0.3 mg		gr $\frac{1}{200}$	300 μg

* Remember that g = Gm or gm; μg = mcg.

† Alternative values.

When solving dosage problems, use whichever equivalent is closer.

EXAMPLE:

Order	Supply	Answer
0.3 g po	gr v tab	1 tab
325 mg po	gr v tab	1 tab
0.06 g po	gr i tab	1 tab
gr i po	65 mg tab	1 tab
gr x po	325 mg tab	2 tab
650 mg po	0.6 g tab	1 tab
gr ii po	60 mg tab	2 tab
0.3 g po	325 mg	1 tab

EXERCISE 6

Practice exercises in solid equivalents. Answers may be found at the end of the chapter.

1. What is the short rule for converting milligrams to grams? _____

    _____

    _____

2. 0.60 mg = _____ g   4. 300 mg = _____ g

3. 0.6 mg = _____ g   5. 500 mg = _____ g

EXERCISE 7

Fill in the blanks.

1. 1000 mg = _____ g
2. 600 mg = _____ g
3. 500 mg = _____ g
4. 300 mg = _____ g
5. 200 mg = _____ g
6. 100 mg = _____ g
7. 60 mg = _____ g

8. 30 mg = _____ g
9. 15 mg = _____ g
10. 10 mg = _____ g
11. 0.6 mg = _____ μg
12. 0.4 mg = _____ μg
13. 0.3 mg = _____ μg
14. 0.25 mg = _____ μg

EXERCISE 8

1. What is the short rule for converting grams to milligrams? _big to smal_

2. 1 g = _1000_ mg
3. 0.01 g = _010_ mg

4. 0.2 g = _200_ mg
5. 0.12 g = _120_ mg

EXERCISE 9

Fill in the table of grams to milligrams.

1. 1 g = _1000_ mg
2. 0.6 g = _600_ mg
3. 0.5 g = _500_ mg
4. 0.3 g = _____ mg
5. 0.2 g = _____ mg

6. 0.1 g = _____ mg
7. 0.06 g = _____ mg
8. 0.03 g = _____ mg
9. 0.015 g = _____ mg
10. 0.01 g = _____ mg

EXERCISE 10

What is the equivalent?

1. 60 mg = gr _1_
2. 30 mg = gr _ss_
3. 15 mg = gr _¼_

4. 0.6 mg = gr _1/100_
5. 0.4 mg = gr _1/150_
6. 0.3 mg = gr _1/200_

EXERCISE 11

Fill in the table of grains to milligrams.

1. gr i = _60_ mg

2. gr $\frac{1}{2}$ = _30_ mg

EXERCISE 11 (Continued)

3. $gr \dfrac{1}{4} =$ _____ mg   **5.** $gr \dfrac{1}{100} =$ _____ mg

4. $gr \dfrac{1}{6} =$ _____ mg   **6.** $gr \dfrac{1}{150} =$ _____ mg

EXERCISE 12

What is the equivalent?

1. 1 g   = gr _____   **6.** 0.03 g = gr _____

2. 0.5 g = gr _____   **7.** 0.015 g = gr _____

3. 0.2 g = gr _____   **8.** 0.01 g = gr _____

4. 0.6 g = gr _____   **9.** 0.06 g = gr _____

5. 0.3 g = gr _____

EXERCISE 13

Fill in the table of grains to grams.

1. gr xv   = _____ g   **5.** gr iii = _____ g

2. gr x   = _____ g   **6.** gr iss = _____ g

3. gr viiss = _____ g

4. gr v   = _____ g

EXERCISE 14

Fill in this table.

1.   1000 mg = _____ g = gr _____

2.   600 mg = _____ g = gr _____

3. _____ mg =   0.5 g = gr _____

4. _____ mg = _____ g = gr iii

5. _____ mg =   0.1 g = gr _____

6.   60 mg = _____ g = gr _____

7. _____ mg =   0.03 g = gr _____

8. _____ mg = _____ g = $gr \dfrac{1}{4}$

9.   10 mg = _____ g = gr _____

10. _____ mg =   0.0006 g = gr _____ = 600 μg

11.   0.4 mg = _____ g = gr _____ = 400 μg

12.   0.3 mg = _____ g = gr _____ = 300 μg

=============== **EXERCISE 15** ===============

Practice exercise in solid equivalents. Express as milligrams.

1. gr $\dfrac{1}{150}$ = _____ mg   5. gr $\dfrac{1}{2}$ = _____ mg

2. 0.03 Gm = _____ mg   6. gr i = _____ mg

3. 0.5 g = _____ mg   7. 0.015 g = _____ mg

4. 1 Gm = _____ mg   8. gr iss = _____ mg

=============== **EXERCISE 16** ===============

Express as grams.

1. 30 mg = _____ g   5. 500 mg = _____ g

2. 100 mg = _____ g   6. gr x = _____ g

3. gr iii = _____ g   7. 0.6 mg = _____ g

4. gr i = _____ g   8. gr xv = _____ g

=============== **EXERCISE 17** ===============

Express as grains.

1. 0.4 mg = gr _____   4. 15 mg = gr _____

2. 0.1 g = gr _____   5. 0.3 g = gr _____

3. 60 mg = gr _____   6. 0.3 mg = gr _____

Liquid Equivalents

The physician's order may not be written in the same system as the supply. In changing from one system to another, conversions may not be exact. Table 4-3 lists common liquid equivalents among the three systems. (See also Fig. 1-3.)

Table 4-3. Common Liquid Metric, Apothecary, and Household Equivalents

Metric	Apothecary	Household
	1 m = 1 gtt	
1 ml*	16 m	
4 ml	ʒi	
5 ml		1 tsp
15 ml	ʒiv	1 tbsp
30 ml	ʒviii	1 oz; 2 tbsp
500 ml		1 pt
1000 ml; 1 L		1 qt; 2 pt

* Remember that 1 ml = 1 cc.

EXERCISE 18

Practice exercises in liquid equivalents. Answers may be found at the end of the chapter.

1. 1 oz = dr _____
2. 1 tbsp = ʒ _____
3. ʒ ss = _____ cc
4. ℥ii = _____ ml
5. 1 ml = m _____

6. 4 dr = _____ oz
7. 1 tsp = _____ ml
8. 1 oz = _____ tbsp
9. 1 oz = _____ ml
10. 1 L   = _____ ml

EXERCISE 19

Express the liquid measure requested.

1. 4 ml = ʒ _____
2. 1 tbsp = _____ ml
3. ʒ i ss = _____ ml
4. 5 ml = _____ tsp
5. 30 ml = _____ oz

6. 30 ml = ʒ _____
7. 1 m = _____ gtt
8. 1 pt = _____ cc
9. 1 qt = _____ ml
10. 1 cc = _____ ml

EXERCISE 20

Fill in the measure requested.

1. ℥ i = _____ cc
2. 1 qt = _____ L
3. 15 ml = _____ tbsp
4. ʒ viii = _____ oz
5. 2 tbsp = _____ oz

6. m xvi = _____ ml
7. 1 L = _____ ml
8. ℥ iv = _____ oz
9. 500 ml = _____ pt
10. 1 kg = _____ lb

===================== **ANSWERS** =====================

EXERCISE 1

1. 300   **3.** 20   **5.** 5000   **7.** 80
2. 1   **4.** 1200   **6.** 400   **8.** 275

EXERCISE 2

1. 0.004   **3.** 0.04   **5.** 0.25   **7.** 0.05
2. 0.12   **4.** 0.075   **6.** 0.001   **8.** 0.6

EXERCISE 3

1. 300   **3.** 20   **5.** 1200   **7.** 5000
2. 1   **4.** 80   **6.** 400   **8.** 700

EXERCISE 4

1. 0.8   **3.** 0.014   **5.** 0.001   **7.** 0.05
2. 0.004   **4.** 0.025   **6.** 0.2   **8.** 0.75

EXERCISE 5

1. 0.0003   **6.** 0.05
2. 30   **7.** 14
3. 0.015   **8.** 0.2
4. 100   **9.** 200
5. 0.1   **10.** 650

EXERCISE 6

1. Divide milligrams by 1000, or move decimal point three places to the left, or use an arrow with the open part facing gram to show movement of decimal point three places.
2. 0.0006 g   **3.** 0.0006 g   **4.** 0.3 g   **5.** 0.5 g

EXERCISE 7

1. 1   **8.** 0.03
2. 0.6   **9.** 0.015
3. 0.5   **10.** 0.01
4. 0.3   **11.** 600
5. 0.2   **12.** 400
6. 0.1   **13.** 300
7. 0.06   **14.** 250

EXERCISE 8

1. Multiply grams by 1000, or move decimal point three places to the right, or use an arrow with the open part toward gram to show movement of decimal point three places.
2. 1000   **3.** 10   **4.** 200   **5.** 120

EXERCISE 9

1. 1000   **6.** 100
2. 600   **7.** 60
3. 500   **8.** 30
4. 300   **9.** 15
5. 200   **10.** 10

EXERCISE 10

1. i   **4.** $\dfrac{1}{100}$
2. s̈s or $\dfrac{1}{2}$ **5.** $\dfrac{1}{150}$
3. $\dfrac{1}{4}$ **6.** $\dfrac{1}{200}$

EXERCISE 11

1.	60	5.	0.6
2.	30	6.	0.4
3.	15		
4.	10		

EXERCISE 12

1. xv
2. viiss̈
3. iii
4. x
5. v
6. $\frac{1}{2}$
7. $\frac{1}{4}$
8. $\frac{1}{6}$
9. i

EXERCISE 13

1.	1	5.	0.2
2.	0.6	6.	0.1
3.	0.5		
4.	0.3		

EXERCISE 14

1. 1; xv
2. 0.6; x
3. 500; vii s̈s
4. 200; 0.2
5. 100; i s̈s
6. 0.06; i
7. 30; $\frac{1}{2}$ or s̈s
8. 15; 0.015
9. 0.01; $\frac{1}{6}$
10. 0.6; $\frac{1}{100}$
11. 0.0004; $\frac{1}{150}$
12. 0.0003; $\frac{1}{200}$

EXERCISE 15

1.	0.4	5.	30
2.	30	6.	60 or 65
3.	500	7.	15
4.	1000	8.	100 (not 90 mg!)

EXERCISE 16

1.	0.03	3.	0.2	5.	0.5	7.	0.0006
2.	0.1	4.	0.06	6.	0.6	8.	1

EXERCISE 17

1. $\frac{1}{150}$
2. is̈s
3. i
4. $\frac{1}{4}$
5. v
6. $\frac{1}{200}$

EXERCISE 18

1. 8 or ʒ viii
2. iv
3. 15
4. 8
5. xvi
6. $\frac{1}{2}$
7. 5
8. 2
9. 30
10. 1000

EXERCISE 19

1.	i	6.	viii
2.	15	7.	1
3.	45	8.	500
4.	1	9.	1000
5.	1	10.	1

EXERCISE 20

1. 30
2. 1
3. 1
4. 1
5. 1
6. 1
7. 1000
8. $\frac{1}{2}$
9. 1
10. 2.2

5

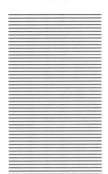

Drug Preparations and Equipment to Measure Doses

Drugs are manufactured in different forms for oral, parenteral, and topical administration. This chapter focuses on the more common drug preparations used in the clinical area and on the equipment that nurses use to prepare accurate doses.

DRUG PREPARATIONS

Oral Route

Oral drug forms are generally the easiest for the patient to take and the most convenient for the nurse to administer.

Tablets are powdered drugs that are compressed or molded into solid shapes. Tablets may contain ingredients that bind the powder or aid in its gastrointestinal absorption (Fig. 5–1A). Plain tablets for oral administration may be crushed if a patient has difficulty swallowing (see Fig. 5–1B).

Scored tablets have a line down the center, such that the tablet can be broken in halves. Unscored tablets should not be broken because there is no certainty that the drug is evenly distributed (see Fig. 5–1C).

Coated tablets or film-coated tablets are smooth and easy to swallow because of their coating. If necessary, these tablets may be crushed.

Enteric-coated tablets dissolve in the less acidic secretions of the intestine, rather than in the highly acidic stomach juices. The enteric coating protects the drug from being inactivated in the stomach and reduces the chance that the drug will irritate the gastric mucosa. Enteric-coated tablets should *not* be crushed.

Prolonged-release or extended-release tablets disintegrate more slowly and have a longer duration of action. The use of these preparations decreases the number of doses needed to only one or two tablets each day. Prolonged-release tablets should not be crushed.

Sublingual tablets dissolve quickly under the tongue. Medication is absorbed through the capillaries and reaches the circulation without passing through the gastrointestinal tract.

Coded tablets have a number or letters, or both, that make them easily identifiable (see Fig. 5–1D).

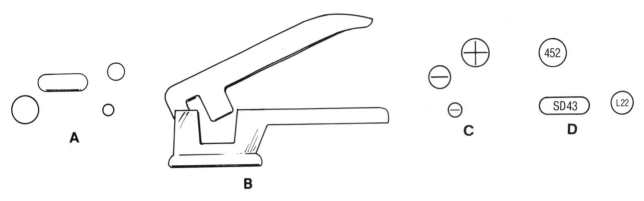

Figure 5-1. (**A**) *Tablets that can be crushed.* (**B**) *Tablet crusher. The tablet is placed in a paper cup on the bottom. A second cup is placed over the pulverizer on top and the tablet is crushed between the two cups.* (**C**) *Scored tablets that can be broken.* (**D**) *Coded tablets—identification of the drug may be by number, letters, or shape.*

Capsules are gelatin containers that hold a drug in solid or liquid form. Nurses should avoid opening capsules; the drug is encased in the capsule for a reason—possibly because contact with gastric juices will decrease its potency, or it may irritate the stomach lining. Occasionally, however, if a patient has difficulty swallowing, the nurse may open a capsule and combine the contents with a semisolid, such as Jello or custard. Before doing this, always check with the pharmacist to find out if the drug is available as a liquid or if there is another alternative (Fig. 5–2A).

Some capsules are enteric-coated. Others (called *spansule, timespan, time-release,* or *sustained-release*) contain particles of the drug that are coated to dissolve at different times. These capsules are long acting and should not be opened (see Fig. 5–2B).

Syrups are solutions of sugar in water, which disguise the taste of an unpleasant medication. Syrups may be contraindicated in patients with diabetes mellitus because they contain sugar.

Elixirs are clear, hydroalcoholic liquids that are sweetened. Elixirs may be contraindicated in patients with a history of alcoholism.

Fluidextracts and *tinctures* are alcoholic, liquid concentrations of a drug; they are potent and, consequently, are ordered in small amounts. Tinctures are ordered in drops. The average dose of a fluidextract is two teaspoons or less. Fluidextracts are the most concentrated of all liquids.

Oral or Parenteral Route

The drug forms for oral or parenteral administration include solutions, suspensions, powders, and others. The term *parenteral* does not indicate a specific route; it is a general term that means *by injection.* Four common parenteral routes are intramuscular (IM), subcutaneous (SC), intravenous (IV), and intravenous piggyback (IVPB).

Solutions are clear liquids that contain a drug dissolved in water for oral or parenteral use. Solutions may be administered by any route.

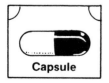

Capsule   A

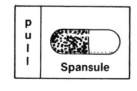

pull   Spansule   B

Figure 5-2. (**A**) *Capsules should not be opened.* (**B**) *Spansules are long-acting capsules.*

Suspensions are solid particles of a drug dispersed in a liquid. The particles settle to the bottom of the container upon standing and must be resuspended to obtain an accurate dose. Oral preparations are shaken; vials for injection are rotated between the hands.

Magmas contain large bulky particles, for example, milk of magnesia.

Gels have small particles, for example, magnesium hydroxide gel.

Emulsions are creamy, white suspensions of fats or oils in an agent that reduces surface tension and makes the oil easier to swallow, for example, emulsified castor oil.

Powders are dry, finely ground drugs that are dissolved for both oral and parenteral use. Powders used parenterally (e.g., IM, IV, IVPB) are reconstituted according to directions and are administered using sterile technique. The nurse who dissolves a powder writes the date, the dilution made, and the nurse's initials on the label and notes the expiration and storage information. The nurse's initials identify the person who dissolved the powder, in the event that a question arises about the dilution.

Antibiotics for the oral route are supplied as powders and reconstituted. Sterile technique is not required. These preparations in liquid form become oral suspensions.

Topical Route

Commonly-ordered preparations include aerosol powders or liquids, creams, ointments, pastes, suppositories, and transdermal medications. The physician's orders will indicate application to the skin, eye, ear, nose, vagina, rectum.

Aerosal powders and liquids are combined with a propellant and used for sprays on the skin, or in nebulizers and inhalers to reach the mucous membranes of the lower respiratory tract.

Powders may be applied to the skin or vagina in dry form.

Creams are semisolid drug preparations applied externally to the skin or mucous membranes. Vaginal creams require a special applicator for insertion.

Ointments are semisolid preparations in a petroleum or lanolin base for topical use. Ointments used for the eye must be labeled "ophthalmic."

Pastes are thick ointments used to protect the skin. They absorb secretions and soften the skin.

Suppositories contain medication molded with a firm base, such as cocoa butter, that melts at body temperature. Suppositories are shaped for insertion into the rectum, vagina, and less commonly into the urethra.

Transdermal medications are drug molecules contained in a unique polymer patch that is applied to the skin, as one would an ordinary plastic bandage. The medication is thus easy to apply and is effective for hours, or days at a time, as it is slowly released and absorbed through the skin.

EXERCISE 1

Match Column A with the letters in Column B to identify the meaning of the terms used for drug preparations. Answers can be found at the end of the chapter.

Column A

Column B

1. _____ Scored tablet

a. Coated drug particles dissolve at different times

2. _____ Enteric-coated

b. The most concentrated of all liquids

(continued)

EXERCISE 1 (Continued)

Column A	Column B
3. _____ Spansule	**c.** Hydroalcoholic liquid ordered in drops
4. _____ Sublingual tablet	**d.** Large particles suspended in a liquid
5. _____ Capsule	**e.** A solid which can be broken in half
6. _____ Syrup	**f.** Route applied to skin or mucous membrane
7. _____ Elixir	**g.** Small particles suspended in a liquid
8. _____ Fluidextract	**h.** Medication dissolves under the tongue
9. _____ Tincture	**i.** Gelatin containers for solid or liquid drug
10. _____ Magma	**j.** Molded solid inserted into the rectum
11. _____ Gel	**k.** Drug dissolves in the less acidic secretions of the intestine
12. _____ Topical	**l.** Sweetened, hydroalcoholic liquid
13. _____ Suppository	**m.** Solution of sugar in water to improve the taste of a drug

EXERCISE 2

Complete these statements related to drug preparation. Answers may be found at the end of the chapter.

1. Elixirs may be contraindicated for patients with a history of _____

    or _____ .

2. The average dose of a fluidextract is _____ .

3. In giving medications parenterally, four common routes are _____ ,

    _____ , _____ , and _____ .

4. When a powder is reconstituted, what three facts must the nurse write on the label?

    a. _____

    b. _____

    c. _____

5. What route(s) require(s) sterile technique in preparing and administering drugs?

    _____ .

6. An example of a drug listed as a magma is _____ .

7. What action must always be carried out before pouring an oral suspension?

    _____ .

8. List 6 drug preparations that can be administered topically.

    _____   _____

    _____   _____

    _____   _____

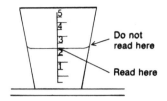

Figure 5-3. *Liquids are poured at eye level. The meniscus (lower curve of the fluid) should be on the line.*

9. List two advantages in using transdermal medications.

_____

_____

10. Define an ointment. _____ .

_____

_____

EQUIPMENT TO MEASURE DOSES

Nurses do not use a scale to weigh oral solid doses such as the gram and the grain. Solids for oral administration come in tablets and capsules. The nurse calculates the number to give and pours the amount needed into a *souffle cup,* a small paper container that is discarded once the medication has been given.

Liquid doses must be measured accurately. Two practices will aid in achieving this goal:

1. *Pour liquids to a line.* Never estimate a dose between two lines.
2. *Pour liquids at eye level.* The surface of a liquid has a natural curve, called the *meniscus.* At eye level, the center of this curve should be on the measurement line. The fluid at the sides of the container will appear to be above the line (Fig. 5-3).

The equipment used most often by nurses to measure liquids are the medicine cup and syringes.

Medicine Cup

The medicine cup is a plastic disposable container that has equivalent measures for metric doses in cubic centimeters, for apothecary doses in drams, and for household doses in tablespoons and teaspoons (Fig. 5-4).

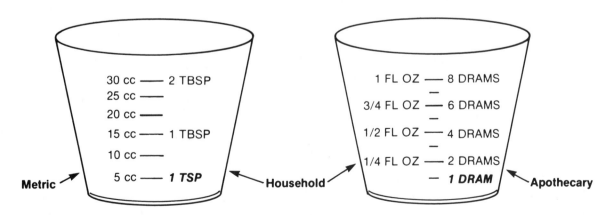

Figure 5-4. *A medicine cup for measurement of metric, apothecary, or household dose units.*

The following exercise will help you apply your knowledge of liquid equivalents.

EXERCISE 3

Look at the medicine cup in Figure 5–4. Two sides are shown. Fill in answers related to this measuring device. Check your answers at the end of the chapter.

1. Find 30 cc. What other measures are equivalent to this?

   _____   _____   _____   _____

2. Find 5 cc. Hold the page of this book up so that the 5 cc line is at eye level. Is a dram equal to 5 cc? _____

3. If an order reads ℥i what line would you use to pour the dose? _____

4. Find 15 cc. What other equivalents equal this?

   _____   _____   _____   _____

5. Consider the following answers to oral liquid dosage problems. What measurement line would you use?

   a. 8 cc   Pour _____

   b. 4 tsp   Pour _____

   c. $\frac{1}{2}$ oz   Pour _____

6. Suppose an answer to an oral liquid problem is 2 ml. Could you pour this dose into a medicine cup? Explain what you would do. _____

   _____

   _____

Syringes

There are four types of syringes used by nurses to prepare routine parenteral doses. Each is different from the others; understanding these differences will help you to prepare doses. The syringes are a 3-ml (cc) syringe, a 1-cc syringe, and two insulin syringes.

3-ml Syringe.   This syringe, which has a 22-gauge needle $1\frac{1}{2}$ inches long, is routinely used for injections (Fig. 5–5). The term *gauge* indicates the diameter (width) of the needle.
Note the following on the 3-ml syringe:

- The markings on one side are in cc (ml) to the nearest tenth. Each line indicates 0.1 ml.
- The markings on the opposite side are in minims. Each line indicates 1 minim.

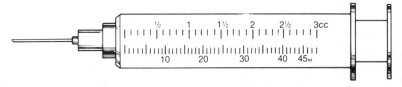

Figure 5-5. *A 3-ml (cc) syringe with metric and apothecary measures.*

- When preparing a dose, the syringe is held with the needle up. The medication is drawn down into the barrel. Suppose a dose was calculated to be 1.1 cc or 18 minims. Look at Figure 5–5, and count the lines to reach the dose.

EXERCISE 4

Use an arrow to indicate these amounts on the 3-ml syringe in Figure 5–5. Check your answers at the end of this chapter.

0.3 ml

25 m

1.2 cc

4 m

2.7 ml

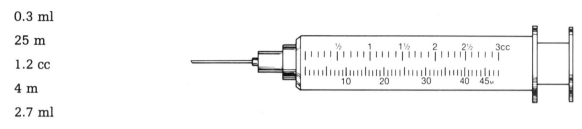

The 3-ml syringe has markings for 0.7 ml and 0.8 ml. What would you do if a dosage answer were 0.75 ml? Nurses do not approximate doses between lines. There are two ways to handle this problem:

1. Round off 0.75 ml to the nearest tenth. The answer would be 0.8 ml, which can be drawn up onto a line. (Rounding off numbers was discussed in Chapter 3, and is discussed again in this chapter.)
2. Use a different syringe with markings to the nearest hundredth. There is a precision syringe that has markings to the nearest hundredth.

1-ml Precision Syringe.   The 1-ml (cc) precision syringe with a 25-gauge, $\frac{5}{8}$-inch needle is the most accurate of the syringes nurses use. It is sometimes called a tuberculin syringe. The syringe is marked in hundredths of a milliliter (cubic centimeter) and in half minims (Fig. 5–6).

Note the following on the 1-ml precision syringe:

- The markings on one side are in minims. There is a short line between each half minim and a long line for a whole minim.
- The markings on the other side are in milliliters (ml; cc). There are nine lines before 0.10. Each line is 0.01 ml.
- To prepare an injection, the syringe is held with the needle up and the medication is drawn down into the barrel. Suppose a dose was calculated to be 0.13 ml or 2 minims. Look at Figure 5–6 and count the lines to reach the dose.

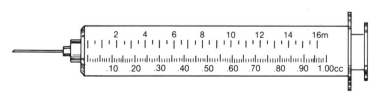

Figure 5-6. A 1-ml (cc) precision syringe with metric and apothecary measures.

LEARNING AID

Whenever you use a syringe, check to be certain that you have chosen the correct line. For 0.13 ml, the nurse would see the longer lines at 0.10 and 0.20. The slightly shorter line between them is 0.15 and two lines below that would be 0.13 ml.

EXERCISE 5

Use arrows to mark the following doses on the 1-ml (cc) precision syringe in Figure 5–6. Check your answers at the end of this chapter.

3 minims

$6\frac{1}{2}$ minims

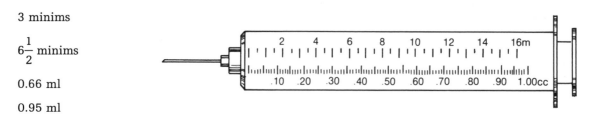

0.66 ml

0.95 ml

ROUNDING OFF NUMBERS IN LIQUID DOSAGE ANSWERS

In solving liquid dosage problems answers are in milliliters, cubic centimeters, or minims. The answer may not be an even number and the nurse must decide the degree of accuracy to be obtained. The degree of accuracy depends on the syringe chosen to give the dose.

Rule for Rounding Off Numbers

1. When the last number is 5 or more, add 1 to the previous number.
2. When the number is 4 or less, drop the number.

> *EXAMPLE:*
>
> | | |
> |---|---|
> | 0.864 becomes 0.86 | 4.562 becomes 4.56 |
> | 1.55 becomes 1.6 | 2.38 becomes 2.4 |
> | 0.33 becomes 0.3 | 0.25 becomes 0.3 |

With the *3-ml syringe* carry out decimals two places and round off to the *nearest tenth for milliliters.* Carry out answers in *minims* to the nearest tenth and round off to the nearest whole number.

With the *1-ml precision syringe,* carry out decimals three places and round off to the *nearest 100th* for milliliters. Carry out answers in *minims* to the nearest 100th and *round off to the nearest tenth.*

EXERCISE 6

The following are possible answers to dosage problems that require use of a 3-ml syringe. Put a check (✔) next to the answer if it is acceptable. If not acceptable, change the answer to a correct form.

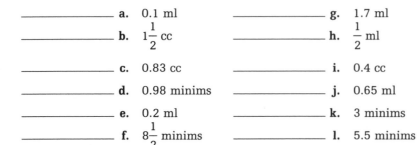

_____ **a.**	0.1 ml	_____ **g.**	1.7 ml
_____ **b.**	$1\frac{1}{2}$ cc	_____ **h.**	$\frac{1}{2}$ ml
_____ **c.**	0.83 cc	_____ **i.**	0.4 cc
_____ **d.**	0.98 minims	_____ **j.**	0.65 ml
_____ **e.**	0.2 ml	_____ **k.**	3 minims
_____ **f.**	$8\frac{1}{2}$ minims	_____ **l.**	5.5 minims

EXERCISE 7

The following are possible answers to dosage problems that require the use of a 1-ml precision syringe. Put a check (✔) next to the answer if it is acceptable. If not acceptable, change the answer to a correct form.

_____ **a.**	0.65 ml	_____ **e.**	0.346 ml
_____ **b.**	12.5 minims	_____ **f.**	0.290 ml
_____ **c.**	0.04 ml	_____ **g.**	0.758 ml
_____ **d.**	12.8 m	_____ **h.**	5 minims

1-cc Insulin Syringe.   The 1-cc insulin syringe (for unit 100 insulin) is marked in units rather than in milliliters or minims. It is used to prepare only U 100 insulins. The physician orders the type of insulin, the strength of insulin, and the number of units (Fig. 5–7).

|| **EXAMPLE:**   Order: 20 units NPH (U 100) insulin qd SC

Look at Figure 5–7. Note that there are four short lines between 10 units and 20 units. This indicates that each line is equal to 2 units on this syringe.

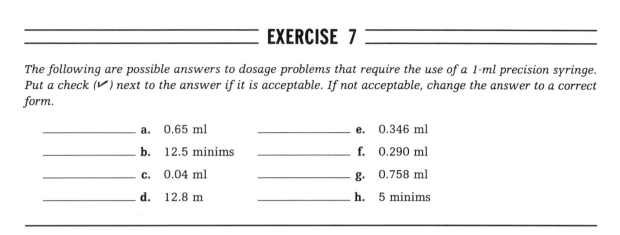

Figure 5-7.   *A 1-ml (cc) insulin syringe (for U 100 insulin).*

EXERCISE 8

Use arrows on the insulin syringe in Figure 5–7 to indicate the following amounts. Check your answers at the end of this chapter.

6 units

34 units

50 units

Odd-numbered insulin doses cannot be drawn up with the syringe in Figure 5–7. Another insulin syringe is used to prepare these doses.

Low-Dose Insulin Syringe.   The low-dose unit 100 insulin syringe with a 28-gauge, $\frac{1}{2}$-inch needle (Fig. 5–8) has four short lines between 10 and 15. This indicates that each line is equal to 1 unit. The syringe is marked for 50 units, so any dose of insulin (U 100) up to 50 units can be drawn up with this syringe.

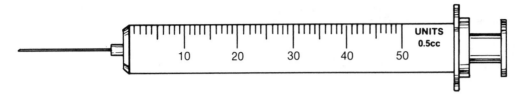

Figure 5-8. *Low-dose insulin syringe for U 100 insulin.*

EXERCISE 9

Use arrows on the insulin syringe in Figure 5–8 to indicate the following amounts. Answers may be found at the end of this chapter.

Units 33

Units 7

Units 40

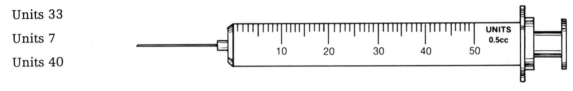

NEEDLES FOR INTRAMUSCULAR AND SUBCUTANEOUS INJECTIONS

Each of the four syringes discussed has a different injection needle.

Syringe	Gauge	Length (inches)
3 ml	22 g	$1\frac{1}{2}$
1 ml	25 g	$\frac{5}{8}$
U 100 insulin	26 g	$\frac{1}{2}$
U 100 low-dose insulin	28 g	$\frac{1}{2}$

Gauge (g) indicates the diameter or width of the needle. *The higher the gauge number, the finer the needle.* In the gauges just given the low-dose insulin syringe has the needle with the smallest diameter (28 gauge) and, hence, is the finest needle in this group. A 15-gauge needle is very wide and has a wide opening. It is used to transfuse blood cells.

The *length* of the needle used depends upon the route of injection. For deep intramuscular injections, a long needle is necessary. A short needle is used for subcutaneous injections.

The nurse determines what type of needle to use for adults and children, depending upon the route of administration, the size and condition of the patient, and the amount of adipose tissue present at the site.

You have now looked at medication orders, types of drug preparations, labels, systems of dosage, and measurement equipment. The next chapter will concentrate on solving dosage problems for the oral and parenteral routes.

ANSWERS

EXERCISE 1

1.	e	**8.**	b
2.	k	**9.**	c
3.	a	**10.**	d
4.	h	**11.**	g
5.	i	**12.**	f
6.	m	**13.**	j
7.	1		

EXERCISE 2

1. Diabetes mellitus; alcoholism
2. Two teaspoons or less
3. SC, IM, IVPB, and IV
4. a. The date; b. the nurse's initials; c. the dilution made
5. Sterile technique is required in preparing and administering drugs parenterally (IM, SC, IV, IVPB).
6. Milk of magnesia
7. Before pouring an oral suspension, the liquid must always be shaken.
8. Aerosol powders; creams; ointments; pastes; suppositories; transdermal medications
9. Ease in administering; prolonged action
10. An ointment is a semisolid preparation in a petroleum or lanolin base for topical use.

EXERCISE 3

1. Other equivalents are 2 tbs, 1 oz, 8 drams, 30 ml. (Remember 1 ml = 1 cc.)
2. No, a dram is slightly less than 5 ml.
3. Use the 1-dram line!
4. 15 cc is equal to 1 tbsp, $\frac{1}{2}$ oz, 4 drams, and 15 ml.
5. a. Pour 2 drams
   b. 4 tsp $\times$ 5 ml = 20 ml; use the 20-cc line
   c. $\frac{1}{2}$ oz. Use the line for $\frac{1}{2}$ oz.
6. No, there is no line for 2 ml. Use a syringe to obtain the 2 ml and then pour the amount into a medicine cup.

EXERCISE 4

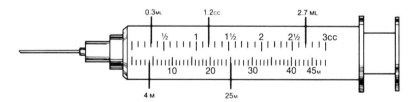

EXERCISE 5

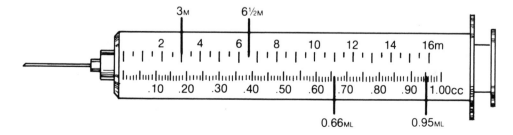

EXERCISE 6

_____✓_____	a.	0.1 ml	_____✓_____	g.	1.7 ml
_____✓_____	b.	$1\frac{1}{2}$ cc	_____✓_____	h.	$\frac{1}{2}$ ml
___0.8 cc___	c.	0.83 cc	_____✓_____	i.	0.4 cc
___1 minim___	d.	0.98 m	___0.7 ml___	j.	0.65 ml
_____✓_____	e.	0.2 ml	_____✓_____	k.	3 minims
___9 m___	f.	$8\frac{1}{2}$ m	___6 minims___	l.	5.5 minims

EXERCISE 7

_____✓_____	a.	0.65 ml	___0.35 ml___	e.	0.346 ml
_____✓_____	b.	12.5 m	___0.29 ml___	f.	0.290 ml
_____✓_____	c.	0.04 ml	___0.76 ml___	g.	0.758 ml
_____✓_____	d.	12.8 m	_____✓_____	h.	5 minims

EXERCISE 8

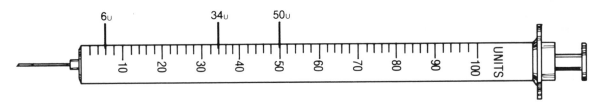

EXERCISE 9

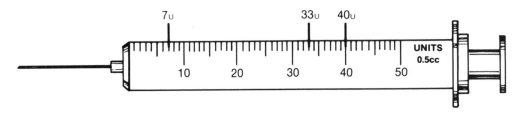

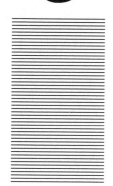

6

Calculation of Oral Medications— Solids and Liquids

Drugs for oral medications are prepared by pharmaceutical companies as solids (tablets, capsules) and liquids. One rule the Desire versus Have rule, can be used to solve these problems:

Rule: $\dfrac{\text{Desire}}{\text{Have}} \times \text{Stock} = \text{Answer}$

ORAL SOLIDS

|| *EXAMPLE:*

Order: tetracycline 0.5 g po q6h

Stock: capsules of 250 mg

Explanation of Rule

Desire is the physician's order.

|| *EXAMPLE:* 0.5 g

Have is the strength of the drug.

|| *EXAMPLE:* 250 mg

   Stock is the unit form of the drug. Because tablets and capsules are single, the stock for solid oral drugs is *always* one (1).
   Answer is how much of the stock to give. For oral solids the *answer* will be the *number* of *capsules* or *tablets* to administer.

Application of the Rule to Oral Solid Problems

Before solving each problem, check to be certain that the order and your supply are in the same weight measure. If they are not, you must convert one or the other to its equivalent. Convert whichever one is easier for you to solve.

EXAMPLE:

Order: tetracycline 0.5 g po q6h

Stock: capsules labeled 250 mg

Equivalent 0.5 g = 500 mg

Rule: $\dfrac{D}{H} \times S = A$

$\dfrac{\overset{2}{\cancel{500 \text{ mg}}}}{\underset{1}{\cancel{250 \text{ mg}}}} \times 1 \text{ cap} = 2$

Give 2 capsules

LEARNING AID
The order is in grams; the stock is in milligrams. Use an equivalent. Review Chapter 4 if necessary.
Note that mg cancel out. The answer is in capsules.

EXAMPLE:

Order: Tylenol 0.6 g po q4h prn

Stock: tablets labeled gr v

Equivalent gr v = 300 mg = 0.3 g

gr x = 600 mg = 0.6 g

Rule: $\dfrac{D}{H} \times S = A$

LEARNING AID
The order is in grams; the stock is in grains. Use an equivalent. Several are possible.

It does not make any difference what equivalent is used. The answer will be the same. If you

Changed to grams	Changed to grains	Changed to milligrams
$\dfrac{\overset{2}{\cancel{0.6 \text{ g}}}}{\underset{1}{\cancel{0.3 \text{ g}}}} \times 1 \text{ tab} = 2 \text{ tabs}$	$\dfrac{\overset{2}{\cancel{\text{gr } 10}}}{\underset{1}{\cancel{\text{gr } 5}}} \times 1 \text{ tab} = 2 \text{ tabs}$	$\dfrac{\overset{2}{\cancel{600 \text{ mg}}}}{\underset{1}{\cancel{300 \text{ mg}}}} \times 1 \text{ tab} = 2 \text{ tabs}$

EXAMPLE:

Order: digoxin 0.125 mg po qd

Stock: scored tablets labeled 0.25 mg

No equivalent is needed.

Rule: $\dfrac{D}{H} \times S = A$

$\dfrac{\overset{1}{\cancel{0.125 \text{ mg}}}}{\underset{2}{\cancel{0.250 \text{ mg}}}} \times 1 \text{ tab} = \dfrac{1}{2} \text{ tab}$

LEARNING AID

$0.25 \overset{0.5}{\overline{\smash{\big)}0.12\,5}}$

See the note following this problem for an easier way to clear the decimal.

Note that there is a quick way to clear decimals in $\dfrac{D}{H}$. When both the numerator and denominator are decimals, add zeros to make the *number of places the same* in both the numerator and denominator.

$$\frac{0.125 \text{ mg}}{0.250 \text{ mg}}$$

In division, remember that the denominator becomes the divisor and is cleared of decimal points. The decimal point in the numerator moves over the same number of places and so is also cleared.

$$\frac{\overset{1}{\cancel{0.125}} \text{ mg}}{\underset{2}{\cancel{0.250}} \text{ mg}} = \frac{1}{2} \text{ tab}$$

EXAMPLE:

Order: Synthroid 37.5 μg po qd

Stock: scored tablets of 0.025 mg

Equivalent 0.025 mg = 25 μg

Rule: $\dfrac{D}{H} \times S = A$

$$\frac{37.5 \ \mu g}{25 \ \ \mu g} \times 1 = A$$

Use the quick way to clear the decimal point.

$$\frac{\overset{3}{\cancel{37.5}}}{\underset{2}{\cancel{25.0}}} \times 1 \text{ tab} = \frac{3}{2}$$

(Divided by 125)

$$\frac{3}{2} = 1\frac{1}{2} \text{ tabs}$$

You can administer $1\dfrac{1}{2}$ tablets because the stock is scored.

> **LEARNING AID**
>
> Remember 1 mg = 1000 μg. If necessary review Chapter 4. The quick rule for converting states that you write the equivalent you want to change first. Then write the conversion you want. Change the mg to μg. To find the equivalent, the open arrow faces the larger measure.
>
> mg > μg
>
> The arrow tells you to move mg three places to the right.
>
> 0.025 mg = 25 μg

EXAMPLE:

Order: Nembutal 0.1 g po hs prn

Stock: Capsules labeled 100 mg

Equivalent 0.1 g = 100 mg

Rule: $\dfrac{D}{H} \times S = A$

$$\frac{\overset{1}{\cancel{100 \text{ mg}}}}{\underset{1}{\cancel{100 \text{ mg}}}} \times 1 \text{ cap} = 1 \text{ cap}$$

EXAMPLE:

Order: Mycostatin 1 million units po tid

Stock: scored tablets labeled 500,000 units

No equivalent needed.

Rule: $\dfrac{D}{H} \times S = A$

$$\frac{\overset{2}{\cancel{1,000,000 \text{ units}}}}{\underset{1}{\cancel{500,000 \text{ units}}}} \times 1 \text{ tab} = 2 \text{ tabs}$$

SELF-TEST 1

Solve these practice problems. Answers may be found at the end of the chapter. Remember the rule:

$$\frac{D}{H} \times S = A$$

1. Order: Decadron 1.5 mg po bid
   Stock: tablets labeled 0.75 mg

2. Order: digoxin 0.25 mg po qd
   Stock: scored tablets labeled 0.5 mg

3. Order: ampicillin 0.5 Gm po q6h
   Stock: capsules labeled 250 mg

4. Order: prednisone 10 mg po tid
   Stock: tablets labeled 2.5 mg

5. Order: aspirin 650 mg po stat
   Stock: tablets labeled 325 mg

6. Order: digitoxin 200 mcg po qd
   Stock: scored tablets labeled 0.1 mg

7. Order: Equanil 0.2 g po q4h
   Stock: scored tablets labeled 400 mg

8. Order: penicillin G potassium 200,000 units po q8h
   Stock: scored tablets labeled 400,000 units

9. Order: digoxin 0.5 mg po qd
   Stock: scored tablets labeled 0.25 mg

10. Order: Lasix 60 mg po qd
    Stock: scored tablets labeled 40 mg

Special Types of Oral Solid Orders

Compounded drugs do not require calculation. These are drugs, such as the over-the-counter (OTC) preparations Rolaids and Tums, or drugs that have a set combination of ingredients. They are ordered by the number to be administered.

EXAMPLE:

> Multivitamin tabs i po qd
>
> Gelusil tabs i po q4h prn

Physicians occasionally specify the weight measure of the drug and the number of tablets to be given. These orders do not require calculation.

EXAMPLE:

> Darvon 65 mg caps ii po hs prn
>
> This is interpreted: Give two capsules of Darvon 65 mg by mouth at the hour of sleep if needed.

EXAMPLE:

> aspirin 325 mg ii po stat
>
> This is interpreted: Give two tablets of aspirin 325 mg by mouth immediately.

ORAL LIQUIDS

Rule: $\dfrac{\text{Desire}}{\text{Have}} \times \text{Stock} = \text{Answer}$

EXAMPLE:

> Order: phenytoin oral suspension 200 mg po bid
>
> Stock: bottle of liquid labeled 125 mg/5 ml

LEARNING AID

Abbreviate the rule:

$\dfrac{D}{H} \times S = A$

Explanation of the Rule

Desire is the physician's order.

|| **EXAMPLE:** 200 mg

Have is the strength of the drug as it comes from the pharmacy.

|| **EXAMPLE:** 125 mg

Stock is the unit form of the drug. Liquid stock varies. The stock above is *5 ml = 125 mg*.

Other examples of different types of stock are

> 250 mg per 5 ml: the unit is 5 ml.
>
> 1 g/ml: the unit is 1 ml.
>
> 100 mg in 2 ml: the unit is 2 ml.

Answer is how much of the stock to give. Because the stock is a liquid, the *answer* will be a *liquid measure* (ml; cc; tsp; tbsp; m; ʒ; ℥).

Application of the Rule to Oral Liquid Problems

Before solving each problem, check to be certain that the order and your supply are in the same measure. If they are not, you must convert one or the other to its equivalent. Convert whichever one is easier for you to solve.

EXAMPLE:

Order: phenytoin oral suspension 200 mg po bid

Stock: bottle of liquid labeled 125 mg/5 ml

No equivalent is needed.

Rule: $\dfrac{D}{H} \times S = A$

$$\frac{\overset{8}{\cancel{200}} \text{ mg}}{\underset{25}{\cancel{125}} \text{ mg}} \times \overset{1}{\cancel{5}} \text{ ml} = 8 \text{ ml}$$

LEARNING AID

There are many ways to solve the math.

$$\frac{\overset{8}{\cancel{200}}}{\underset{5}{\cancel{125}}} \times \overset{1}{\cancel{5}} = 8 \text{ ml}$$

$$200 \times 5 = \frac{\cancel{1000}}{125} \quad 125\overline{)1000.}^{\,8.}$$
$$\underline{1000}$$
$$0$$

EXAMPLE:

Order: Dimetane Susp. 15 mg po bid

Stock: liquid labeled 10 mg/4 ml

No equivalent needed

Rule: $\dfrac{D}{H} \times S = A$

$$\frac{15 \text{ mg}}{10 \text{ mg}} \times 4 \text{ ml} = \frac{\cancel{60}}{\cancel{10}} = 6 \text{ ml}$$

LEARNING AID

There are different ways to solve the math.

EXAMPLE:

Order: Septra Susp. 0.1 g po qd

Stock: liquid labeled 200 mg/10 ml

Equivalent 0.1 g = 100 mg

Rule: $\dfrac{D}{H} \times S = A$

$$\frac{\overset{1}{\cancel{100}} \text{ mg}}{\underset{2}{\cancel{200}} \text{ mg}} \times \overset{5}{\cancel{10}} \text{ ml} = 5 \text{ ml}$$

EXAMPLE:

Order: Elixir Feosol 600 mg po qd

Stock: liquid labeled gr v per tsp

Equivalents: gr v = 300 mg

1 tsp = 5 ml

Rule: $\dfrac{D}{H} \times S = A$

$$\frac{\overset{2}{\cancel{600}} \text{ mg}}{\underset{1}{\cancel{300}} \text{ mg}} \times 5 \text{ ml} = 10 \text{ ml or 2 tsp}$$

EXAMPLE:

Order: Mysoline oral susp. 0.45 g po qid

Stock: liquid in a bottle with a calibrated dropper

labeled 0.3 g/ml

No equivalent is necessary.

Rule: $\dfrac{D}{H} \times S = A$

$$\frac{0.\overset{3}{\cancel{45}}\ \cancel{gm}}{0.\underset{2}{\cancel{30}}\ \cancel{gm}} \times 1\ ml = \frac{3}{2} = 1.5\ ml$$

LEARNING AID

Because the drug comes in a bottle with a dropper you are alerted that your answer will be a small amount. This is typical of a pediatric problem.

LEARNING AID

$$0.3\,\overline{)0.4\,5}\ \ ^{1.5}$$
$$\underline{\ \ 3\ \ }$$
$$1\ 5$$
$$\underline{1\ 5}$$
$$0$$

═══════════════ **SELF-TEST 2** ═══════════════

Solve these oral liquid problems. Answers may be found at the end of the chapter.

1. Order: erythromycin susp. 0.75 g po qid
   Stock: liquid labeled 250 mg/5 ml

2. Order: ampicillin susp. 500 mg po q8h
   Stock: liquid labeled 250 mg/5 ml

3. Order: Cephalex in oral suspension 0.35 Gm po q6h
   Stock: liquid labeled 125 mg/5 ml

4. Order: cyclosporine 150 mg po stat and qd
   Stock: liquid labeled 100 mg/ml in a bottle with a calibrated dropper

5. Order: sulfasoxizole susp. 300 mg po qid
   Stock: liquid labeled 250 mg/5 ml

6. Order: digoxin 0.02 mg po qd
   Stock: pediatric elixir 0.05 mg/ml in a bottle with a dropper marked in tenths of a milliliter

7. Order: potassium chloride 30 mEq po qd
   Stock: liquid labeled 20 mEq/15 ml

(continued)

========== SELF-TEST 2 (*Continued*) ==========

8. Order: elixir Digoxin 0.25 mg via nasogastric tube qd
        Stock: liquid labeled 0.5 mg/10 ml

9. Order: hydrocortisone cypionate oral susp. 30 mg po q6h
        Stock: liquid labeled 10 mg/5 ml

10. Order: promethazine HCl syrup 12.5 mg po tid
         Stock: liquid labeled 6.25 mg/5 ml

Special Types of Oral Liquid Problems

Compounded drugs do not require calculation. These are drugs, such as OTC preparations, liquid multivitamin preparations, or drugs that have a set combination of ingredients. They are ordered by the amount to be given.

> *EXAMPLE:*
>
>   Order: terpin hydrate elixir ℨii q 4 h prn po
>
>   Stock: liquid labeled Terpin hydrate elixir
>
>   No calculation is needed. Pour 2 drams every 4 hours by mouth if necessary.
>
> *EXAMPLE:*
>
>   Order: milk of magnesia 30 cc hs tonight po
>
>   Stock: liquid labeled milk of magnesia
>
>   No calculation is required. Pour 30 cc of milk of magnesia and give tonight by mouth.

MENTAL DRILL FOR ORAL SOLID AND LIQUID PROBLEMS

As you develop proficiency in solving problems, you will be able to calculate many answers without written work. This drill combines your knowledge of equivalents and dosage.

========== SELF-TEST 3 ==========

Solve the problems mentally and write only the amount to be given. Answers will be found at the end of the chapter. Keep the rule in mind as you solve each problem.

Order	Stock (Scored Tablets)	Answer
1. 20 mg	10 mg	_____
2. 0.125 mg	0.25 mg	_____

Order	Stock (Scored Tablets)	Answer
3. 0.25 mg	0.125 mg	_____
4. 200,000 units	100,000 units	_____
5. 0.5 mg	0.25 mg	_____
6. 0.2 Gm	400 mg	_____
7. 1 Gm	gr xv	_____
8. 0.1 Gm	100 mg	_____
9. 0.01 Gm	20 mg	_____
10. gr x	325 mg	_____
11. grs vii s̈s	250 mg	_____
12. gr ii	60 mg	_____
13. 50 mg	0.1 Gm	_____
14. 4 mg	2 mg	_____

══ SELF-TEST 4 ══

Order	Stock	Answer
1. 20 mg	10 mg per 5 ml	_____
2. 10 mg	2 mg/5 cc	_____
3. 0.5 Gm	250 mg/5 ml	_____
4. 0.1 Gm	200 mg per 10 ml	_____
5. 250 mg	0.1 g per 6 ml	_____
6. 100 mg	50 mg/10 cc	_____
7. 12 mg	4 mg/5 ml	_____
8. 15 mg	30 mg/10 ml	_____
9. 15 mg	10 mg per 4 ml	_____
10. 0.25 mg	0.5 mg/5 ml	_____

══ PROFICIENCY TEST 1 ══

For liquid answers draw a line on the medicine cup indicating the amount you would pour. Answers may be found at the end of the chapter. Aim for 100% accuracy!

1. Order: KCl elixir 20 mEq po bid
    Stock: liquid labeled 30 mEq/15 ml

   Answer   _____

(continued)

PROFICIENCY TEST 1 (Continued)

2. Order: Dilantin Susp. 150 mg po tid
    Stock: liquid labeled 75 mg/7.5 ml

    Answer _____

3. Order: elixir Digoxin 0.125 mg po qd
    Stock: liquid labeled 0.25 mg/10 ml

    Answer _____

4. Order: Dilantin oral suspension 150 mg po tid
    Stock: liquid labeled 75 mg/6 ml

    Answer _____

5. Order: Proximyl 10 mg po bid
    Stock: liquid labeled 2 mg/5 ml

    Answer _____

6. Order: digoxin 0.5 mg po qd
    Stock: tablets labeled 0.25 mg

    Answer _____

7. Order: Lanoxin 10 µg qd po
    Stock: 0.02 mg scored tablets

    Answer _____

8. Order: Zyloprim 250 mg po qd
    Stock: scored tablets 100 mg

    Answer _____

9. Order: ampicillin 0.5 g po q6h
    Stock: capsules labeled 250 mg

    Answer _____

10. Order: Synthroid 0.3 mg po qd
    Stock: tablets labeled 300 µg scored

    Answer _____

Medicine cup markings:

30 cc — 2 TBSP
25 cc —
20 cc —
15 cc — 1 TBSP
10 cc —
5 cc — *1 TSP*

1 FL OZ — 8 DRAMS
—
3/4 FL OZ — 6 DRAMS
—
1/2 FL OZ — 4 DRAMS
—
1/4 FL OZ — 2 DRAMS
— *1 DRAM*

PROFICIENCY TEST 2

For liquid answers draw a line on the medicine cup indicating the amount you would pour. Answers may be found at the end of the chapter. Aim for 100% accuracy!

1. Order: ibuprofen 0.8 gm po tid
    Stock: tablets labeled 400 mg

    Answer _____

2. Order: isoniazid 0.3 Gm po qd
   Stock: tablets labeled 300 mg

   Answer _____

3. Order: ethambutal HCl 600 mg po qd
   Stock: tablets scored and labeled 400 mg

   Answer _____

4. Order: acetaminophen 0.65 Gm po q4h
   Stock: tablets labeled 325 mg

   Answer _____

5. Order: ascorbic acid 250 mg po bid
   Stock: tablets scored and labeled 500 mg

   Answer _____

6. Order: colistin sulfate oral suspension 80 mg po tid
   Stock: liquid labeled 25 mg/tsp

   Answer _____

7. Order: oxacillin sodium 0.75 Gm po q6h
   Stock: liquid labeled 250 mg/5 ml

   Answer _____

8. Order: penicillin V potassium 600 mg po q6h
   Stock: liquid labeled 250 mg/5 ml

   Answer _____

9. Order: Mylanta II 30 ml q4h prn
   Stock: liquid labeled Mylanta II

   Answer _____

10. Order: Elixophyllin 160 mg po q6h
   Stock: liquid labeled 80 mg/15 ml

   Answer _____

1 FL OZ —— 8 DRAMS
—
3/4 FL OZ —— 6 DRAMS
—
1/2 FL OZ —— 4 DRAMS
—
1/4 FL OZ —— 2 DRAMS
— *1 DRAM*

30 cc —— 2 TBSP
25 cc ——
20 cc ——
15 cc —— 1 TBSP
10 cc ——
5 cc —— *1 TSP*

ANSWERS

SELF-TEST 1

1. Rule: $\dfrac{D}{H} \times S = A$

   No equivalent needed

   $$\dfrac{\overset{2}{\cancel{1.50}} \text{ mg}}{\underset{1}{\cancel{0.75}} \text{ mg}} \times 1 \text{ tab} = 2 \text{ tablets}$$

<blockquote>
LEARNING AID

$$0.75\,)\overline{1.50}\quad\dfrac{2.}{}$$
$$\underline{1\ 50}$$
$$0$$
</blockquote>

2. No equivalent necessary

   $$\dfrac{\cancel{0.25} \text{ mg}}{\cancel{0.50} \text{ mg}} \times 1 \text{ tab} = \dfrac{1}{2} \text{ tablet}$$

<blockquote>
LEARNING AID

$$0.5\,)\overline{0.2.5}\quad\dfrac{0.5}{}\ \text{or}\ \dfrac{1}{2}$$
$$\underline{2}$$
$$0$$
</blockquote>

3. Equivalent 0.5 Gm = 500 mg

   $$\dfrac{\overset{2}{\cancel{500} \text{ mg}}}{\underset{1}{\cancel{250} \text{ mg}}} \times 1 \text{ tab} = 2 \text{ tablets}$$

<blockquote>
LEARNING AID

$$250\,)\overline{500.}\quad\dfrac{2.}{}$$
$$\underline{500}$$
$$0$$
</blockquote>

4. No equivalent necessary

   $$\dfrac{\cancel{10.0} \text{ mg}}{\cancel{2.5} \text{ mg}} \times 1 \text{ tab} = 4 \text{ tablets}$$

<blockquote>
LEARNING AID

$$2.5\,)\overline{10.0}\quad\dfrac{4.}{}$$
</blockquote>

5. No equivalent necessary

   $$\dfrac{\overset{2}{\cancel{650} \text{ mg}}}{\underset{1}{\cancel{325} \text{ mg}}} \times 1 \text{ tab} = 2 \text{ tablets}$$

<blockquote>
LEARNING AID

$$325\,)\overline{650.}\quad\dfrac{2.}{}$$
$$\underline{650}$$
$$0$$
</blockquote>

6. Equivalent 1 mg = 1000 mcg

   mg > mcg

   0.1 mg = 100 mcg

   $$\dfrac{\overset{2}{\cancel{200} \text{ mcg}}}{\underset{1}{\cancel{100} \text{ mcg}}} \times 1 \text{ tab} = 2 \text{ tablets}$$

<blockquote>
LEARNING AID

Move decimal three places to the right.

$$0.100\, = 100 \text{ mcg}$$
</blockquote>

7. Equivalent 0.2 g = 200 mg

$$g > mg$$

$$\frac{\overset{1}{\cancel{200}\ \text{mg}}}{\underset{2}{\cancel{400}\ \text{mg}}} \times 1\ \text{tab} = \frac{1}{2}\ \text{tablet}$$

LEARNING AID

Move decimal point three places to the right.

0.200 = 200 mg

Important! Do *not* invert the numbers in the answer. The answer is $\frac{1}{2}$ tablet, *not* 2 tablets.

8. No equivalent necessary

$$\frac{\overset{1}{\cancel{200,000}\ \text{units}}}{\underset{2}{\cancel{400,000}\ \text{units}}} = \frac{1}{2}\ \text{tablet}$$

9. No equivalent necessary

$$\frac{\overset{2}{\cancel{0.50}\ \text{mg}}}{\underset{1}{\cancel{0.25}\ \text{mg}}} \times 1\ \text{tab} = 2\ \text{tablets}$$

LEARNING AID

$$0.25\ )\overline{0.50}\quad \frac{2.}{}$$
$$\underline{50}$$
$$0$$

10. No equivalent necessary

$$\frac{\cancel{60}\ \text{mg}}{\cancel{40}\ \text{mg}} \times 1\ \text{tab} = 1\frac{1}{2}\ \text{tablets}$$

LEARNING AID

$$40\ )\overline{60.0}\quad \frac{1.5}{}$$
$$\underline{40}$$
$$200$$
$$\underline{200}$$
$$0$$

SELF-TEST 2

1. Rule: $\dfrac{D}{H} \times S = A$

Equivalent 0.75 g = 750 mg

$$\frac{\overset{3}{\cancel{750}\ \text{mg}}}{\underset{1}{\cancel{250}\ \text{mg}}} \times 5\ \text{ml} = 15\ \text{ml}$$

LEARNING AID

Calculations may be done in different ways. Answers should be the same regardless of the method chosen to solve the problem.

2. No equivalent necessary

$$\frac{\overset{2}{\cancel{500}\ \text{mg}}}{\underset{1}{\cancel{250}\ \text{mg}}} \times 5\ \text{ml} = 10\ \text{ml}$$

LEARNING AID

500 × 5 = 2500

$$250\ )\overline{2500.}\quad \frac{10.}{}$$
$$\underline{250}$$
$$0$$

3. Equivalent 0.35 Gm = 350 mg

$$\frac{\overset{14}{\cancel{350}}\text{ mg}}{\underset{\cancel{25}}{\cancel{125}\text{ mg}}} \times \overset{1}{\cancel{5}}\text{ml} = 14 \text{ ml}$$

$$1$$

LEARNING AID

350 × 5 = 1750

$$\begin{array}{r} 14. \\ 125 \overline{)1750.} \\ \underline{125} \\ 500 \\ \underline{500} \\ 0 \end{array}$$

4. No equivalent necessary

$$\frac{\overset{3}{\cancel{150}\text{ mg}}}{\underset{2}{\cancel{100}\text{ mg}}} \times 1 \text{ ml} = \frac{3}{2} = 1.5 \text{ ml}$$

LEARNING AID

$$\begin{array}{r} 1.5 \\ 100 \overline{)150.0} \\ \underline{100} \\ 500 \\ \underline{500} \end{array}$$

5. No equivalent necessary

$$\frac{\overset{6}{\cancel{300}\text{ mg}}}{\underset{\cancel{50}}{\cancel{250}\text{ mg}}} \times \overset{1}{\cancel{5}}\text{ml} = 6 \text{ ml}$$

$$1$$

LEARNING AID

300 × 5 = 1500

$$\begin{array}{r} 6. \\ 250 \overline{)1500.} \\ \underline{1500} \\ 0 \end{array}$$

6. No equivalent necessary

$$\frac{0.02\text{ mg}}{0.05\text{ mg}} \times 1 \text{ ml} = \frac{2}{5} = 0.4 \text{ ml}$$

LEARNING AID

$$\begin{array}{r} .4 \\ 0.05 \overline{)0.02.0} \\ \underline{20} \\ 0 \end{array}$$

7. No equivalent necessary

$$\frac{\overset{3}{\cancel{30}\text{ mEq}}}{\underset{2}{\cancel{20}\text{ mEq}}} \times 15 \text{ ml} = \frac{45}{2} \overline{)45.0}^{22.5} = 22.5 \text{ ml}$$

8. No equivalent necessary

$$\frac{\overset{1}{\cancel{0.25}\text{ mg}}}{\underset{\cancel{2}}{\cancel{0.50}\text{ mg}}} \times \overset{5}{\cancel{10}} \text{ ml} = 5 \text{ ml}$$

$$1$$

LEARNING AID

0.25 × 10 = 2.5

$$\begin{array}{r} 5. \\ 0.5 \overline{)2.5} \\ \underline{25} \end{array}$$

9. No equivalent necessary

$$\frac{\cancel{30 \text{ mg}}}{\cancel{10 \text{ mg}}} \times 5 \text{ ml} = 15 \text{ ml}$$

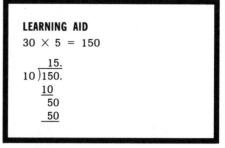

10. No equivalent necessary

$$\frac{12.5 \text{ mg}}{6.25 \text{ mg}} \times 5 \text{ ml} = 10 \text{ ml}$$

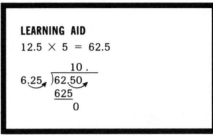

SELF-TEST 3

1.	2 tablets	**8.**	1 tablet
2.	$\frac{1}{2}$ tablet	**9.**	$\frac{1}{2}$ tablet
3.	2 tablets	**10.**	2 tablets
4.	2 tablets	**11.**	2 tablets
5.	2 tablets	**12.**	2 tablets
6.	$\frac{1}{2}$ tablet	**13.**	$\frac{1}{2}$ tablet
7.	1 tablet	**14.**	2 tablets

SELF-TEST 4

1.	10 ml	**6.**	20 cc
2.	25 cc	**7.**	15 ml
3.	10 ml	**8.**	5 ml
4.	5 ml	**9.**	6 ml
5.	15 ml	**10.**	2.5 ml

PROFICIENCY TEST 1

1.

$$\frac{\cancel{20 \text{ mEq}}^{1}}{\cancel{30 \text{ mEq}}_{1}} \times \cancel{15}^{5} \text{ ml} = 10 \text{ ml}$$

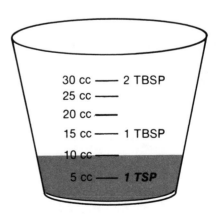

2.

$$\frac{\overset{2}{\cancel{150} \text{ mg}}}{\underset{1}{\cancel{75} \text{ mg}}} \times 7.5 \text{ ml} = 15 \text{ ml}$$

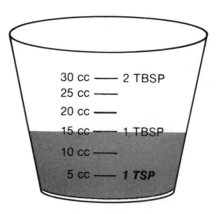

3.

$$\frac{\overset{1}{\cancel{0.125} \text{ mg}}}{\underset{\underset{1}{\cancel{2}}}{\cancel{0.250} \text{ mg}}} \times \overset{5}{\cancel{10}} \text{ ml} = 5 \text{ ml}$$

Alternate arithmetic

$$0.25\,)\overline{0.12\,5} \overset{.5}{} \times 10 \text{ ml} = 5 \text{ ml}$$
$$12\ 5$$

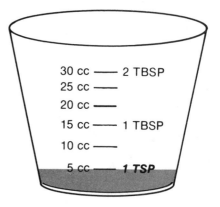

4.

$$\frac{\overset{2}{\cancel{150} \text{ mg}}}{\underset{1}{\cancel{75} \text{ mg}}} \times 6 \text{ ml} = 12 \text{ ml} = ʒiii$$

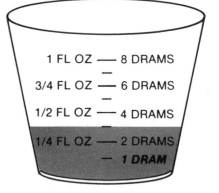

5.

$$\frac{\overset{5}{\cancel{10} \text{ mg}}}{\underset{1}{\cancel{2} \text{ mg}}} \times 5 \text{ ml} = 25 \text{ ml}$$

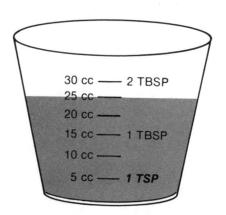

6. Rule: $\dfrac{D}{H} \times S = A$

$$\frac{0.50 \text{ mg}}{0.25 \text{ mg}} \times 1 \text{ tab} = \quad 0.25 \overline{)0.50} \quad \text{2 tablets}$$

7. Equivalent 0.02 mg = 20 µg

$$\frac{\overset{1}{10} \text{ µg}}{\underset{2}{20} \text{ µg}} \times 1 \text{ tab} = \frac{1}{2} \text{ tablet}$$

8.

$$\frac{\overset{5}{250} \text{ mg}}{\underset{2}{100} \text{ mg}} \times 1 \text{ tab} = \frac{5}{2} = 2\frac{1}{2} \text{ tablets}$$

9. Equivalent 0.5 g = 500 mg

$$\frac{\overset{2}{500} \text{ mg}}{\underset{1}{250} \text{ mg}} \times 1 \text{ tab} = 2 \text{ tablets}$$

10. Equivalent 0.3 mg = 300 µg

$$\frac{\overset{1}{300 \text{µg}}}{\underset{1}{300 \text{µg}}} \times 1 \text{ tab} = 1 \text{ tablet}$$

PROFICIENCY TEST 2

1. Rule: $\dfrac{D}{H} \times S = A$

Equivalent 0.8 gm = 800 mg

$$\frac{\overset{2}{800} \text{ mg}}{\underset{1}{400} \text{ mg}} \times 1 \text{ tab} = 2 \text{ tablets}$$

2. Equivalent 0.3 Gm = 300 mg

$$\frac{\overset{1}{300} \text{ mg}}{\underset{1}{300} \text{ mg}} \times 1 \text{ tab} = 1 \text{ tablet}$$

3.

$$\frac{\overset{3}{\cancel{600\ mg}}}{\underset{2}{\cancel{400\ mg}}} \times 1\ tablet = \frac{3}{2} = 1.5\ or\ 1\frac{1}{2}\ tablets$$

4.   0.65 Gm = 650 mg

$$\frac{\overset{2}{\cancel{650\ mg}}}{\underset{1}{\cancel{325\ mg}}} \times 1\ tablet = 2\ tablets$$

5.

$$\frac{\overset{1}{\cancel{250\ mg}}}{\underset{2}{\cancel{500\ mg}}} \times 1\ tablet = \frac{1}{2}\ tablet$$

6.   Equivalent 1 tsp = 5 ml

$$\frac{\overset{16}{\cancel{80\ mg}}}{\underset{1}{\underset{5}{\cancel{25\ mg}}}} \times \overset{1}{\cancel{5}}\ ml = 16\ ml = \mathfrak{Z}iv$$

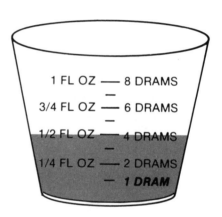

Alternate arithmetic

80 × 5 = 400

$$\begin{array}{r} 16. \\ 25\overline{)400.} \\ \underline{25} \\ 150 \\ \underline{150} \\ 0 \end{array}$$

7.   Equivalent 0.75 Gm = 750 mg

$$\frac{\overset{3}{\cancel{750\ mg}}}{\underset{1}{\cancel{250\ mg}}} \times 5\ ml = 15\ ml$$

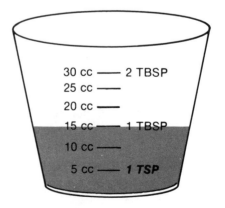

8.

$$\frac{\overset{12}{\cancel{600}\text{ mg}}}{\underset{\underset{1}{\cancel{50}}}{\cancel{250}\text{ mg}}} \times \overset{1}{\cancel{5}}\text{ ml} = 12 \text{ ml}$$

Alternate arithmetic

$600 \times 5 = 3000$

$$\begin{array}{r} 12. \\ 250\overline{)3000.} \\ \underline{250} \\ 500 \\ \underline{500} \\ 0 \end{array}$$ $12 \text{ ml} = 3 \text{ drams}$

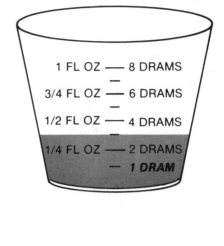

9. No arithmetic necessary
Compounded drug. Pour 30 ml

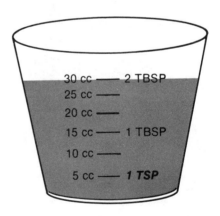

10.

$$\frac{\overset{2}{\cancel{160}\text{ mg}}}{\underset{1}{\cancel{80}\text{ mg}}} \times 15 \text{ ml} = 30 \text{ ml}$$

7

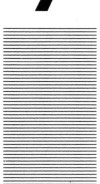

Liquids for Injection

Liquid drugs for injection are prepared by pharmaceutical companies as sterile solutions or suspensions. Sterile techniques are used to prepare and administer them. As with oral medications, the nurse may be required to calculate the correct dosage.

RULE AND EXPLANATION

The rule used to solve liquid injection problems is the same as that for oral solids and liquids.

$$\frac{\text{Desire}}{\text{Have}} \times \text{Stock} = \text{Answer}$$

> **EXAMPLE:**
>
> Order: Demerol HCl 75 mg IM q4h prn
>
> Stock: vial labeled 100 mg/2 ml

Desire is the order.

> **EXAMPLE:** 75 mg

Have is the strength of the drug supplied.

> **EXAMPLE:** 100 mg

Stock is the unit form of the drug. In the example it is *2 ml* = 100 mg.
Answer is how much liquid to give by injection. The answer is a liquid measure, usually milliliters (ml) or minims.

CALCULATING INJECTION PROBLEMS

The degree of accuracy in calculating injection answers depends on the syringe used. Figure 7-1 shows a 3-cc (3 ml) syringe marked in milliliters to the nearest tenth and in minims to the nearest

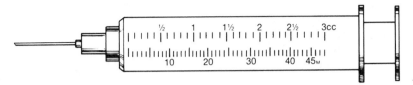

Figure 7-1. A 3-cc (3-ml) syringe.

whole number. To calculate milliliter answers for this 3-ml syringe, the arithmetic is carried out to the hundredth place and the answer is rounded off to the nearest tenth.

| | **EXAMPLE:** 1.25 ml becomes 1.3 ml

To calculate minims on the 3-ml syringe, the arithmetic is carried out to the tenth place and the answer is rounded off to the nearest whole number.

| | **EXAMPLE:** 19.7 minims becomes 20 minims

Figure 7-2 shows a 1-cc (1 ml) precision syringe marked in milliliters to the nearest hundredth and in minims to the nearest half-minim. To calculate milliliters when the 1-ml syringe is used, the arithmetic is carried out to the thousandth place and the answer is rounded off to the nearest hundredth.

| | **EXAMPLE:** 0.978 ml becomes 0.98 ml

To calculate minims for the 1-ml syringe, the arithmetic is carried out to the nearest hundredth and the answer is reported as the closest half minim.

||| **EXAMPLE:**

14.28 minims becomes 14 minims. (The answer 14.28 rounds off to 14.3. Because 0.3 is less than 0.5, it is dropped.)

A syringe is provided for each of the practice problems that follow. Calculate milliliters and minims to the accuracy required by the order given. Calculation of minims is provided as an exercise; because these are apothecary measures and are not exact, you are urged to use only metric milliliter or cubic centimeter calculations. Draw a line on the syringe indicating the answer for *milliliter* only.

|| **EXAMPLE:**

Order: Demerol HCl 75 mg IM q4h prn

Stock: ampule labeled 100 mg/2 ml

Rule: $\dfrac{D}{H} \times S = A$

$$\frac{\overset{3}{\cancel{75}} \text{ mg}}{\underset{4}{\cancel{100}} \text{ mg}} \times \overset{1}{\cancel{2}} \text{ ml} = \frac{3}{2} = 1.5 \text{ ml}$$

Give: 1.5 ml (or 24 m) IM

LEARNING AID

16 minims = 1 ml

To obtain minims, multiply the ml answer by 16.

$$\begin{array}{r} 1.5 \text{ ml} \\ \times\ 16 \text{ m} \\ \hline 90 \\ 15 \\ \hline 24.0 \text{ m} \end{array}$$

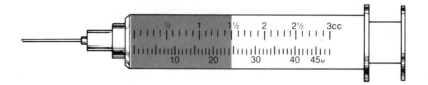

EXAMPLE:

Order: Kantrex 0.75 g IM q12h

Stock: vial labeled 1 g/3 ml

Rule: $\dfrac{D}{H} \times S = A$

$\dfrac{0.75\ \cancel{g}}{1\ \cancel{g}} \times 3\ \text{ml} = \begin{array}{r} 0.75 \\ \times\ \ 3 \\ \hline 2.25\ \text{ml} \end{array}$

Give: 2.3 ml (or 36 m) IM

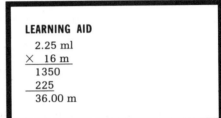

```
      LEARNING  AID
        2.25 ml
      ×  16 m
      ────────
        1350
         225
      ────────
       36.00 m
```

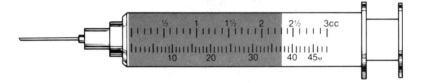

Note: You are using a 3-ml syringe. Round off the answer to the nearest tenth.

EXAMPLE:

Order: Lanoxin 0.125 mg IM qd

Stock: ampule labeled 0.25 mg/ml

Rule: $\dfrac{D}{H} \times S = A$

$\dfrac{\overset{1}{\cancel{0.125}}\ \cancel{mg}}{\underset{2}{\cancel{0.250}}\ \cancel{mg}} \times 1\ \text{ml} = \dfrac{1}{2}\ \text{ml or } 0.5\ \text{ml}$

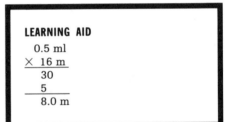

```
      LEARNING  AID
        0.5 ml
      ×  16 m
      ────────
         30
          5
      ────────
        8.0 m
```

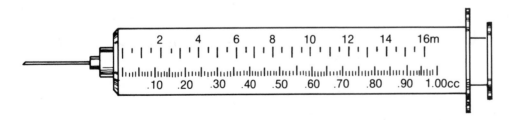

Figure 7-2. *A 1-cc (1-ml) syringe.*

Give: 0.5 ml (or 8 m) IM

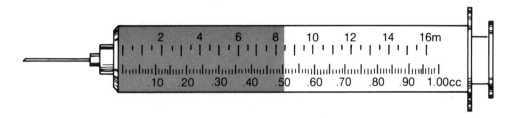

Note: You are using a 1-ml precision syringe.

EXAMPLE:

Order: Gantrisin 400 mg IM q12h

Stock: vial labeled 2 g/5 ml

Logic: You have milligrams in the order and grams in the stock. Use an equivalent (2 g = 2000 mg).

Rule: $\dfrac{D}{H} \times S = A$

$$\frac{\overset{1}{\cancel{400}\text{ mg}}}{\underset{5}{\cancel{2000}\text{ mg}}} \times \overset{1}{\cancel{5}}\text{ ml} = 1\text{ ml}$$

$$1\text{ ml} = 16\text{ m}$$

Give: 1 ml (or 16 m) IM

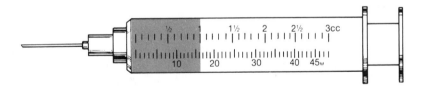

═══ SELF-TEST 1 ═══

Practice calculation of injections from a liquid. Solve these problems. Report your answer in both milliliters (ml) and minims (m), but mark the syringe in milliliters. Answers may be found at the end of the chapter.

1. Order: cleocin 0.3 Gm IM q6h
      Stock: liquid in a vial labeled 300 mg/2 ml

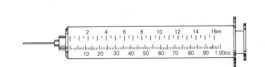

2. Order: morphine SO$_4$ 12 mg SC stat
      Stock: vial of liquid labeled gr $\dfrac{1}{4}$ /ml

(continued)

SELF-TEST 1 (*Continued*)

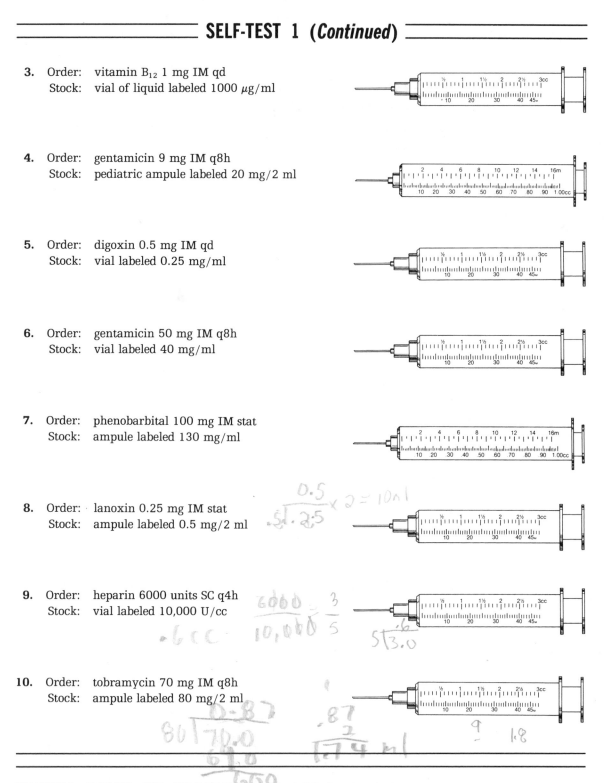

3. Order: vitamin B$_{12}$ 1 mg IM qd
     Stock: vial of liquid labeled 1000 μg/ml

4. Order: gentamicin 9 mg IM q8h
     Stock: pediatric ampule labeled 20 mg/2 ml

5. Order: digoxin 0.5 mg IM qd
     Stock: vial labeled 0.25 mg/ml

6. Order: gentamicin 50 mg IM q8h
     Stock: vial labeled 40 mg/ml

7. Order: phenobarbital 100 mg IM stat
     Stock: ampule labeled 130 mg/ml

8. Order: lanoxin 0.25 mg IM stat
     Stock: ampule labeled 0.5 mg/2 ml

9. Order: heparin 6000 units SC q4h
     Stock: vial labeled 10,000 U/cc

10. Order: tobramycin 70 mg IM q8h
     Stock: ampule labeled 80 mg/2 ml

SPECIAL TYPES OF PROBLEMS IN INJECTIONS FROM A LIQUID

When Stock Is a Ratio

Labels may state the strength of a drug as a ratio.

|| **EXAMPLE:**   Adrenalin 1:1000

Ratios are always interpreted in the metric system as grams per milliliters. In the example given, 1:1000 means 1 g in 1000 ml. Ratios may be stated in three ways:

1 g per 1000 ml

1 g = 1000 ml

1 g/1000 ml

====================== **EXERCISE 1** ======================

Write the following ratios in three ways. Answers may be found at the end of the chapter.

1. 1:20 _____ _____ _____

2. 2:15 _____ _____ _____

3. 1:500 _____ _____ _____

Some nurses have difficulty understanding the meaning of ratio in relation to drugs. A deductive line of reasoning may help to make this clear.

Figure 7-3 shows an ampule of epinephrine that is labeled 2 ml and is a 1:1000 solution. You know that 1:1000 means 1 g in 1000 ml. You also know that 1 g is equivalent to 1000 mg. Therefore, the solution can be interpreted as 1000 mg = 1000 ml. Logic tells you that if there are 1000 mg in 1000 ml, then there is 1 mg in 1 ml.

$$\frac{\cancel{1000}\ mg}{\cancel{1000}\ ml} = \frac{1\ mg}{1\ ml}$$

Because the ampule has 2 ml, the ampule contains 2 mg of the drug. Be careful reading and writing milligram (mg) and milliliter (ml)! Remember milligram is the solid measure; milliliter is the liquid measure.

> **EXAMPLE:**
>
> Order: epinephrine 1 mg SC stat
>
> Stock: ampule labeled 1:1000
>
> Equivalents: 1:1000 means
>
>   1 g in 1000 ml
>
>   1 g = 1000 mg
>
> Stock is 1000 mg in 1000 ml
>
> Rule: $\dfrac{D}{H} \times S = A$
>
> $$\frac{1\ \cancel{mg}}{\underset{1}{\cancel{1000}\ \cancel{mg}}} \times \overset{1}{\cancel{1000}}\ ml = 1\ ml$$
>
> Give: 1 ml SC

> **EXAMPLE:**
>
> Order: isoproterenol HCl 0.2 mg IM stat
>
> Stock: ampule labeled 1:5000
>
> Equivalents: 1:5000 means
>
>   1 g in 5000 ml
>
>   1 g = 1000 mg

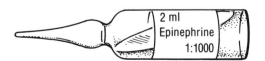

Figure 7-3. *A 2-ml ampule of epinephrine 1:1000.*

Therefore, the solution is 1000 mg/5000 ml.

Rule: $\dfrac{D}{H} \times S = A$

$$\frac{0.2\ \cancel{mg}}{\cancel{1000}\ \cancel{mg}} \times \overset{5}{\cancel{5000}}\ ml = \begin{array}{r} 5 \\ \times\ 0.2 \\ \hline 1.0\ ml \end{array}$$

Give: 1 ml IM

====================== **EXERCISE 2** ======================

Solve these problems involving ratios. Answers may be found at the end of the chapter.

1. Order: neostigmine 0.5 mg SC
      Stock: ampule labeled 1:2000

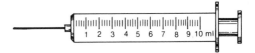

2. Order: Isuprel 1 mg; add to IV
      Stock: vial labeled 1:5000
             A 10-ml syringe is available.

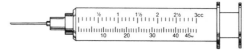

3. Order: ponthaline 50 mg IM
      Stock: ampule labeled 1:20

When Stock Is a Percent

Labels may state the strength of a drug as a percent. Percent means parts per hundred. *Percentages are always interpreted in the metric system as grams per 100 ml.*

|| **EXAMPLE:**   Lidocaine 2% (2 g in 100 ml)

Percents may be stated in three ways:

    2 g per 100 ml

    2 g = 100 ml

    2 g/100 ml

EXERCISE 3

Write the following percentages in three ways. Answers may be found at the end of the chapter.

1. 0.9% ───────────── ───────────── ─────────────

2. 10% ───────────── ───────────── ─────────────

3. 0.45% ───────────── ───────────── ─────────────

Percent problems can be solved by applying the meaning of ratio.

> **EXAMPLE:**
>
> Order: Lidocaine 30 mg for injection before suturing wound
>
> Stock: ampule labeled 2%
>
> Equivalents: 2% means
>
> 2 g in 100 ml
>
> 1 g = 1000 mg
>
> 2 g = 2000 mg
>
> Stock is 2000 mg in 100 ml
>
> Rule: $\dfrac{D}{H} \times S = A$
>
> $\dfrac{\cancel{30}\ \cancel{mg}}{\cancel{2000}\ \cancel{mg}} \times \overset{1}{\cancel{100}}\ ml = \dfrac{3}{2}$ $\quad 2\overline{)3.0}^{\;1.5}$
>
> Prepare: 1.5 ml for physician

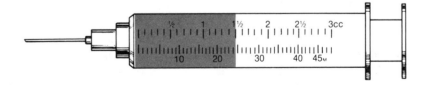

> **EXAMPLE**
>
> Order: calcium gluconate 1 g; add to IV stat
>
> Stock: vial of liquid labeled 10%
>
> Equivalents: 10% means 10 g in 100 ml
>
> Rule: $\dfrac{D}{H} \times S = A$

$$\frac{1 \overset{10}{\cancel{g}}}{\underset{1}{\cancel{10\,g}}} \times 10\cancel{0}\ \text{ml} = 10\ \text{ml}$$

Add: 10 ml to IV (Amount is correct. The route is IV, not IM.)

=================== **EXERCISE 4** ===================

Solve these problems involving percentages. Answers may be found at the end of the chapter. Answers in milliliters (ml).

1. Order: epinephrine 5 mg SC stat
    Stock: ampule labeled 1%

    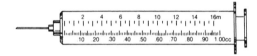

2. Order: mesterin 2.5 mg IM
    Stock: ampule labeled 0.5%

3. Order: phenylephrine HCl 3 mg SC stat
    Stock: ampule labeled 1%

INSULIN INJECTIONS

Types of Insulin

Insulin is a hormone that regulates glucose metabolism. It is measured in units and is administered by injection. Insulin is supplied in 10-ml vials containing 100 units per milliliter. There are many types of insulin currently available. Because onset of action, time of peak activity, and duration of action vary, *nurses must be careful to choose the correct insulin.* The following are examples of insulin labels:

Regular insulin U 100/ml

Lente insulin U 100/ml

Semilente insulin U 100/ml

NPH insulin U 100/ml

Humulin insulin U 100/ml (This is regular insulin made from recombinant DNA.)

Regular insulin should appear clear and colorless; it is the only insulin that may be given IV. Other insulins appear cloudy. Insulin vials should be gently rotated between the hands to resuspend the particles. *Never shake insulin vials.* This may result in the formation of bubbles or froth and interfere with accurate measurement of the dose ordered.

Types of Insulin Syringes

Insulin doses are administered subcutaneously with an insulin syringe. Two standard syringes are available to measure U 100 insulin. The first measures doses up to 100 units (Fig. 7-4). The second, called a low-dose insulin syringe, is used when the dose is 50 units or less (Fig. 7-5).

Preparing an Injection Using an Insulin Syringe

No calculation is required to prepare an insulin dose. The physician's order is in units; the stock comes in 100 units/ml, and both syringes are calibrated (lined) for 100 units/ml

EXAMPLE:

    Order: units 60 NPH SC qd

    Stock: NPH insulin U 100/ml

    Ask yourself three questions:

        1.   What is the order? NPH units 60
        2.   What is the stock? NPH U 100/ml
        3.   Is a U 100 insulin syringe available? Yes.

    Draw up the amount required into the syringe using sterile technique.

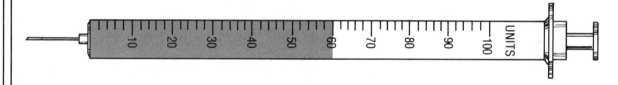

EXAMPLE:

    Order: U 35 regular insulin SC stat

    Stock: U 100/ml regular insulin

    Ask yourself three questions:

        1.   What is the order? Regular insulin U 35
        2.   What is the stock? U 100/ml regular insulin
        3.   What syringe should be used? Low-dose insulin syringe

    Draw up the amount required into the syringe using sterile technique.

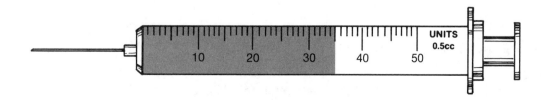

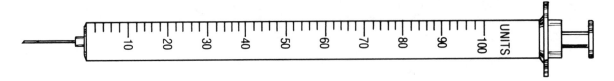

Figure 7-4. *Syringe for 100 units of insulin. Each line equals 2 units.*

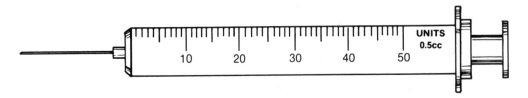

Figure 7-5. *Low-dose insulin syringe. Each line equals 1 unit.*

Mixing Two Insulins in One Syringe

Sometimes the physician will order regular insulin to be mixed with another insulin and injected together at the same site. The method of preparing two medications in one syringe is handled later in this book. For now, remember two facts:

1. The regular insulin is always drawn up first into the syringe.
2. The total number of units in the syringe will be the addition of the two insulin orders.

EXAMPLE:

Order: regular insulin U 15 ⎫
                                                ⎬ qd SC
     NPH insulin U 10 ⎭

Stock: regular insulin U 100/ml
      NPH insulin U 100/ml

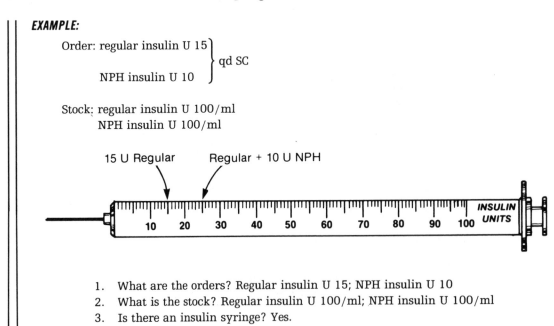

1. What are the orders? Regular insulin U 15; NPH insulin U 10
2. What is the stock? Regular insulin U 100/ml; NPH insulin U 100/ml
3. Is there an insulin syringe? Yes.
4. What will be the total units in the syringe? 25 U

Preparing an Insulin Injection When No Insulin Syringe Is Available

When an insulin syringe is not available, it is possible to calculate and administer an insulin dose. Handle the order as an injection from a liquid and use a 1-ml precision syringe.

EXAMPLE:

Order: Lente insulin units 40 SC qd

Stock: Lente insulin U 100/ml

Rule: $\dfrac{D}{H} \times S = A$

$$\dfrac{\overset{2}{\cancel{40 \text{ Units}}}}{\underset{5}{\cancel{100 \text{ Units}}}} \times 1 \text{ ml} = \dfrac{2}{5} \bigg) \overset{0.4}{2.0}$$

Give: 0.4 ml SC

EXERCISE 5

Solve these insulin problems. Draw a line on the syringe to indicate the dose you would prepare. Answers may be found at the end of the chapter.

1. Order: regular insulin U 25 SC stat
   Stock: vial of regular insulin U 100/ml and a low-dose insulin syringe

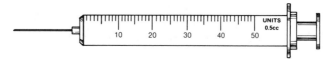

2. Order: U 56 semilente insulin SC at 10 AM
   Stock: vial of semilente insulin U 100/ml and an insulin syringe

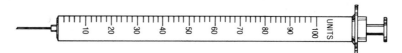

3. Order: 22 units of NPH 100 qd SC at 7:30 AM
   Stock: vial of NPH insulin U 100/ml and an insulin syringe

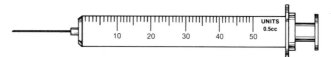

4. Order: 5 U regular insulin U 100 and 10 U NPH insulin U 100 SC qd 7 AM
   Stock: vials of regular insulin U 100 and NPH insulin U 100

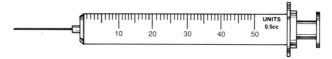

PROFICIENCY TEST 1

Solve these injection problems. Draw a line on the syringe indicating the amount you would prepare in milliliters (ml). Answers may be found at the end of the chapter. Aim for 100% accuracy!

(continued)

PROFICIENCY TEST 1 (Continued)

1. Order: Sodium Amytal 0.1 Gm IM at 7 AM
   Stock: ampule of liquid labeled 200 mg/3 ml

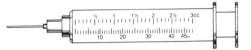

2. Order: morphine sulfate 5 mg SC stat
   Stock: vial of liquid labeled 15 mg/ml

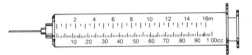

3. Order: Benadryl 25 mg IM q4h prn
   Stock: ampule of liquid labeled 50 mg (2-cc size)

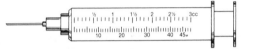

4. Order: NPH insulin 15 units and Humulin insulin 5
           units SC qd 7 AM

   Stock: vials of NPH insulin U 100 and Humulin in-
           sulin U 100

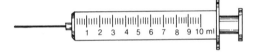

5. Order: add 20 mEq potassium chloride to IV stat
   Stock: vial of liquid labeled 40 mEq (3 g) per 20 ml

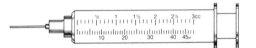

6. Order: scopolamine 0.6 mg SC stat
   Stock: vial labeled 0.4 mg/ml

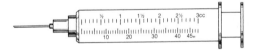

7. Order: atropine sulfate 0.8 mg IM at 7 AM
   Stock: vial labeled 0.4 mg/ml

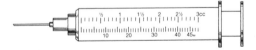

8. Order: add 0.5 Gm dextrose 25% to IV stat
   Stock: vial of liquid labeled Infant 25% Dextrose In-
           jection 250 mg/ml

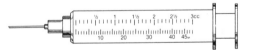

9. Order: ascorbic acid 200 mg IM bid
   Stock: ampule labeled 500 mg/2 ml

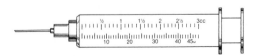

10. Order: epinephrine 7.5 mg SC stat
    Stock: ampule labeled 1:100

PROFICIENCY TEST 2

Solve these problems in injections from a liquid. Draw a line on the syringe indicating the amount you would prepare in milliliters (ml). Answers may be found at the end of the chapter. Aim for 100% accuracy!

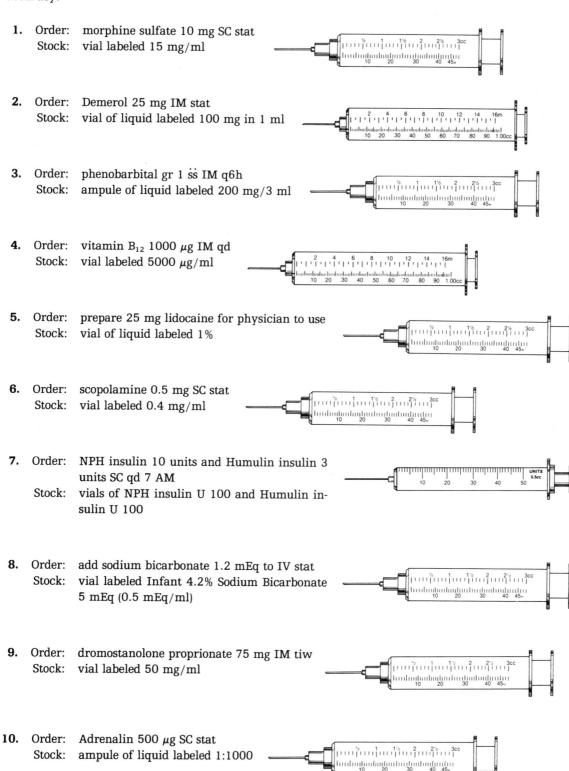

1. Order: morphine sulfate 10 mg SC stat
    Stock: vial labeled 15 mg/ml

2. Order: Demerol 25 mg IM stat
    Stock: vial of liquid labeled 100 mg in 1 ml

3. Order: phenobarbital gr 1 ss IM q6h
    Stock: ampule of liquid labeled 200 mg/3 ml

4. Order: vitamin B$_{12}$ 1000 μg IM qd
    Stock: vial labeled 5000 μg/ml

5. Order: prepare 25 mg lidocaine for physician to use
    Stock: vial of liquid labeled 1%

6. Order: scopolamine 0.5 mg SC stat
    Stock: vial labeled 0.4 mg/ml

7. Order: NPH insulin 10 units and Humulin insulin 3
    units SC qd 7 AM
    Stock: vials of NPH insulin U 100 and Humulin in-
    sulin U 100

8. Order: add sodium bicarbonate 1.2 mEq to IV stat
    Stock: vial labeled Infant 4.2% Sodium Bicarbonate
    5 mEq (0.5 mEq/ml)

9. Order: dromostanolone proprionate 75 mg IM tiw
    Stock: vial labeled 50 mg/ml

10. Order: Adrenalin 500 μg SC stat
    Stock: ampule of liquid labeled 1:1000

═══ MENTAL DRILL IN LIQUIDS FOR INJECTION PROBLEMS ═══

As you develop proficiency in solving problems, you will be able to calculate many answers without written work. This drill combines your knowledge of equivalents and dosages. Solve these problems mentally and write only the amount to give. Answers will be found at the end of the chapter. Keep the rule in mind as you solve each problem.

Order		Stock	Give
1.	0.5 g IM	250 mg/ml	2 tab
2.	10 mEq IV	40 mEq/20 ml	
3.	0.5 mg IM	0.25 mg/ml	2 ml
4.	100 mg IM	0.2 Gm per 2 ml	10 ml → 1.0 ml
5.	50 mg IM	100 mg = 1 ml	.5 ml
6.	0.25 mg IM	0.5 mg per 2 ml	1.0 ml
7.	0.3 mg SC	0.4 mg/ml	.75 ml
8.	1 mg SC	1:1000 solution	
9.	1 g IV	5% solution	
10.	0.1 g IM	200 mg/5 ml	2.5 ml
11.	400,000 units IM	500,000 U/ml	.8 ml
12.	0.5 mg IM	0.5 mg per 2 ml	2 ml
13.	1 g IV	50% solution	
14.	75 mg IM	100 mg per 2 ml	1.5 ml
15.	15 mg IM	1:100 solution	
16.	35 mg IM	100 mg/ml	.35 ml
17.	0.6 mg SC	0.4 mg per ml	1.5 ml
18.	0.15 g IM	0.2 g/2 ml	15 ml 1.6 ml

ANSWERS

SELF-TEST 1

1. Equivalent 0.3 Gm = 300 mg

$$\frac{\overset{1}{\cancel{300}\ \text{mg}}}{\underset{1}{\cancel{300}\ \text{mg}}} \times 2\ \text{ml} = 2\ \text{ml} \qquad \begin{array}{r} 16\ \text{m} \\ \times\ 2\ \text{ml} \\ \hline 32\ \text{m} \end{array}$$

Give 2 ml (or 32 m) IM

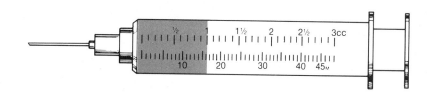

2. Equivalent gr $\frac{1}{4}$ = 15 mg

$$\frac{\overset{4}{\cancel{12}\ \text{mg}}}{\underset{5}{\cancel{15}\ \text{mg}}} \times 1\ \text{ml} = \frac{4}{5} \overset{.8}{\overline{)4.0}} \qquad \begin{array}{r} 16\ \text{m} \\ \times\ 0.8 \\ \hline 12.8\ \text{m} \end{array}$$

Give 0.8 ml (or 13 m) SC

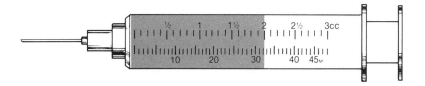

3. Equivalent 1 mg = 1000 μg

$$\frac{\overset{1}{\cancel{1000}\ \cancel{\mu g}}}{\underset{1}{\cancel{1000}\ \cancel{\mu g}}} \times 1\ \text{ml} = 1\ \text{ml} \qquad 1\ \text{ml} = 16\ \text{m}$$

Give 1 ml (or 16 m) IM

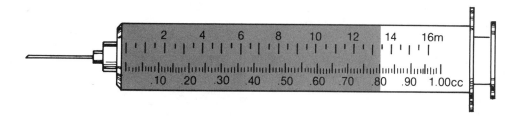

4. $\dfrac{9 \text{ mg}}{20 \text{ mg}} \times 2 \text{ ml} = \dfrac{18}{20}$ $\begin{array}{r} .9 \\ 20\overline{)18.0} \\ \underline{18.0} \end{array}$ $\begin{array}{r} 16 \text{ m} \\ \times\, 0.9 \text{ ml} \\ \hline 14.4 \end{array}$

Give 0.9 ml (or 14.5 m) IM. You are using a 1-ml precision syringe so minims are decided to the closest *half* minim.

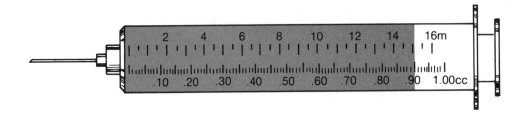

5. $\dfrac{0.50 \text{ mg}}{0.25 \text{ mg}} \times 1 \text{ ml} = 2 \text{ ml}$ $\begin{array}{l} \\ 2 \text{ ml} = 32 \text{ m} \end{array}$

Give 2 ml (or 32 m) IM

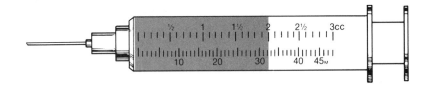

6. $\dfrac{50 \text{ mg}}{40 \text{ mg}} \times 1 \text{ ml} = \dfrac{5}{4}$ $\begin{array}{r} 1.25 \\ 4\overline{)5.00} \\ \underline{4} \\ 1\ 0 \\ \underline{\ 8} \\ 20 \\ \underline{20} \end{array}$ $\begin{array}{r} 1.25 \text{ ml} \\ \times\ 16 \text{ m} \\ \hline 750 \\ \underline{125} \\ 20.00 \text{ m} \end{array}$

Give 1.3 ml (or 20 m) IM

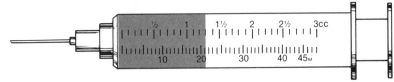

7. $\dfrac{100 \text{ mg}}{130 \text{ mg}} \times 1 \text{ ml} = \dfrac{10}{13}$ $\begin{array}{r} .769 \\ 13\overline{)10.000} \\ \underline{9\ 1} \\ 90 \\ \underline{78} \\ 120 \\ \underline{117} \\ 3 \end{array}$ $\begin{array}{r} .769 \text{ ml} \\ \times\ 16 \text{ m} \\ \hline 4614 \\ \underline{769} \\ 12.304 \end{array}$

Give 0.77 ml (or 12.5 m) IM. You are using a 1-ml precision syringe, hence, milliliters to the nearest hundredth and minims to the nearest $\frac{1}{2}$ minim.

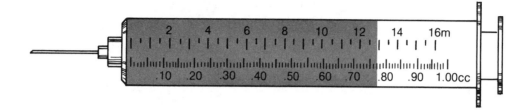

8. $\dfrac{0.25\ \text{mg}}{0.50\ \text{mg}} \times 2\ \text{ml} = 1\ \text{ml}$

$1\ \text{ml} = 16\ \text{m}$

Give 1 ml (or 16 m) IM.

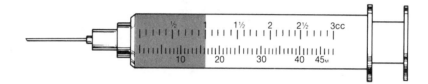

9. $\dfrac{6000\ \text{units}}{10000\ \text{units}} \times 1\ \text{cc} = \dfrac{6}{10} = 0.6$

$\begin{array}{r} 16\ \text{m} \\ \times\ 0.6 \\ \hline 9.6\ \text{m} \end{array}$

Give 0.6 ml (or 10 m) SC

10. $\dfrac{70\ \text{mg}}{80\ \text{mg}} \times 2\ \text{ml} = \dfrac{7}{4}$

$\begin{array}{r} 1.75 \\ 4\,\overline{)7.00} \\ \underline{4} \\ 3\,0 \\ \underline{2\,8} \\ 20 \\ \underline{20} \end{array}$

$\begin{array}{r} 1.75\ \text{ml} \\ \times\ 16\ \text{m} \\ \hline 1050 \\ 175 \\ \hline 28.00\ \text{m} \end{array}$

Give 1.8 ml (or 28 m) IM

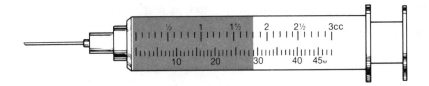

EXERCISE 1

1.   1 g per 20 ml; 1 g = 20 ml; 1 g/20 ml
2.   2 g per 15 ml; 2 g = 15 ml; 2 g/15 ml
3.   1 g per 500 ml; 1 g = 500 ml; 1 g/500 ml

EXERCISE 2

1.   Equivalent 1:2000 means
                        1 g in 2000 ml
                        1 g = 1000 mg

Hence, the solution is 1000 mg/2000 ml.

$$\frac{0.5 \text{ mg}}{1000 \text{ mg}} \times \overset{2}{2000} \text{ ml} = \begin{array}{r} 0.5 \\ \times 2 \\ \hline 1.0 \end{array}$$

Give 1 ml (or 16 m) SC

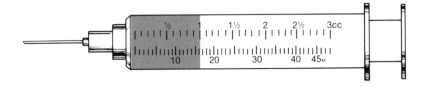

2.   Equivalent 1:5000 means
                        1 g in 5000 ml
                        1 g = 1000 mg

Hence, the solution is 1000 mg/5000 ml.

$$\frac{1 \text{ mg}}{1000 \text{ mg}} \times \overset{5}{5000} \text{ ml} = 5 \text{ ml}$$

Add 5 ml to IV (This is correct because route is IV, not IM.)

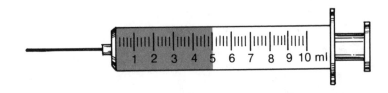

3. Equivalent 1:20 means
$$1 \text{ g in } 20 \text{ ml}$$
$$1 \text{ g} = 1000 \text{ mg}$$

Hence, the solution is 1000 mg/20 ml.

$$\frac{\overset{1}{\cancel{50 \text{ mg}}}}{\underset{20}{\cancel{1000 \text{ mg}}}} \times \overset{1}{\cancel{20}} \text{ ml} = 1 \text{ ml}$$

$$1 \text{ ml} = 16 \text{ m}$$

Give 1 ml (or 16 m) IM

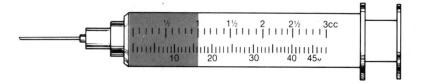

EXERCISE 3

1. 0.9 g per 100 ml; 0.9 g = 100 ml; 0.9 g/100 ml
2. 10 g per 100 ml; 10 g = 100 ml; 10 g/100 ml
3. 0.45 g per 100 ml; 0.45 g = 100 ml; 0.45 g/100 ml

EXERCISE 4

1. Equivalent 1%   1 g in 100 ml
$$1 \text{ g} = 1000 \text{ mg}$$

Hence, the solution is 1000 mg/100 ml.

$$\frac{\overset{1}{\cancel{5 \text{ mg}}}}{\underset{\underset{2}{\cancel{10}}}{\cancel{1000 \text{ mg}}}} \times \overset{1}{\cancel{100}} \text{ ml} = \frac{1}{2} \text{ ml or } 0.5 \text{ ml}$$

$$\begin{array}{r} 16 \text{ m} \\ \hline 0.5 \text{ ml} \\ \hline 8.0 \text{ m} \end{array}$$

Give 0.5 ml (or 8 m) SC

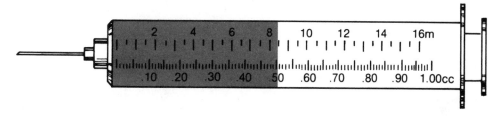

2. Equivalent 0.5%   0.5 g in 100 ml
$$0.5 \text{ g} = 500 \text{ mg}$$

Hence, the solution is 500 mg/100 ml.

$$\frac{2.5 \text{ mg}}{\underset{5}{\cancel{500 \text{ mg}}}} \times \overset{1}{\cancel{100}} \text{ ml} = \frac{2.5}{5} \quad 5\overline{)2.5}^{0.5}$$

$$\begin{array}{r} 16 \text{ m} \\ \hline 0.5 \text{ ml} \\ \hline 8.0 \end{array}$$

Give 0.5 ml (or 8 m) IM

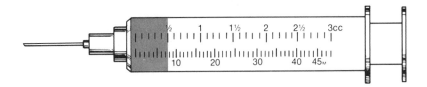

3. Equivalent 1%   1 g in 100 ml

   1 g = 1000 mg

Hence, the solution is 1000 mg per 100 ml.

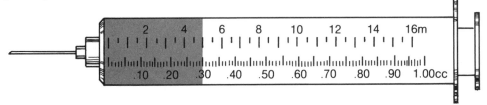

$$\frac{3 \text{ mg}}{1000 \text{ mg}} \times 100 \text{ ml} = \frac{3}{10} = 0.3 \text{ ml} \qquad \begin{array}{r} 16 \text{ m} \\ \times\, 0.3 \text{ ml} \\ \hline 4.8 \text{ m} \end{array}$$

Give 0.3 ml (or 5 m) SC

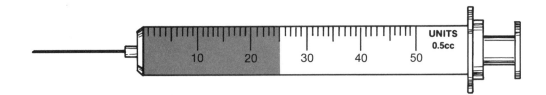

EXERCISE 5

1.

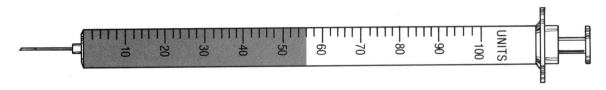

2.

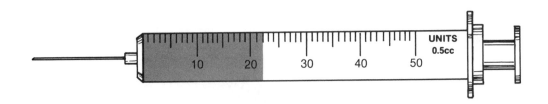

3.

4.

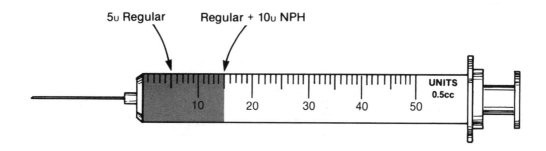

5ᵤ Regular   Regular + 10ᵤ NPH

PROFICIENCY TEST 1

1. Equivalent 0.1 Gm = 100 mg

$$\frac{\overset{1}{\cancel{100\ mg}}}{\underset{2}{\cancel{200\ mg}}} \times 3\ ml = \frac{3}{2} \overset{1.5}{\overline{)3.0}}$$

Give 1.5 ml IM

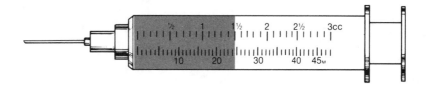

2. $\frac{\overset{1}{\cancel{5\ mg}}}{\underset{3}{\cancel{15\ mg}}} \times 1\ ml = \frac{1}{3} \overset{.333}{\overline{)1.000}}$

Give 0.33 ml SC

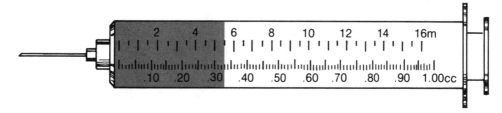

3. $\frac{\overset{1}{\cancel{25\ mg}}}{\underset{1}{\underset{\cancel{2}}{\cancel{50\ mg}}}} \times \overset{1}{\cancel{2}}\ cc = 1\ cc$

Give 1 cc IM

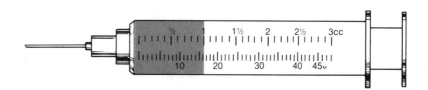

4. 20 units. Remember that Humulin insulin is a type of regular insulin and so must be drawn up first into the syringe!

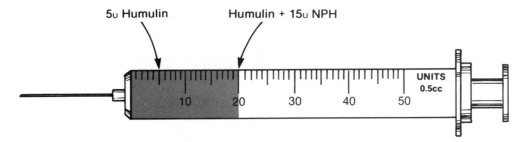

5$_U$ Humulin   Humulin + 15$_U$ NPH

5.
$$\frac{\overset{1}{\cancel{20}\ \cancel{mEq}}}{\underset{2}{\cancel{40}\ \cancel{mEq}}} \times \overset{10}{\cancel{20}}\ ml = 10\ ml$$

Add 10 ml to IV

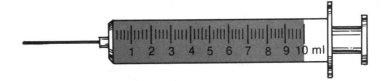

6.
$$\frac{\overset{3}{\cancel{0.8}\ \cancel{mg}}}{\underset{2}{\cancel{0.4}\ \cancel{mg}}} \times 1\ ml = \frac{3}{2}\overset{1.5}{\overline{)3.0}}$$

Give 1.5 ml SC

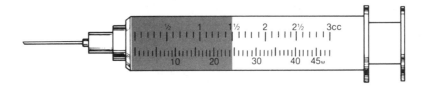

7.
$$\frac{\overset{2}{\cancel{0.8}\ \cancel{mg}}}{\underset{1}{\cancel{0.4}\ \cancel{mg}}} \times 1\ ml = 2\ ml$$

Give 2 ml IM

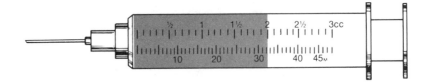

8. Equivalent 0.5 Gm = 500 mg

$$\frac{\overset{2}{\cancel{500}\ \cancel{mg}}}{\underset{1}{\cancel{250}\ \cancel{mg}}} \times 1\ ml = 2\ ml$$

Add 2 ml to IV. Were you confused by the 25%? No reason to use it to solve this problem!

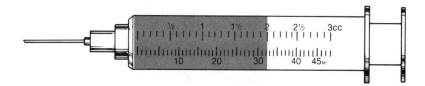

9. $\dfrac{200 \text{ mg}}{500 \text{ mg}} \times 2 \text{ ml} = \dfrac{4}{5} \overline{)\dfrac{.8}{4.0}}$

Give 0.8 ml IM

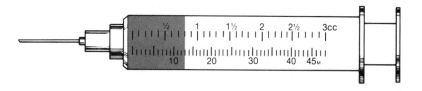

10. Equivalent 1:100 means 1 g in 100 ml

$$1 \text{ g} = 1000 \text{ mg}$$

Hence, the solution is 1000 mg/100 ml.

$$\dfrac{7.5 \text{ mg}}{1000 \text{ mg}} \times 100 \text{ ml} = \dfrac{7.5}{10} \overline{)\dfrac{.75}{7.50}}$$

$$\begin{array}{r} 7\ 0 \\ \hline 50 \\ 50 \\ \hline \end{array}$$

Give 0.8 ml SC

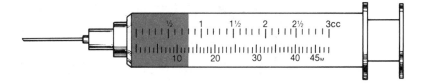

PROFICIENCY TEST 2

1. $\dfrac{\overset{2}{10 \text{ mg}}}{\underset{3}{15 \text{ mg}}} \times 1 \text{ ml} = \dfrac{2}{3} \overline{)\dfrac{.66}{2.00}}$

Give 0.7 ml SC

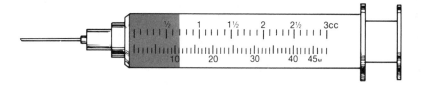

2. $\dfrac{\overset{1}{25 \text{ mg}}}{\underset{4}{100 \text{ mg}}} \times 1 \text{ ml} = \dfrac{1}{4} \overline{)\dfrac{.25}{1.00}}$

Give 0.25 ml. You are using a 1-ml precision syringe; therefore, the answer is the nearest hundredth.

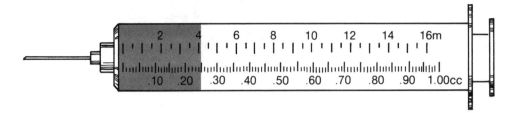

3. Equivalent gr 1 s̈s̈ = 100 mg

$$\frac{\overset{1}{\cancel{100\ mg}}}{\underset{2}{\cancel{200\ mg}}} \times 3\ ml = \frac{3}{2} \overset{1.5}{)3.0}$$

Give 1.5 ml IM

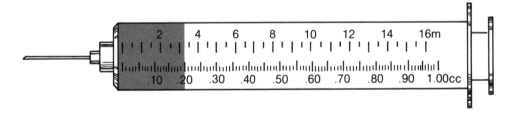

4. $\dfrac{\overset{1}{\cancel{1000\ \mu g}}}{\underset{5}{\cancel{5000\ \mu g}}} \times 1\ ml = \dfrac{1}{5} \overset{.2}{)1.0}$

Give 0.2 ml IM

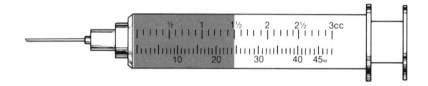

5. Equivalent 1% means 1 g in 100 ml

1 g = 1000 mg

Hence, the solution is 1000 mg in 100 ml

$$\frac{\overset{5}{\cancel{25\ mg}}}{\underset{\underset{2}{\cancel{10}}}{\cancel{1000\ mg}}} \times \overset{1}{\cancel{100}}\ ml = \frac{5}{2} \overset{2.5}{)5.0}$$

Prepare 2.5 ml for the physician

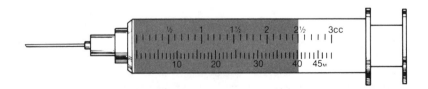

6. $\dfrac{0.5 \text{ mg}}{0.4 \text{ mg}} \times 1 \text{ ml} = \dfrac{5}{4} \overline{)\dfrac{1.25}{5.00}}$

Give 1.3 ml SC

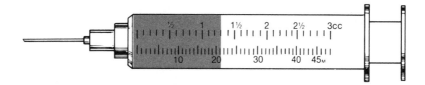

7. 13 units. Remember that Humulin insulin is a type of regular insulin and so must be drawn up first into the syringe!

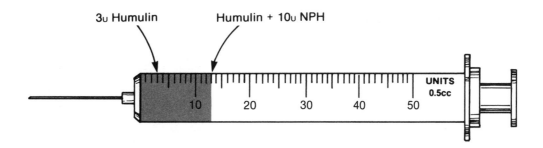

3ᵤ Humulin   Humulin + 10ᵤ NPH

UNITS 0.5cc

8. $\dfrac{1.2 \text{ mEq}}{0.5 \text{ mEq}} \times 1 \text{ ml} = \dfrac{1.2}{0.5} \overline{)\dfrac{2.4}{1.2\,0}}$

Add 2.4 ml to the IV stat

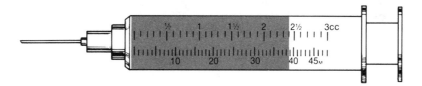

9. $\dfrac{\overset{3}{75} \text{ mg}}{\underset{2}{50} \text{ mg}} \times 1 \text{ ml} = \dfrac{3}{2} \overline{)\dfrac{1.5}{3.0}}$

Give 1.5 ml IM

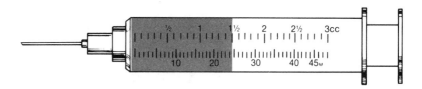

10. Equivalent 1:1000 means 1 g in 1000 ml
1 g = 1000 mg

Hence, the solution is 1000 mg in 1000 ml

$500 \ \mu g = 0.5 \ mg$

$$\frac{0.5 \ \cancel{mg}}{\underset{1}{\cancel{1000} \ \cancel{mg}}} \times \cancel{1000} \ ml = 0.5 \ ml$$

Give 0.5 ml SC stat

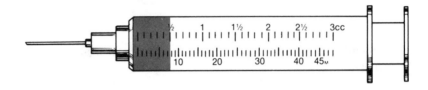

MENTAL DRILL IN LIQUIDS FOR INJECTION PROBLEMS

1. 2 ml IM	**7.** 0.8 ml SC	**13.** 2 ml IV
2. 5 ml IV	**8.** 1 cc SC	**14.** 1.5 ml IM
3. 2 ml IM	**9.** 20 ml IV	**15.** 1.5 ml IM
4. 1 ml IM	**10.** 2.5 ml IM	**16.** 0.35 ml or 0.4 ml IM
5. 0.5 ml IM	**11.** 0.8 ml IM	**17.** 1.5 ml SC
6. 1 ml IM	**12.** 2 ml IM	**18.** 1.5 ml IM

8

Injections From Powders

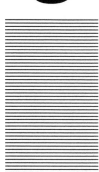

Some medications are prepared in a dry form, because in solution they lose stability over time. To prepare injections from powders the nurse must carry out several steps.

1. Read the directions to reconstitute the drug.
2. Dissolve the drug according to the directions.
3. Label the vial with the date, the strength of solution made, and the nurse's initials.
4. Prepare and administer the injection.
5. Store the vial following the manufacturer's recommendations.

RULE AND EXPLANATION

The rule used to solve injection from powder problems is the same as that for oral medications and for injection from a liquid, because the powdered drug *becomes a liquid* once the powder is dissolved.

$$\frac{Desire}{Have} \times Stock = Answer$$

EXAMPLE:

Order: ceftizoxime sodium 270 mg IM q6h

Supply: 1 g powder

Label directions: Add 3.0 ml of sterile water for injection. Shake well. Provides a volume of 3.7 ml (270 mg/ml). Stable for 24 hours at room temperature or 96 hours if refrigerated (Fig. 8-1).

Desire: The order in the example is 270 mg IM.

Have: The strength of the drug supplied. In the example it is 1 g as a dry powder; when it is reconstituted, it is 270 mg/ml. Remember that the manufacturer gives the solution strength; the nurse does not have to determine it.

(continued)

(continued)

Stock: The fluid portion of the solution made: in this example it is *1 ml = 270* mg.

Answer: How much liquid to give (stated as ml, cc, or minims). In the example given, the nurse has a solution of 270 mg/ml and an order for 270 mg IM. The answer is obvious: give 1 ml IM. The remaining solution is stored in the refrigerator. The vial is labeled with the date, the solution made, and the nurse's initials.

DISTINCTIVE FEATURES OF INJECTIONS FROM POWDERS

Sterile technique is used to prepare and administer the medication, which is given parenterally (usually IM, IV, or IVPB). The dry drug is supplied in vials of powder or crystals and may come in different strengths. Because powders deteriorate in solution, choose the strength closest to the amount ordered.

The powder is usually diluted with one of the following:

Sterile water for injection

Bacteriostatic water for injection that has a preservative added

Normal saline for injection (0.9% sodium chloride)

Directions will state which fluids may be used. Read this information carefully because some fluids may be incompatible (i.e., unsuitable) as diluents. When the powder goes into solution, *displacement* occurs. This means that the *volume* added to the vial is *increased* by the powder as it is dissolved. There is no uniformity in the way powders go into solution.

Refer to the label in Figure 8-1 again. The manufacturer tells the nurse to add 3.0 ml of sterile water to provide an approximate volume of 3.7 ml. In this example 0.7 ml is the displacement volume. This volume is not important in solving powder problems.

Injections from powder problems are solved by using the solution made. This information is provided by the manufacturer. Three pieces of information are necessary to solve injection from powder problems:

- The type of fluid needed to dissolve the powder
- The amount of fluid to add
- The solution made

WHERE TO FIND INFORMATION ABOUT RECONSTITUTION OF POWDERS

Information about reconstitution of powders may be found from

- The label on the vial of powder
- The package insert that comes with the vial of powder
- Nursing drug handbooks and other references

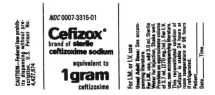

Figure 8-1. Label of ceftizoxime sodium (Cefizox). (Courtesy of Smith Kline & French Laboratories.)

Package Inserts

The package insert is a reference used by many health care professionals, including physicians, nurses, microbiologists, laboratory workers, pharmacists, and toxicologists; consequently, it contains much information. The reader skims the material for the specific facts needed.

The package insert information concerning cefoperazone sodium (Cefobid) injection is reproduced in Figure 8-2. Practice Exercise 1 is designed to provide the reader with the opportunity to become familiar with the types of information that can be obtained. Reconstitution directions will be discussed in the next section.

===================== PRACTICE EXERCISE 1 =====================

After scanning the insert on cefoperazone sodium (Cefobid) in Figure 8–2, answer the following questions. Answers will be found at the end of the chapter.

1. What is the class of cefoperazone? _____

   _____

2. By what routes may this drug be administered? _____

3. What is the main route of excretion for cefoperazone? _____

4. List three classes of microorganisms against which this drug is effective. _____

   _____ ; _____ ; and _____

5. How does cefoperazone act? (see Microbiology) _____

   _____

6. List four diseases for which cefoperazone is indicated

   _____ ; _____ ;

   _____ ; and _____ ;

7. For whom is the drug contraindicated? _____

   _____

8. List three warnings the nurse should heed in administering cefoperazone:

   a. _____

   b. _____

   c. _____

9. What does the manufacturer state about the use of cefoperazone in

   a. pregnancy _____

   b. nursing mothers _____

   c. pediatrics _____

10. What is the usual adult dose of cefoperazone? _____

    _____

(continued)

=========== PRACTICE EXERCISE 1 (*Continued*) ===========

11. List five types of adverse reactions that might occur, and give one symptom for each reaction.

a. _____

b. _____

c. _____

d. _____

e. _____

70-4169-00-2

CEFOBID®
cefoperazone sodium
and
cefoperazone sodium injection
For Intravenous or Intramuscular Use

DESCRIPTION

CEFOBID (cefoperazone sodium) is a sterile, semisynthetic, broad-spectrum, parenteral cephalosporin antibiotic for intravenous or intramuscular administration. It is the sodium salt of 7-[D(-)-α-(4-ethyl-2,3-dioxo-1-piperazinecarboxamido)-α-(4-hydroxyphenyl) acetamido]-3-[(1-methyl-1H-tetrazol-5-yl)thiomethyl]-3-cephem-4-carboxylic acid. Its chemical formula is $C_{25}H_{26}N_9NaO_8S_2$ with a molecular weight of 667.65. The structural formula is given below:

CEFOBID contains 34 mg sodium (1.5 mEq) per gram. CEFOBID is a white powder which is freely soluble in water. The pH of a 25% (w/v) freshly reconstituted solution varies between 4.5–6.5 and the solution ranges from colorless to straw yellow depending on the concentration.
   CEFOBID in crystalline form is supplied in vials equivalent to 1 g or 2 g of cefoperazone and in Piggyback Units for intravenous administration equivalent to 1 g or 2 g cefoperazone. CEFOBID is also supplied premixed as a frozen, sterile, nonpyrogenic, iso-osmotic solution equivalent to 1 g or 2 g cefoperazone in plastic containers. After thawing, the solution is intended for intravenous use.
   The plastic container is fabricated from specially formulated polyvinyl chloride. Solutions in contact with the plastic container can leach out certain of its chemical components in very small amounts within the expiration period, e.g., di 2-ethylhexyl phthalate (DEHP), up to 5 parts per million. However, the safety of the plastic has been confirmed in tests in animals according to the USP biological tests for plastic containers, as well as by tissue culture toxicity studies.

CLINICAL PHARMACOLOGY

High serum and bile levels of CEFOBID are attained after a single dose of the drug. Table 1 demonstrates the serum concentrations of CEFOBID in normal volunteers following either a single 15-minute constant rate intravenous infusion of 1, 2, 3 or 4 grams of the drug, or a single intramuscular injection of 1 or 2 grams of the drug.

TABLE 1. Cefoperazone Serum Concentrations

Dose/Route	Mean Serum Concentrations (mcg/ml)						
	0*	0.5 hr	1 hr	2 hr	4 hr	8 hr	12 hr
1 g IV	153	114	73	38	16	4	0.5
2 g IV	252	153	114	70	32	8	2
3 g IV	340	210	142	89	41	9	2
4 g IV	506	325	251	161	71	19	6
1 g IM	32**	52	65	57	33	7	1
2 g IM	40**	69	93	97	58	14	4

*Hours post-administration, with 0 time being the end of the infusion.
**Values obtained 15 minutes post-injection.

The mean serum half-life of CEFOBID is approximately 2.0 hours, independent of the route of administration.
   In vitro studies with human serum indicate that the degree of CEFOBID reversible protein binding varies with the serum concentration from 93% at 25 mcg/ml of CEFOBID to 90% at 250 mcg/ml and 82% at 500 mcg/ml.
   CEFOBID achieves therapeutic concentrations in the following body tissues and fluids:

Tissue or Fluid	Dose	Concentration
Ascitic Fluid	2 g	64 mcg/ml
Cerebrospinal Fluid	50 mg/kg	1.8 mcg/ml to 8.0 mcg/ml
(in patients with inflamed meninges)		
Urine	2 g	3,286 mcg/ml
Sputum	3 g	6.0 mcg/ml
Endometrium	2 g	74 mcg/g
Myometrium	2 g	54 mcg/g
Palatine Tonsil	1 g	8 mcg/g
Sinus Mucous Membrane	1 g	8 mcg/g
Umbilical Cord Blood	1 g	25 mcg/ml
Amniotic Fluid	1 g	4.8 mcg/ml
Lung	1 g	28 mcg/g
Bone	2 g	40 mcg/g

Figure 8-2. Portion of the package insert for cefoperazone (Cefobid). (Courtesy of Roerig-Pfizer Laboratories.)

(*continued*)

CEFOBID is excreted mainly in the bile. Maximum bile concentrations are generally obtained between one and three hours following drug administration and exceed concurrent serum concentrations by up to 100 times. Reported biliary concentrations of CEFOBID range from 66 mcg/ml at 30 minutes to as high as 6000 mcg/ml at 3 hours after an intravenous bolus injection of 2 grams.

Following a single intramuscular or intravenous dose, tne urinary recovery of CEFOBID over a 12-hour period averages 20–30%. No significant quantity of metabolites has been found in the urine. Urinary concentrations greater than 2200 mcg/ml have been obtained following a 15-minute infusion of a 2 g dose. After an IM injection of 2 g, peak urine concentrations of almost 1000 mcg/ml have been obtained, and therapeutic levels are maintained for 12 hours.

Repeated administration of CEFOBID at 12-hour intervals does not result in accumulation of the drug in normal subjects. Peak serum concentrations, areas under the curve (AUC's), and serum half-lives in patients with severe renal insufficiency are not significantly different than those in normal volunteers. In patients with hepatic dysfunction, the serum half-life is prolonged and urinary excretion is increased. In patients with combined renal and hepatic insufficiencies, CEFOBID may accumulate in the serum.

CEFOBID has been used in pediatrics, but the safety and effectiveness in children have not been established. The half-life of CEFOBID in serum is 6–10 hours in low birth-weight neonates.

Microbiology
CEFOBID is active *in vitro* against a wide range of aerobic and anaerobic, gram-positive and gram-negative pathogens. The bactericidal action of CEFOBID results from the inhibition of bacterial cell wall synthesis. CEFOBID has a high degree of stability in the presence of beta-lactamases produced by most gram-negative pathogens. CEFOBID is usually active against organisms which are resistant to other beta-lactam antibiotics because of beta-lactamase production. CEFOBID is usually active against the following organisms *in vitro* and in clinical infections:

Gram-Positive Aerobes:
Staphylococcus aureus, penicillinase and non-penicillinase-producing strains
Staphylococcus epidermidis
Streptococcus pneumoniae (formerly *Diplococcus pneumoniae*)
Streptococcus pyogenes (Group A beta-hemolytic streptococci)
Streptococcus agalactiae (Group B beta-hemolytic streptococci)
Enterococcus (*Streptococcus faecalis*, *S. faecium* and *S. durans*)

Gram-Negative Aerobes:

Escherichia coli	*Providencia stuartii*
Klebsiella species (including *K. pneumoniae*)	*Providencia rettgeri*
Enterobacter species	(formerly *Proteus rettgeri*)
Citrobacter species	*Serratia marcescens*
Haemophilus influenzae	*Pseudomonas aeruginosa*
Proteus mirabilis	*Pseudomonas* species
Proteus vulgaris	Some strains of *Acinetobacter calcoaceticus*
Morganella morganii (formerly *Proteus morganii*)	*Neisseria gonorrhoeae*

Anaerobic Organisms:
Gram-positive cocci (including *Peptococcus* and *Peptostreptococcus*)
Clostridium species
Bacteroides fragilis
Other *Bacteroides* species

CEFOBID is also active *in vitro* against a wide variety of other pathogens although the clinical significance is unknown. These organisms include: *Salmonella* and *Shigella* species, *Serratia liquefaciens*, *N. meningitidis*, *Bordetella pertussis*, *Yersinia enterocolitica*, *Clostridium difficile*, *Fusobacterium* species, *Eubacterium* species and beta-lactamase producing strains of *H. influenzae* and *N. gonorrhoeae*.

SUSCEPTIBILITY TESTING
Diffusion Technique. For the disk diffusion method of susceptibility testing, a 75 mcg CEFOBID diffusion disk should be used. Organisms should be tested with the CEFOBID 75 mcg disk since CEFOBID has been shown *in vitro* to be active against organisms which are found to be resistant to other beta-lactam antibiotics.

Tests should be interpreted by the following criteria:

Zone Diameter	Interpretation
Greater than or equal to 21 mm	Susceptible
16–20 mm	Moderately Susceptible
Less than or equal to 15 mm	Resistant

Quantitative procedures that require measurement of zone diameters give the most precise estimate of susceptibility. One such method which has been recommended for use with the CEFOBID 75 mcg disk is the NCCLS approved standard. (Performance Standards for Antimicrobic Disk Susceptibility Tests. Second Information Supplement Vol. 2 No. 2 pp. 49-69. Publisher–National Committee for Clinical Laboratory Standards, Villanova, Pennsylvania.)

A report of "susceptible" indicates that the infecting organism is likely to respond to CEFOBID therapy and a report of "resistant" indicates that the infecting organism is not likely to respond to therapy. A "moderately susceptible" report suggests that the infecting organism will be susceptible to CEFOBID if a higher than usual dosage is used or if the infection is confined to tissues and fluids (e.g., urine or bile) in which high antibiotic levels are attained.

Dilution Techniques. Broth or agar dilution methods may be used to determine the minimal inhibitory concentration (MIC) of CEFOBID. Serial twofold dilutions of CEFOBID should be prepared in either broth or agar. Broth should be inoculated to contain 5×10^5 organisms/ml and agar "spotted" with 10^4 organisms.

MIC test results should be interpreted in light of serum, tissue, and body fluid concentrations of CEFOBID. Organisms inhibited by CEFOBID at 16 mcg/ml or less are considered susceptible, while organisms with MIC's of 17–63 mcg/ml are moderately susceptible. Organisms inhibited at CEFOBID concentrations of greater than or equal to 64 mcg/ml are considered resistant, although clinical cures have been obtained in some patients infected by such organisms.

INDICATIONS AND USAGE
CEFOBID is indicated for the treatment of the following infections when caused by susceptible organisms:

Respiratory Tract Infections caused by *S. pneumoniae*, *H. influenzae*, *S. aureus* (penicillinase and non-penicillinase producing strains), *S. pyogenes* (Group A beta-hemolytic streptococci), *P. aeruginosa*, *Klebsiella pneumoniae*, *E. coli*, *Proteus* species (indole-positive and indole-negative), and *Enterobacter species*.

Peritonitis and Other Intra-abdominal Infections caused by *E. coli*, *P. aeruginosa*, enterococci, anaerobic gram-positive cocci, and anaerobic gram-positive and gram-negative bacilli (including *Bacteroides fragilis*).

Bacterial Septicemia caused by *S. pneumoniae*, *S. pyogenes*, *S. agalactiae*, *S. aureus*, enterococci, *H. influenzae*, *Pseudomonas aeruginosa*, *E. coli*, *Klebsiella* spp., *Proteus* species (indole-positive and indole-negative), *Clostridium* spp. and anaerobic gram-positive cocci.

Infections of the Skin and Skin Structures caused by *S. aureus* (penicillinase and non-penicillinase producing strains), *S. pyogenes* and *P. aeruginosa*.

Pelvic Inflammatory Disease, Endometritis, and Other Infections of the Female Genital Tract caused by *N. gonorrhoeae*, *S. aureus* and *S. epidermidis*, *S. agalactiae*, *E. coli*, *Clostridium* spp., *Bacteroides* species (including *Bacteroides fragilis*) and anaerobic gram-positive cocci.

Urinary Tract Infections caused by *Enterococcus*, *Escherichia coli*, and *Pseudomonas aeruginosa*.

Susceptibility Testing
Before instituting treatment with CEFOBID, appropriate specimens should be obtained for isolation of the causative organism and for determination of its susceptibility to the drug. Treatment may be started before results of susceptibility testing are available.

Combination Therapy
Synergy between CEFOBID and aminoglycosides has been demonstrated with many gram-negative bacilli. However, such enhanced activity of these combinations is not predictable. If such therapy is considered, *in vitro* susceptibility tests should be performed to determine the activity of the drugs in combination, and renal function should be monitored carefully. (See PRECAUTIONS, and DOSAGE AND ADMINISTRATION sections).

CONTRAINDICATIONS
CEFOBID is contraindicated in patients with known allergy to the cephalosporin-class of antibiotics.

WARNINGS
BEFORE THERAPY WITH CEFOBID IS INSTITUTED, CAREFUL INQUIRY SHOULD BE MADE TO DETERMINE WHETHER THE PATIENT HAS HAD PREVIOUS HYPERSENSITIVITY REACTIONS TO CEPHALOSPORINS, PENICILLINS OR OTHER DRUGS. THIS PRODUCT SHOULD BE GIVEN CAUTIOUSLY TO PENICILLIN-SENSITIVE PATIENTS. ANTIBIOTICS SHOULD BE ADMINISTERED WITH CAUTION TO ANY PATIENT WHO HAS DEMONSTRATED SOME FORM OF ALLERGY, PARTICULARLY TO DRUGS. SERIOUS ACUTE HYPERSENSITIVITY REACTIONS MAY REQUIRE THE USE OF SUBCUTANEOUS EPINEPHRINE AND OTHER EMERGENCY MEASURES.

Figure 8-2. (*continued*)

PSEUDOMEMBRANOUS COLITIS HAS BEEN REPORTED WITH THE USE OF CEPHALOSPORINS (AND OTHER BROAD-SPECTRUM ANTIBIOTICS); THEREFORE, IT IS IMPORTANT TO CONSIDER ITS DIAGNOSIS IN PATIENTS WHO DEVELOP DIARRHEA IN ASSOCIATION WITH ANTIBIOTIC USE.

Treatment with broad-spectrum antibiotics alters normal flora of the colon and may permit overgrowth of clostridia. Studies indicate a toxin produced by *Clostridium difficile* is one primary cause of antibiotic-associated colitis. Cholestyramine and colestipol resins have been shown to bind the toxin *in vitro*.

Mild cases of colitis may respond to drug discontinuance alone.

Moderate to severe cases should be managed with fluid, electrolyte, and protein supplementation as indicated.

When the colitis is not relieved by drug discontinuance or when it is severe, oral vancomycin is the treatment of choice for antibiotic-associated pseudomembranous colitis produced by *C. difficile*. Other causes of colitis should also be considered.

PRECAUTIONS

Although transient elevations of the BUN and serum creatinine have been observed, CEFOBID alone does not appear to cause significant nephrotoxicity. However, concomitant administration of aminoglycosides and other cephalosporins has caused nephrotoxicity.

CEFOBID is extensively excreted in bile. The serum half-life of CEFOBID is increased 2–4 fold in patients with hepatic disease and/or biliary obstruction. In general, total daily dosage above 4 g should not be necessary in such patients. If higher dosages are used, serum concentrations should be monitored.

Because renal excretion is not the main route of elimination of CEFOBID (see CLINICAL PHARMACOLOGY), patients with renal failure require no adjustment in dosage when usual doses are administered. When high doses of CEFOBID are used, concentrations of drug in the serum should be monitored periodically. If evidence of accumulation exists, dosage should be decreased accordingly.

The half-life of CEFOBID is reduced slightly during hemodialysis. Thus, dosing should be scheduled to follow a dialysis period. In patients with both hepatic dysfunction and significant renal disease, CEFOBID dosage should not exceed 1–2 g daily without close monitoring of serum concentrations.

As with other antibiotics, vitamin K deficiency has occurred rarely in patients treated with CEFOBID. The mechanism is most probably related to the suppression of gut flora which normally synthesize this vitamin. Those at risk include patients with a poor nutritional status, malabsorption states (e.g., cystic fibrosis), alcoholism, and patients on prolonged hyper-alimentation regimens (administered either intravenously or via a naso-gastric tube). Prothrombin time should be monitored in these patients and exogenous vitamin K administered as indicated.

A disulfiram-like reaction characterized by flushing, sweating, headache, and tachycardia has been reported when alcohol (beer, wine) was ingested within 72 hours after CEFOBID administration. Patients should be cautioned about the ingestion of alcoholic beverages following the administration of CEFOBID. A similar reaction has been reported with other cephalosporins.

Prolonged use of CEFOBID may result in the overgrowth of nonsusceptible organisms. Careful observation of the patient is essential. If superinfection occurs during therapy, appropriate measures should be taken.

CEFOBID should be prescribed with caution in individuals with a history of gastrointestinal disease, particularly colitis.

Drug Laboratory Test Interactions

A false-positive reaction for glucose in the urine may occur with Benedict's or Fehling's solution.

Carcinogenesis, Mutagenesis, Impairment of Fertility

Long term studies in animals have not been performed to evaluate carcinogenic potential. The maximum duration of CEFOBID animal toxicity studies is six months. In none of the *in vivo* or *in vitro* genetic toxicology studies did CEFOBID show any mutagenic potential at either the chromosomal or subchromosomal level. CEFOBID produced no impairment of fertility and had no effects on general reproductive performance or fetal development when administered subcutaneously at daily doses up to 500 to 1000 mg/kg prior to and during mating, and to pregnant female rats during gestation. These doses are 10 to 20 times the estimated usual single clinical dose. CEFOBID had adverse effects on the testes of prepubertal rats at all doses tested. Subcutaneous administration of 1000 mg/kg per day (approximately 16 times the average adult human dose) resulted in reduced testicular weight, arrested spermatogenesis, reduced germinal cell population and vacuolation of Sertoli cell cytoplasm. The severity of lesions was dose dependent in the 100 to 1000 mg/kg per day range; the low dose caused a minor decrease in spermatocytes. This effect has not been observed in adult rats. Histologically the lesions were reversible at all but the highest dosage levels. However, these studies did not evaluate subsequent development of reproductive function in the rats. The relationship of these findings to humans is unknown.

Usage in Pregnancy

Pregnancy Category B: Reproduction studies have been performed in mice, rats, and monkeys at doses up to 10 times the human dose and have revealed no evidence of impaired fertility or harm to the fetus due to CEFOBID. There are, however, no adequate and well controlled studies in pregnant women. Because animal reproduction studies are not always predictive of human response, this drug should be used during pregnancy only if clearly needed.

Usage in Nursing Mothers

Only low concentrations of CEFOBID are excreted in human milk. Although CEFOBID passes poorly into breast milk of nursing mothers, caution should be exercised when CEFOBID is administered to a nursing woman.

Pediatric Use

Safety and effectiveness in children have not been established. For information concerning testicular changes in prepubertal rats (see Carcinogenesis, Mutagenesis, Impairment of Fertility).

ADVERSE REACTIONS

In clinical studies the following adverse effects were observed and were considered to be related to CEFOBID therapy or of uncertain etiology:

Hypersensitivity: As with all cephalosporins, hypersensitivity manifested by skin reactions (1 patient in 45), drug fever (1 in 260), or a change in Coombs' test (1 in 60) has been reported. These reactions are more likely to occur in patients with a history of allergies, particularly to penicillin.

Hematology: As with other beta-lactam antibiotics, reversible neutropenia may occur with prolonged administration. Slight decreases in neutrophil count (1 patient in 50) have been reported. Decreased hemoglobins (1 in 20) or hematocrits (1 in 20) have been reported, which is consistent with published literature on other cephalosporins. Transient eosinophilia has occurred in 1 patient in 10.

Hepatic: Of 1285 patients treated with cefoperazone in clinical trials, one patient with a history of liver disease developed significantly elevated liver function enzymes during CEFOBID therapy. Clinical signs and symptoms of nonspecific hepatitis accompanied these increases. After CEFOBID therapy was discontinued, the patient's enzymes returned to pre-treatment levels and the symptomatology resolved. As with other antibiotics that achieve high bile levels, mild transient elevations of liver function enzymes have been observed in 5–10% of the patients receiving CEFOBID therapy. The relevance of these findings, which were not accompanied by overt signs or symptoms of hepatic dysfunction, has not been established.

Gastrointestinal: Diarrhea or loose stools has been reported in 1 in 30 patients. Most of these experiences have been mild or moderate in severity and self-limiting in nature. In all cases, these symptoms responded to symptomatic therapy or ceased when cefoperazone therapy was stopped. Nausea and vomiting have been reported rarely.

Symptoms of pseudomembranous colitis can appear during or for several weeks subsequent to antibiotic therapy (see WARNINGS).

Renal Function Tests: Transient elevations of the BUN (1 in 16) and serum creatinine (1 in 48) have been noted.

Local Reactions: CEFOBID is well tolerated following intramuscular administration. Occasionally, transient pain (1 in 140) may follow administration by this route. When CEFOBID is administered by intravenous infusion some patients may develop phlebitis (1 in 120) at the infusion site.

DOSAGE AND ADMINISTRATION

The usual adult daily dose of CEFOBID is 2 to 4 grams per day administered in equally divided doses every 12 hours.

In severe infections or infections caused by less sensitive organisms, the total daily dose and/or frequency may be increased. Patients have been successfully treated with a total daily dosage of 6–12 grams divided into 2, 3 or 4 administrations ranging from 1.5 to 4 grams per dose.

In a pharmacokinetic study, a total daily dose of 16 grams was administered to severely immunocompromised patients by constant infusion without complications. Steady state serum concentrations were approximately 150 mcg/ml in these patients.

When treating infections caused by *Streptococcus pyogenes*, therapy should be continued for at least 10 days.

Solutions of CEFOBID and aminoglycoside should not be directly mixed, since there is a physical incompatibility between them. If combination therapy with CEFOBID and an aminoglycoside is contemplated (see INDICATIONS) this can be accomplished by sequential intermittent intravenous infusion provided that separate secondary intravenous tubing is used, and that the primary intravenous tubing is adequately irrigated with an approved diluent between doses. It is also suggested that CEFOBID be administered prior to the aminoglycoside. *In vitro* testing of the effectiveness of drug combination(s) is recommended.

Figure 8-2. (continued)

DIRECTIONS FOR USE OF CEFOBID (cefoperazone sodium) INJECTION IN PLASTIC CONTAINERS
CEFOBID supplied premixed as a frozen, sterile, iso-osmotic solution in plastic containers is to be administered either as continuous or intermittent infusion.

Thaw container at room temperature. After thawing, check for minute leaks by squeezing bag firmly. If leaks are found, discard solution as sterility may be impaired. Additives should not be introduced into this solution. Do not use if the solution is cloudy or precipitated or if the seal is not intact.

After thawing, the solution is stable for 10 days if stored under refrigeration (5°C) and for 48 hours at room temperature. DO NOT REFREEZE. Use sterile equipment.

CAUTION: Do not use plastic container in series connections. Such use could result in air embolism due to residual air being drawn from the primary container before administration of the fluid from the secondary container is complete.

Preparation for administration
1. Suspend container from eyelet support.
2. Remove plastic protector from outlet port at bottom of container.
3. Attach administration set. Refer to complete directions accompanying set.

Figure 8-2. (*continued*)

INTERPRETING DILUTION DIRECTIONS

Directions for reconstitution may be found under the headings Preparation of Solutions; Dosage and Administration; or Reconstitution.

Part of the package insert related to the IM administration of cefoperazone is reproduced in Figure 8–3. Examine this information with the intention of solving the following problem:

Order: cefoperazone 0.5 g IM q12h

Supply: vial of powder labeled 1 g

1. Table 1 gives *Solutions for Initial Reconstitution:* sterile water for injection, bacteriostatic water for injection, and 0.9% sodium chloride injection. Choose one.
2. The heading *Preparation for Intramuscular Injection* states that when a concentration of 250 mg or more is to be administered, a 2% lidocaine solution should be used together with sterile water for injection in a two-step dilution.
3. Two tables are given. The upper table has the two-step dilution, the lower one does not. Because the order requires two steps, use the directions in the top table.
4. Two strengths of powder are listed in the upper table. Look at the extreme left. They are 1-g vial and 2-g vial. Our supply is a 1-g vial. Follow directions for 1 g.
5. The next heading is *Final Cefoperazone Concentration.* Two possibilities are given for the dilution: 333 mg/ml and 250 mg/ml. Because the order calls for 0.5 g, choose 250 mg/ml. This concentration makes the arithmetic easy. Do you see that the answer will be 2 ml?
6. To make the solution of 250 mg/ml, the following are added: 2.8 ml of sterile water and 1.0 ml of 2% lidocaine.
7. The last column to the right is headed *Withdrawable Volume* and lists 4 ml. Ignore this column; it does not affect the answer. When you add 2.8 ml and 1.0 ml, you expect to have 3.8 ml. The package insert states you will end up with 4 ml. The manufacturer is giving the displacement.
8. You now have all the information needed to prepare the dose ordered.

Use the following outline of steps to solve injection from powder problems. With practice you will remember the steps and they will help you choose the information needed.

EXAMPLE:

Order: cefoperazone 0.5 g IM = 500 mg

Stock powder: 1 g

RECONSTITUTION

The following solutions may be used for the initial reconstitution of CEFOBID sterile powder:

Table 1. Solutions for Initial Reconstitution

5% Dextrose Injection (USP)	0.9% Sodium Chloride Injection (USP)
5% Dextrose and 0.9% Sodium Chloride Injection (USP)	Normosol* M and Dextrose Injection
5% Dextrose and 0.2% Sodium Chloride Injection (USP)	Normosol* R
10% Dextrose Injection (USP)	Sterile Water for Injection*
Bacteriostatic Water for Injection [Benzyl Alcohol or Parabens] (USP)*†	

*Not to be used as a vehicle for intravenous infusion
†Preparations containing Benzyl Alcohol should not be used in neonates.

Preparation for Intramuscular Injection

Any suitable solution listed above may be used to prepare CEFOBID sterile powder for intramuscular injection. When concentrations of 250 mg/ml or more are to be administered, a lidocaine solution should be used. These solutions should be prepared using a combination of Sterile Water for Injection and 2% Lidocaine Hydrochloride Injection (USP) that approximates a 0.5% Lidocaine Hydrochloride Solution. A two-step dilution process as follows is recommended: First, add the required amount of Sterile Water for Injection and agitate until CEFOBID powder is completely dissolved. Second, add the required amount of 2% lidocaine and mix.

	Final Cefoperazone Concentration	Step 1 Volume of Sterile Water	Step 2 Volume of 2% Lidocaine	Withdrawable Volume*†
1 g vial	333 mg/ml	2.0 ml	0.6 ml	3 ml
	250 mg/ml	2.8 ml	1.0 ml	4 ml
2 g vial	333 mg/ml	3.8 ml	1.2 ml	6 ml
	250 mg/ml	5.4 ml	1.8 ml	8 ml

When a diluent other than Lidocaine HCl Injection (USP) is used reconstitute as follows:

	Cefoperazone Concentration	Volume of Diluent to be Added	Withdrawable Volume*
1 g vial	333 mg/ml	2.6 ml	3 ml
	250 mg/ml	3.8 ml	4 ml
2 g vial	333 mg/ml	5.0 ml	6 ml
	250 mg/ml	7.2 ml	8 ml

*There is sufficient excess present to allow for withdrawal of the stated volume.
†Final lidocaine concentration will approximate that obtained if a 0.5% Lidocaine Hydrochloride Solution is used as diluent

STORAGE AND STABILITY

CEFOBID sterile powder is to be stored at or below 25°C (77°F) and protected from light prior to reconstitution. After reconstitution, protection from light is not necessary.

The following parenteral diluents and approximate concentrations of CEFOBID provide stable solutions under the following conditions for the indicated time periods. (After the indicated time periods, unused portions of solutions should be discarded.)

Controlled Room Temperature (15°–25°C/59°–77°F)

24 Hours	Approximate
Bacteriostatic Water for Injection [Benzyl Alcohol or Parabens] (USP)	300 mg/ml
5% Dextrose Injection (USP)	2 mg to 50 mg/ml
5% Dextrose and Lactated Ringer's Injection	2 mg to 50 mg/ml
5% Dextrose and 0.9% Sodium Chloride Injection (USP)	2 mg to 50 mg/ml
5% Dextrose and 0.2% Sodium Chloride Injection (USP)	2 mg to 50 mg/ml
10% Dextrose Injection (USP)	2 mg to 50 mg/ml
Lactated Ringer's Injection (USP)	2 mg/ml
0.5% Lidocaine Hydrochloride Injection (USP)	300 mg/ml
0.9% Sodium Chloride Injection (USP)	2 mg to 300 mg/ml
Normosol* M and 5% Dextrose Injection	2 mg to 50 mg/ml
Normosol* R	2 mg to 50 mg/ml
Sterile Water for Injection	300 mg/ml

Reconstituted CEFOBID solutions may be stored in glass or plastic syringes, or in glass or flexible plastic parenteral solution containers.

Refrigerator Temperature (2°–8°C/36°–46°F)

5 Days	Approximate Concentrations
Bacteriostatic Water for Injection [Benzyl Alcohol or Parabens] (USP)	300 mg/ml
5% Dextrose Injection (USP)	2 mg to 50 mg/ml
5% Dextrose and 0.9% Sodium Chloride Injection (USP)	2 mg to 50 mg/ml
5% Dextrose and 0.2% Sodium Chloride Injection (USP)	2 mg to 50 mg/ml
Lactated Ringer's Injection (USP)	2 mg/ml
0.5% Lidocaine Hydrochloride Injection (USP)	300 mg/ml
0.9% Sodium Chloride Injection (USP)	2 mg to 300 mg/ml
Normosol* M and 5% Dextrose Injection	2 mg to 50 mg/ml
Normosol* R	2 mg to 50 mg/ml
Sterile Water for Injection	300 mg/ml

Reconstituted CEFOBID solutions may be stored in glass or plastic syringes, or in glass or flexible plastic parenteral solution containers.

Figure 8-3. *Reconstitution directions for cefoperazone sodium (Cefobid). (Courtesy of Roerig-Pfizer Laboratories.)*

Diluting fluid and number of milliliters

Step 1. Add 2.8 ml sterile water

Step 2. Add 1 ml 2% lidocaine

Solution and new stock: 250 mg/ml

Rule and arithmetic: $\dfrac{D}{H} \times S = A$

$$\dfrac{\overset{2}{\cancel{500} \text{ mg}}}{\underset{1}{\cancel{250} \text{ mg}}} \times 1 \text{ ml} = 2 \text{ ml}$$

Answer: Give 2 ml IM

Write on label: 250 mg/ml; date; initials

Storage: Refer to Figure 8–3. Under the heading *Storage and Stability,* the reconstituted drug is stable in the refrigerator for 5 days. Refrigerate the remaining solution.

EXAMPLE:

Order: streptomycin sulfate 0.1 gm IM qd (Fig. 8–4)

Stock powder: 1 g

1. You are told to dissolve the powder in water for injection or sodium chloride injection. Choose one.
2. The first column is headed *Approx. Conc. (mg/ml).* Three dilutions are possible. Think what the amount of injection would be for each of these and choose one.

   200 mg/ml: would need 0.5 ml
   250 mg/ml: would need 0.4 ml
   400 mg/ml: would need 0.3 ml

   Choose 200 mg/ml $\left(\dfrac{1}{2} \text{ ml is an adequate amount for injection}\right)$.
3. The second column is headed *Volume (ml) of Solvent.* Below this are listed 1-g vial and 5-g vial. Your stock powder is 1 g. Read down that column and across to 200 mg/ml. Note that you need to add 4.2 ml to the vial. You are ready to solve the problem.

Order: streptomycin sulfate 0.1 g = 100 mg

Stock powder: 1 g

Diluting fluid and number of milliliters: Add 4.2 ml sterile water for injection

Solution and new stock: 200 mg/ml

Rule: $\dfrac{D}{H} \times S = A$

$$\frac{\overset{1}{\cancel{100 \text{ mg}}}}{\underset{2}{\cancel{200 \text{ mg}}}} \times 1 \text{ ml} = \frac{1}{2} \overline{)1.0}^{\,0.5}$$

Answer: Give 0.5 ml

Write on label: 200 mg/ml; date; initials

The dry powder is dissolved by adding Water for Injection, USP or Sodium Chloride Injection, USP in an amount to yield the desired concentration as indicated in the following table:

Approx. Conc. (mg/ml)	Volume (ml) of Solvent 1 g Vial	5 g Vial
200	4.2	—
250	3.2	—
400	1.8	9.0

Sterile reconstituted solutions should be protected from light and may be stored at room temperature for four weeks without significant loss of potency.

Figure 8-4. *Reconstitution directions for streptomycin sulfate. (Courtesy of Roerig-Pfizer Laboratories.)*

EXAMPLE:

Order: penicillin G potassium 1 million units IM q6h (Fig. 8–5)

Stock powder: 5 million unit vial

Diluting fluid and number of milliliters: Use sterile water for injection. The reconstitution directions are difficult to read. The word "respectively" at the end of the sentence means "in order." Write out the directions for the 5 million unit vial (stock).

23 ml will provide 200,000 U/ml
18 ml will provide 250,000 U/ml
8 ml will provide 500,000 U/ml
3 ml will provide 1 million U/ml

Choose 3 ml to dilute the powder.

Solution and new stock: 1 million units/ml

Rule: not needed because

$$\frac{D}{H} \times S = A$$

$$\frac{1 \text{ million units}}{1 \text{ million units}} \times 1 \text{ ml} = 1 \text{ ml}$$

Write on label: 1 million units/ml; date; initials

Storage: refrigerate remaining solution

Note: This solution may be so concentrated that it is painful to the patient. The nurse could decide to dilute the powder with 8 ml to make 500,000 U/ml and give 2 ml to the patient. This more dilute solution may be less painful.

Here are a few tips before you begin Practice Exercise 2.

Preparation of Solutions

Solutions of penicillin should be prepared as follows: Loosen powder. Hold vial horizontally and rotate it while *slowly* directing the stream of diluent against the wall of the vial. Shake vial vigorously after all the diluent has been added. Depending on the route of administration, use Sterile Water for Injection USP, isotonic Sodium Chloride Injection USP, or Dextrose Injection USP. NOTE: Penicillins are rapidly inactivated in the presence of carbohydrate solutions at alkaline pH.

RECONSTITUTION: 1,000,000 u vial—add 9.6 ml, 4.6 ml, or 3.6 ml diluent to provide 100,000 u, 200,000 u, or 250,000 u per ml, respectively: 5,000,000 u vial—add 23 ml, 18 ml, 8 ml, or 3 ml diluent to provide 200,000 u, 250,000 u, 500,000 u, or 1,000,000 u per ml, respectively. *For IV infusion only:* 10,000,000 u vial—add 15.5 ml or 5.4 ml diluent to provide 500,000 u or 1,000,000 u per ml,

respectively: 20,000,000 u vial—add 31.6 ml diluent to provide 500,000 u per ml.

HOW SUPPLIED

Penicillin G Potassium for Injection USP is available in vials providing 1, 5, 10 and 20 million u of crystalline penicillin G potassium.

Storage

The dry powder is relatively stable and may be stored at room temperature without significant loss of potency. Sterile solutions may be kept in the refrigerator one week without significant loss of potency. Solutions prepared for intravenous infusion are stable at room temperature for at least 24 hours.

Figure 8-5. *Preparation of solution for the 5-million-unit vial of penicillin G potassium. (Package insert used by permission of E. R. Squibb & Sons, Inc., copyright owner.)*

- When you read the directions for reconstitution, look first at the solutions you can make. Think the problem through mentally and choose one dilution. This provides a focus as you read.
- If your answer is more than 3 ml for an IM injection, consider using two syringes and injecting in two different sites.
- Experience will guide you in choosing the concentration of the solution. Stronger concentrations, although smaller in volume, may be more painful; a more dilute solution may be more suitable despite its larger volume.
- Each powder problem is unique. Read the directions carefully!
- Choose one diluting fluid—generally sterile water or 0.9% sodium chloride for injection. Do not list all of them in your answer.
- For the following practice problems and self-tests, assume that the doses ordered and the order are correct. Chapter 12 discusses the nurse's responsibilities in drug knowledge. Dosages for infants and children are discussed in Chapter 10.

PRACTICE EXERCISE 2

Solve the following problems in injections from powders and write your answers using the steps. Answers are found at the end of the chapter.

1. Order: carbenicillin disodium 1 g IM q6h (for an adult) (Fig. 8-6)
   Stock: vial of powder labeled 2 g

   a. Diluting fluid and number of milliliters:

   b. Solution and new stock:

   c. Rule and arithmetic:

   d. Answer:

   e. Write on label:

   f. Storage:

2. Order: ceftazidime 1 g IM q6h (Fig. 8-7)
   Stock: 1 g powder

   a. Diluting fluid and number of milliliters:

   b. Solution and new stock:

(continued)

For Intramuscular Use: The 2 g vial should be reconstituted with 4.0 ml of Sterile Water for Injection, 0.5% Lidocaine Hydrochloride (without epinephrine), or Bacteriostatic Water containing 0.9% benzyl alcohol. (Preparations containing benzyl alcohol should not be used in neonates.) In order to facilitate reconstitution up to 7.2 ml of diluent can be used.

Amount of Diluent to be Added to the 2 g Vial	Volume to be Withdrawn for a 1 g Dose
4.0 ml	2.5 ml
5.0 ml	3.0 ml
7.2 ml	4.0 ml

The 5 g vial should be reconstituted with 7.0 ml of Sterile Water for Injection, 0.5% Lidocaine Hydrochloride (without epinephrine), or Bacteriostatic Water containing 0.9% benzyl alcohol. (Preparations containing benzyl alcohol should not be used in neonates.) In order to facilitate reconstitution, up to 17 ml of diluent can be used.

Amount of Diluent to be Added to the 5 g Vial	Volume to be Withdrawn for a 1 g Dose
7.0 ml	2.0 ml
9.5 ml	2.5 ml
12.0 ml	3.0 ml
17.0 ml	4.0 ml

After reconstitution, no significant loss of potency occurs for up to 24 hours at room temperature, and for 72 hours if refrigerated. Any of these unused solutions should be discarded.

Figure 8-6. *Preparation of solution of carbenicillin sodium (Geopen). (Courtesy of Roerig-Pfizer Laboratories.)*

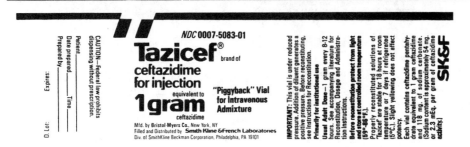

RECONSTITUTION

Single Dose Vials:

For I.M. injection, I.V. direct (bolus) injection, or I.V. infusion, reconstitute with Sterile Water for Injection according to the following table. The vacuum may assist entry of the diluent. SHAKE WELL.

Table 5

Vial Size	Diluent to Be Added	Approx. Avail. Volume	Approx. Avg. Concentration
Intramuscular or Intravenous Direct (bolus) Injection			
1 gram	3.0 ml.	3.6 ml.	280 mg./ml.
Intravenous Infusion			
1 gram	10 ml.	10.6 ml.	95 mg./ml.
2 gram	10 ml.	11.2 ml.	180 mg./ml.

Withdraw the total volume of solution into the syringe (the pressure in the vial may aid withdrawal). The withdrawn solution may contain some bubbles of carbon dioxide.

NOTE: As with the administration of all parenteral products, accumulated gases should be expressed from the syringe immediately before injection of 'Tazicef'.

These solutions of 'Tazicef' are stable for 18 hours at room temperature or seven days if refrigerated (5°C.). Slight yellowing does not affect potency.

Figure 8-7. *Label (top) and reconstitution directions (left) for ceftazidime (Tazicef) 1 g. (Courtesy of Smith Kline & French Laboratories.)*

For dilution of 500-mg, 1-gram, and 2-gram vials, dissolve contents of a vial with the amount of Sterile water for Injection, USP, or Bacteriostatic Water for Injection, USP, listed in the table below:

Label Claim	Recommended Amount of Diluent	Withdrawable Volume	Concentration in mg/ml
500 mg	1.8 ml	2.0 ml	250 mg
1.0 gram	3.4 ml	4.0 ml	250 mg
2.0 gram	6.8 ml	8.0 ml	250 mg

While the 1-gram and 2-gram vials are primarily for intravenous use, they may be administered intramuscularly when the 250-mg or 500-mg vials are unavailable. In such instances, dissolve in 3.4 or 6.8 ml Sterile Water for Injection, USP, or Bacteriostatic Water for Injection, USP, to give a final concentration of 250 mg/ml

The above solutions must be used within one hour after reconstitution.

Figure 8-8. *Reconstitution directions for ampicillin sodium (Omnipen). (Courtesy of Wyeth–Ayerst Laboratories, Philadelphia, PA.)*

================ **PRACTICE EXERCISE 2 (*Continued*)** ================

   c. Rule and arithmetic:

   d. Answer:

   e. Write on label:

   f. Storage:

3. Order: Omnipen 250 mg IM q6h (Fig. 8-8)
      Stock: 500-mg vial of powder

   a. Diluting fluid and number of milliliters:

   b. Solution and new stock:

   c. Rule and arithmetic:

   d. Answer:

   e. Write on label:

   f. Storage:

================ **PRACTICE EXERCISE 3** ================

Solve the following problems in injections from powders using the steps. Answers can be found at the end of the chapter.

1. Order: Ancef 225 mg IM q6h (Fig. 8-9)
      Stock: On the shelf there are three vial sizes of powder: 250 mg, 500 mg, 1 g

   a. Stock chosen:

   b. Diluting fluid and number of milliliters:

   c. Solution and new stock:

   d. Rule and arithmetic:

   e. Answer:

   f. Write on label:

   g. Storage:

(*continued*)

RECONSTITUTION
Preparation of Parenteral Solution
Parenteral drug products should be SHAKEN WELL when reconstituted, and inspected visually for particulate matter prior to administration. If particulate matter is evident in reconstituted fluids, the drug solutions should be discarded. When reconstituted or diluted according to the instructions below, Ancef (sterile cefazolin sodium, SK&F) is stable for 24 hours at room temperature or for 96 hours if stored under refrigeration. Reconstituted solutions may range in color from pale yellow to yellow without a change in potency.
Single-Dose Vials
For I.M. injection, I.V. direct (bolus) injection, or I.V. infusion, reconstitute with Sterile Water for Injection according to the following table. SHAKE WELL.

Vial Size	Amount of Diluent	Approximate Concentration	Approximate Available Volume
250 mg.	2.0 ml.	125 mg./ml.	2.0 ml.
500 mg.	2.0 ml.	225 mg./ml.	2.2 ml.
1 gram	2.5 ml.	330 mg./ml.	3.0 ml.

Figure 8-9. *Dosage and administration directions for cefazolin sodium (Ancef). (Courtesy of Smith Kline & French Laboratories.)*

Directions: For intramuscular use reconstitute with sterile water for injection or bacteriostatic water for injection. Reconstituted solution stable for 24 hours at room temperature, 5 days if refrigerated.

Label Claim	Amount Diluent	Withdrawal Volume	Concentration (mg/ml)
125 mg	0.7 ml	1 ml	125 mg
250 mg	0.9 ml	1 ml	250 mg
500 mg	1.5 ml	2 ml	250 mg
1 g	3.2 ml	4 ml	250 mg
2 g	6.5 ml	8 ml	250 mg

Figure 8-10. *Reconstitution directions for ampicillin N in a hypothetical table.*

PRACTICE EXERCISE 3 (*Continued*)

2. Order: ampicillin N 200 mg IM q4h (Fig. 8-10)
    Stock: vials of powder of 125 mg, 250 mg, 500 mg, 1 Gm and 2 Gm

    a. Stock chosen:

    b. Diluting fluid and number of milliliters:

    c. Solution and new stock:

    d. Rule and arithmetic:

    e. Answer:

    f. Write on label:

    g. Storage:

3. Order: cefazolin sodium 0.5 g IM q8h (see Fig. 8-9)
    Stock: vial of powder labeled 1 Gm

    a. Diluting fluid and number of milliliters:

    b. Solution made and new stock:

    c. Rule and arithmetic:

    d. Answer:

    e. Write on label:

    f. Storage:

SELF-TEST 1

Solve these problems. Check your answers at the end of the chapter.

1. Order: cefoxitin sodium 200 mg IM q4h (Fig. 8-11)
    Stock: vial of powder labeled 1 g

    a. Diluting fluid and number of milliliters:

    b. Solution made and new stock:

    c. Rule and arithmetic:

    d. Answer:

    e. Write on label:

    f. Storage:

Table 3 — Preparation of Solution			
Strength	Amount of Diluent to be Added (mL) + +	Approximate Withdrawable Volume (mL)	Approximate Average Concentration (mg/mL)
1 gram Vial	2 (Intramuscular)	2.5	400
2 gram Vial	4 (Intramuscular)	5	400
1 gram Vial	10 (IV)	10.5	95
2 gram Vial	10 or 20 (IV)	11.1 or 21.0	180 or 95
1 gram Infusion Bottle	50 or 100 (IV)	50 or 100	20 or 10
2 gram Infusion Bottle	50 or 100 (IV)	50 or 100	40 or 20
10 gram Bulk	43 or 93 (IV)	49 or 98.5	200 or 100
+ + Shake to dissolve and let stand until clear.			

Intramuscular
MEFOXIN, as constituted with Sterile Water for Injection, Bacteriostatic Water for Injection, or 0.5 percent or 1 percent lidocaine hydrochloride solution (without epinephrine), maintains satisfactory potency for 24 hours at room temperature, for one week under refrigeration (below 5°C), and for at least 30 weeks in the frozen state.

Figure 8-11. *Directions to reconstitute cefoxitin sodium (Mefoxin). (Courtesy of Merck Sharp & Dohme.)*

2. Order: oxacillin sodium 750 mg IM q4h (Fig. 8-12)
   Stock: oxacillin sodium in dry form. Vials of 250 mg, 500 mg, 1 g, 2 g, and 4 g

   a. Stock chosen:

   b. Diluting fluid and number of milliliters:

   c. Solution made and new stock:

   d. Rule and arithmetic:

   e. Answer:

   f. Write on label:

   g. Storage:

3. Order: Claforan 800 mg IM q12h (Fig. 8-13)
   Stock: vials of powder 1 g, and 2 g

   a. Stock chosen:

   b. Diluting fluid and number of milliliters:

   c. Solution made and new stock:

   d. Rule and arithmetic:

   e. Answer:

   f. Write on label:

   g. Storage:

4. Order: invincimycin 0.5 g IM q6h (a hypothetical drug) (Fig. 8-14)
   Stock: 1-g vial available as a powder

(continued)

For intramuscular injection: To obtain a solution containing 250 mg of drug in 1.5 ml of solution, add sterile water for injection as follows:

Vial	Diluent
250 mg	1.1 ml
500 mg	2.1 ml
1 g	5.1 ml
2 g	11.1 ml
4 g	23.0 ml

Stable in the refrigerator for 5 days.

Figure 8-12. *Hypothetical directions for reconstitution of oxacillin sodium.*

PREPARATION OF CLAFORAN STERILE

Claforan for IM or IV administration should be reconstituted as follows:

Strength	Diluent (mL)	Withdrawable Volume (mL)	Approximate Concentration (mg/mL)
1g vial (IM)*	3	3.4	300
2g vial (IM)*	5	6.0	330
1g vial (IV)*	10	10.4	95
2g vial (IV)*	10	11.0	180
1g infusion	50-100	50-100	20-10
2g infusion	50-100	50-100	40-20
10g bottle	47	52.0	200
10g bottle	97	102.0	100

(*) in conventional vials

Shake to dissolve; inspect for particulate matter and discoloration prior to use. Solutions of Claforan range from very pale yellow to light amber, depending on concentration, diluent used, and length and condition of storage.

For Intramuscular use: Reconstitute VIALS with Sterile Water for Injection or Bacteriostatic Water for Injection as described above.

COMPATIBILITY AND STABILITY

Solutions of Claforan Sterile reconstituted as described above (**Preparation of Claforan Sterile**) maintain satisfactory potency for 24 hours at room temperature (at or below 22°C), 10 days under refrigeration (at or below 5°C), and for at least 13 weeks frozen.

Figure 8-13. *Preparation of solution of cefotaxime sodium (Claforan). (Courtesy of Hoechst–Roussel Pharmaceuticals.)*

Intramuscular use: Add Sterile Water for Injection, USP in the amounts indicated below. The entire contents should be withdrawn.

Potency	Recommended Amount of Sterile Water for Injection, USP	Available Volume	Concentration (mg/ml)
500 mg	1.8 ml	2.0 ml	250 mg
1 g	3.5 ml	4.0 ml	250 mg
	or 7.5 ml	8.0 ml	125 mg
2 g	6.8 ml	8.0 ml	250 mg

Figure 8-14. *Directions for reconstitution of hypothetical drug invincimycin.*

SELF-TEST 1 (Continued)

a. Stock used:

b. Diluting fluid and number of milliliters:

c. Solution made and new stock:

d. Rule and arithmetic:

e. Answer:

f. Write on label:

g. Storage:

SELF-TEST 2

Solve these problems. Write the steps. Answers can be found at the end of the chapter.

Directions: To obtain a concentration of 500 mg/ml:

Add 1.8 ml diluent to the 1 g vial
Add 5.8 ml diluent to the 4 g vial
Add 8.8 ml diluent to the 6 g vial
Diluting solutions: sterile water for injection;
0.9% sodium chloride
Solutions are stable for 24 hours at room temperature and 5 days if refrigerated.

Figure 8-15. *Directions to reconstitute gracilimycin, a hypothetical drug.*

1. Order: penicillin G potassium 300,000 U IM q3h (see Fig. 8-5)
   Stock: vial of powder labeled 1,000,000 units

2. Order: gracilimycin 1 g IM q6h (a hypothetical drug) (Fig. 8-15)
   Stock: vials of 1 g, 4 g, and 6 g powder

3. Order: Amytal sodium 250 mg IM stat
   Stock: ampule of crystals labeled 0.5 g
   Directions: To derive a 20% solution, add 2.5 ml of sterile water for injection

4. Order: Velosef 350 mg IM q8h (Fig. 8-16)
   Stock: vial of powder labeled 1 g for injection

===== MENTAL DRILL IN INJECTION FROM POWDER PROBLEMS =====

*As you develop proficiency in solving these problems, you will be able to calculate many answers without written work. Here are two drills to sharpen your skill. The first drill **should be easy** because the*

(continued)

VELOSEF FOR INJECTION
(Cephradine for Injection USP)

IM DILUTION TABLE

Vial Size	Volume of Diluent	Approximate Available Volume	Approximate Available Concentration
250 mg	1.2 mL	1.2 mL	208 mg/mL
500 mg	2.0 mL	2.2 mL	227 mg/mL
1 g	4.0 mL	4.5 mL	222 mg/mL

For I.M. Use.—Aseptically add Sterile Water for Injection or Bacteriostatic Water for Injection (containing 0.9% [w/v] benzyl alcohol, or 0.12% methylparaben and 0.014% propylparaben) according to the following table [i.e., the table entitled "IM Dilution Table" below].

Intramuscular solutions should be used within two hours at room temperature; if stored in the refrigerator at 5° C., solutions retain full potency for 24 hours. Constituted solutions may vary in color from light straw to yellow; however, this does not affect the potency.

Figure 8-16. *Directions to reconstitute cephradine (Velosef) for IM injection. (Package insert used by permission of E. R. Squibb & Sons, Inc., copyright owner.)*

‾MENTAL DRILL IN INJECTION FROM POWDER PROBLEMS (*Continued*)‾

specific directions needed are given to you. In the second exercise you must choose the direction you need. Aim for 100%! Here is the way the answers will appear at the end of the chapter. We will not indicate storage directions.

      a.   Diluting fluid and number of milliliters:
      b.   Solution made and new stock:
      c.   Answer:
      d.   Label:

Set A

1.   Order: penicillin G 300,000 units IM
     Stock: powder labeled 1 million units
     Directions: dissolve with 4.6 ml sterile water for injection to make 200,000 units/ml.

2.   Order: acetazolamide sodium 200 mg IM
     Stock: vial of powder labeled 500 mg
     Directions: dissolve powder with 5 cc sterile water for injection. Each cc = 100 mg.

3.   Order: hydrocortisone sodium succinate 100 mg IM
     Stock: vial of powder labeled 100 mg and an ampule of 2 ml diluent
     Directions: add diluent to powder. Each 2 ml = 100 mg.

4.   Order: penicillin G 400,000 units IM
     Stock: vial of powder labeled 1 million units
     Directions: dissolve powder with 4.6 ml sterile water for injection to make 200,000 U/ml.

5.   Order: acetazolamide 150 mg IM
     Stock: vial of powder labeled 500 mg
     Directions: reconstitute powder with 5 ml sterile water for injection. Solution will be 100 mg/ml.

6.   Order: Amytal sodium 200 mg IM
     Stock: ampule of crystals labeled 250 mg
     Directions: add 5 ml sterile water for injection to make a solution of 50 mg/ml, or add 2.5 ml sterile water for injection to make a solution of 100 mg/ml.

7.   Order: colycillin 250 mg IM (a hypothetical drug)
     Stock: vial of powder labeled 1 g.
     Directions: add 1.5 ml sterile water for injection to prepare a solution of 500 mg/cc.

8.   Order: phenytoin sodium 100 mg IM
     Stock: vial of powder labeled 250 mg
     Directions: add 3.5 ml sterile water for injection. Solution will be 75 mg/ml.

9. Order: ampicillin 400 mg IM
   Stock: vial of powder labeled 500 mg
   Directions: add 1.8 ml sterile water for injection to make a solution of 250 mg/ml.

10. Order: cefazolin sodium 150 mg IM
    Stock: vial of powder labeled 250 mg
    Directions: Add 2 ml sterile water for injection to make a solution of 125 mg/ml.

Set B

Choose the directions you need to give the ordered dose. Aim for 100%.

1. Order: ceftizoxime sodium 90 mg IM q12h
   Stock: vial of powder labeled Cefizox 1 gram. (Fig. 8-17)

2. Order: carbenicillin disodium 0.5 Gm q8h
   Stock: vial of powder labeled Geopen 2 grams (see Fig. 8-6)

3. Order: penicillin G potassium 40,000 units q4h IM
   Stock: vial of powder labeled Pfizerpen 1,000,000 U (Fig. 8-18)

4. Order: cefazolin sodium 0.45 g IM q12h
   Stock: vial of powder labeled Kefzol 500 mg (Fig. 8-19)

5. Order: ticarcillin disodium 0.5 g IM
   Stock: vial of powder labeled Ticar 1 gram (Fig. 8-20)

6. Order: cefotaxime sodium 1 g IM 1 hr before surgery
   Stock: vial of powder labeled Claforan 1 gram (see Fig. 8-13)

7. Order: cephradine 500 mg IM q6h
   Stock: vial of powder labeled 500 mg (see Fig. 8-16)

(continued)

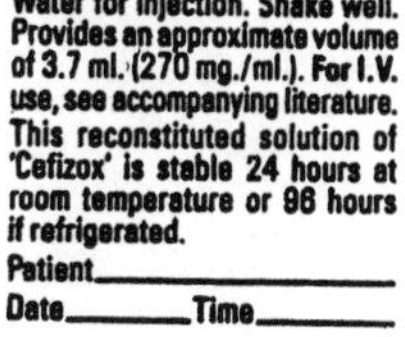

For I.M. or I.V. use

Usual Adult Dose: See accompanying literature.
For I.M. use, add 3.0 ml. Sterile Water for Injection. Shake well. Provides an approximate volume of 3.7 ml. (270 mg./ml.). For I.V. use, see accompanying literature. This reconstituted solution of 'Cefizox' is stable 24 hours at room temperature or 96 hours if refrigerated.

Patient_____
Date_____Time_____

Figure 8-17. *Directions for reconstitution of ceftizoxime sodium (Cefizox). (Courtesy of Smith Kline & French Laboratories.)*

Pfizerpen

Approx. Desired Concentration (units/ml)	Approx. Volume (ml) 1,000,000 units	Solvent for Vial of 5,000,000 units	Infusion Only 20,000,000 units
50,000	20.0	. . .	. . .
100,000	10.0	. . .	. . .
250,000	4.0	18.2	75.0
500,000	1.8	8.2	33.0
750,000	. . .	4.8	. . .
1,000,000	. . .	3.2	11.5

(1) Intramuscular Injection: Keep total volume of injection small. The intramuscular route is the preferred route of administration. Solutions containing up to 100,000 units of penicillin per ml of diluent may be used with a minimum of discomfort. Greater concentration of penicillin G per ml is physically possible and may be employed where therapy demands. When large dosages are required, it may be advisable to administer solutions of penicillin by means of continuous intravenous drip.

Buffered Pfizerpen (penicillin G potassium) for Injection is highly water soluble. It may be dissolved in small amounts of Water for Injection, or Sterile Isotonic Sodium Chloride Solution for Parenteral Use. All solutions should be stored in a refrigerator. When refrigerated, penicillin solutions may be stored for seven days without significant loss of potency. Buffered Pfizerpen (penicillin G potassium) for Injection may be given intramuscularly or by continuous intravenous drip for dosages of 500,000, 1,000,000, or 5,000,000 units.

Figure 8-18. *Preparation of solution of penicillin G potassium (Pfizerpen). (Courtesy of Roerig–Pfizer Laboratories.)*

Vial Size	Diluent to Be Added	Approximate Available Volume	Approximate Average Concentration
250 mg	2 ml	2 ml	125 mg/ml
500 mg	2 ml	2.2 ml	225 mg/ml
1 g*	2.5 ml	3 ml	330 mg/ml

* The 1-g vial should be reconstituted only with Sterile Water for Injection or Bacteriostatic Water for Injection.

STABILITY
Reconstituted Kefzol (cefazolin sodium, Lilly) and dilutions of Kefzol in the recommended intravenous fluids are stable for 24 hours at room temperature and for 96 hours stored under refrigeration (5°C).

Figure 8-19. *Dilution table for cefazolin sodium (Kefzol). (Courtesy of Eli Lilly & Company.)*

DIRECTIONS FOR USE
—1 Gm, 3 Gm and 6 Gm Standard Vials—
INTRAMUSCULAR USE: (Concentration of approximately 385 mg/ml).
For initial reconstitution use Sterile Water for Injection, USP, Sodium Chloride Injection, USP or 1% Lidocaine Hydrochloride solution* (without epinephrine).
Each gram of Ticarcillin should be reconstituted with 2 ml of Sterile Water for Injection, U.S.P., Sodium Chloride Injection, U.S.P. or 1% Lidocaine Hydrochloride solution* (without epinephrine) and **used promptly.** Each 2.6 ml of the resulting solution will then contain 1 Gm of Ticarcillin.
* [For full product information, refer to manufacturer's package insert for Lidocaine Hydrochloride.]
As with all intramuscular preparations, TICAR (Ticarcillin Disodium) should be injected well within the body of a relatively large muscle, using usual techniques and precautions.

Figure 8-20. *Directions for use of ticarcillin disodium (Ticar). (Courtesy of Beecham Laboratories.)*

⁻MENTAL DRILL IN INJECTION FROM POWDER PROBLEMS (*Continued*)⁻

8. Order: cefoxitin sodium 0.5 gm IM q12h
   Stock: vial of powder labeled Mefoxin 1 gram (see Fig. 8-11)

9. Order: cefazolin sodium 150 mg IM q8h
   Stock: vial of powder labeled 250 mg (see Fig. 8-9)

10. Order: penicillin G potassium 250,000 U IM q8h
    Stock: vial of powder labeled 5 million units (see Fig. 8-5)

===== **ANSWERS** =====

PRACTICE EXERCISE 1

1. A broad-spectrum cephalosporin antibiotic
2. IVPB, IV, and IM
3. In the bile
4. Gram-positive aerobes, gram-negative aerobes, anaerobic organisms
5. It is bactericidal. It inhibits bacterial cell wall synthesis.
6. Respiratory infections; peritonitis and other intra-abdominal infections; infections of the skin and skin structures; pelvic inflammatory disease. (Others are bacterial septicemia, endometritis, and infections of the female genital tract.)
7. Patients with known allergy to cephalosporin antibiotics
8. a. Ask the patient if he has any known reaction to cephalosporins, penicillins, or other drugs.
   b. Patients with some form of allergy, particularly to drugs, may experience a severe reaction requiring emergency treatment. Check with the patient.
   c. Patients who develop diarrhea during therapy should be monitored for pseudomembranous colitis, which has been reported with this drug.
9. a. Used only if clearly indicated. There are no adequate or well-controlled studies to indicate that the drug is safe.
   b. Exercise caution in giving this drug. Low concentrations are excreted in milk.
   c. Safety and effectiveness in children have not been established.
10. 2–4g/day, administered in equally divided doses every 12 hours
11. a. Hypersensitivity—drug-related fever, skin reaction
    b. Hematology (blood)—neutropenia (decrease in white cells)
    c. Hepatic—elevation of liver enzymes
    d. Gastrointestinal—diarrhea
    e. Renal function—elevation of blood urea nitrogen (BUN)
    f. Local reactions—phlebitis; pain at the site of injection

PRACTICE EXERCISE 2

1. There are two ways to prepare carbenicillin. We could make a solution of

   1 g = 2.5 ml

   or

   1 g = 3.0 ml

   Either one is correct. Both are shown. The last dilution 1 g = 4.0 ml is too much. It would require two syringes.

   a. 4 ml sterile water   a. 5 ml sterile water
   b. 1 g = 2.5 ml   b. 1 g = 3 ml
   c. Not necessary   c. Not necessary
   d. Give 2.5 ml   d. Give 3 ml
   e. 1 g = 2.5 ml, date, initials   e. 1 g = 3 ml, date, initials
   f. Refrigerate remaining solution   f. Refrigerate remaining solution

2. You want 1 g. The stock is 1 g. When you dilute the powder, you will give the whole amount of fluid, *whatever the amount is.* The manufacturer states it will be 3.6 ml/1 g. If you solve the arithmetic you have:

$$\frac{D}{H} \times S = A$$

$$\frac{1000 \text{ mg}}{280 \text{ mg}} \times 1 \text{ ml} = \frac{100}{28}$$

$$
\begin{array}{r}
3.57 \\
28\overline{)100.00} = 3.6 \text{ ml} \\
\underline{84} \\
160 \\
\underline{140} \\
200 \\
\underline{196}
\end{array}
$$

    a.   3 ml sterile water for injection
    b.   1 g in 3.6 ml, 280 mg/ml
    c.   Not necessary
    d.   Give 3.6 ml in two syringes
    e.   Nothing! Discard the vial; it is empty.
    f.   Discard the vial in appropriate receptacle.

3. a.   1.8 ml sterile water for injection
    b.   250 mg/ml

    c. $\dfrac{D}{H} \times S = A$

$$\frac{250 \text{ mg}}{250 \text{ mg}} \times 1 \text{ ml} = 1 \text{ ml}$$

    d.   Give 1 ml IM
    e.   Nothing! Read the last line: "The above solutions must be used within 1 hour after reconstitution."
        You must discard the remaining fluid!
    f.   None

PRACTICE EXERCISE 3

1. a.   Choose 500 mg powder (Can you see why?)
    b.   Add 2 ml sterile water for injection
    c.   225 mg/ml
    d.   Not necessary: you want 225 mg; you made 225 mg/ml
    e.   Give 1 ml IM
    f.   225 mg/ml, date, initials
    g.   Refrigerator (you have another dose ready)

2. a.   Choose 250 mg. It is closest to the amount you need
    b.   Add 0.9 ml sterile water for injection
    c.   250 mg/ml

    d. $\dfrac{D}{H} \times S = A$ $\dfrac{\overset{4}{200 \text{ mg}}}{\underset{5}{250 \text{ mg}}} \times 1 \text{ ml} = \dfrac{4}{5}\overset{0.8}{\overline{)4.0}}$

    e.   Give 0.8 ml IM
    f.   250 mg/ml, date, initials
    g.   Refrigerator. If this vial were labeled *Single Dose* you would have to discard the remainder of
        the drug.

3. a.   2.5 ml sterile water for injection
    b.   330 mg/ml
    c.   0.5 g = 500 mg

$$\frac{D}{H} \times S = A \qquad \frac{500 \text{ mg}}{33\cancel{0} \cancel{\text{mg}}} \times 1 \text{ ml} = \frac{50}{33} \begin{array}{r} 1.51 \\ \overline{)50.00} \\ \underline{33} \\ 170 \\ \underline{165} \\ 50 \\ \underline{33} \\ 17 \end{array}$$

    d. Give 1.5 ml IM
    e. 330 mg/ml, date, initials
    f. Refrigerator

SELF-TEST 1

1. a. Add 2 ml of sterile water for injection
    b. 400 mg/ml

    c. $\dfrac{D}{H} \times S = A \qquad \dfrac{\overset{1}{\cancel{200}} \cancel{\text{mg}}}{\underset{4}{\cancel{400}} \cancel{\text{mg}}} \times 1 \text{ ml} = \dfrac{1}{2} \text{ ml or 0.5 ml}$

    d. Give $\dfrac{1}{2}$ ml (0.5 ml)

    e. 400 mg/ml, date, initials
    f. Refrigerator

2. a. Choose 1 g. It is closest to the amount needed.
    b. Add 5.1 ml sterile water for injection
    c. 250 mg/1.5 ml

    d. $\dfrac{D}{H} \times S = A \qquad \dfrac{\overset{3}{\cancel{750}} \cancel{\text{mg}}}{\underset{1}{\cancel{250}} \cancel{\text{mg}}} \times 1.5 \text{ ml} = 4.5 \text{ ml}$

    e. Give 4.5 ml IM in two separate syringes at two different injection sites.
    f. 250 mg/1.5 ml, date, initials
    g. Refrigerator

3. a. Choose 1 g. It is closest to the order.
    b. Add 3 ml of sterile water for injection
    c. 300 mg/ml
    d. $\dfrac{D}{H} \times S = A \qquad \dfrac{800 \cancel{\text{mg}}}{300 \cancel{\text{mg}}} \times 1 \text{ ml} = \dfrac{8}{3} \begin{array}{r} 2.66 \\ \overline{)8.00} \end{array}$

    e. Give 2.7 ml IM
    f. 300 mg/ml, date, initials
    g. Refrigerator

4. a. 1 g powder (you want the 500 mg, but do not have it)
    b. You must choose 3.5 ml to make 250 mg/ml. (If you choose 7.4 ml you would have 4 ml as an answer.)
    c. 250 mg/ml

d. $\dfrac{D}{H} \times S = A \qquad \dfrac{\overset{2}{\cancel{500}\ \cancel{mg}}}{\underset{1}{\cancel{250}\ \cancel{mg}}} \times 1\ ml = 2\ ml$

e. Give 2 ml IM
f. Nothing! Directions say entire contents should be withdrawn, so you cannot save the remaining solution. Discard the vial.
g. No—discard in a suitable receptacle.

SELF-TEST 2

1. Actually all three ways to dilute the powder are possible! (A) If you made 100,000 U/ml—give 3 ml. (B) If you made 200,000 U/ml—give 1.5 ml. (C) If you made 250,000 U/ml—give 1.2 ml. The steps for all three ways are shown.

	A	B	C
Diluting fluid and no. ml	9.6 ml sterile water	4.6 ml sterile water	3.6 ml sterile water
Solution made	100,000 U/ml	200,000 U/ml	250,000 U/ml
Rule (and arithmetic)			
$\dfrac{D}{H} \times S = A$	$\dfrac{300{,}000\ U}{100{,}000\ U} \times 1\ ml = 3\ ml$	$\dfrac{300{,}000\ U}{200{,}000\ U} \times 1\ ml =$	$\dfrac{\overset{6}{\cancel{300{,}000\ U}}}{\underset{5}{\cancel{250{,}000\ U}}} \times 1\ ml =$
		$\begin{array}{r} 3\ \ 1.5 \\ 2\overline{)3.0} \end{array}$	$\begin{array}{r} 6\ \ 1.2 \\ 5\overline{)6.0} \end{array}$
Answer	Give 3 ml IM	Give 1.5 ml IM	Give 1.2 ml IM
Write on label	100,000 U/ml, date, initials	200,000 U/ml, date, initials	250,000 U/ml, date, initials
Storage	Refrigeration	Refrigeration	Refrigeration

2.
a. Stock chosen: Choose vial of 1 g
b. Diluting fluid and number of milliliters: Add 1.8 ml sterile water for injection
c. Solution made and new stock: 500 mg/ml
d. Rule and arithmetic:

$$\dfrac{D}{H} \times S = A \qquad \dfrac{\overset{2}{\cancel{1000}\ \cancel{mg}}}{\underset{1}{\cancel{500}\ \cancel{mg}}} \times 1\ ml = 2\ ml$$

e. Answer: Give 2 ml IM (you could say: give the entire amount.)
f. Write on label: Nothing! Needed 1 g; used 1 g.
g. Storage: Discard in proper receptacle.

3.
a. Diluting fluid and number of milliliters: Add 2.5 ml sterile water for injection
b. Solution made and new stock: 20% solution means

$$20\ g = 100\ ml \text{ or reducing that } \dfrac{\overset{1}{\cancel{20}}\ g}{\underset{5}{\cancel{100}}\ ml} = \dfrac{1\ g}{5\ ml}$$

New stock: 1 g = 5 ml; 1 g = 1000 mg; therefore, 1000 mg = 5 ml

c. Rule and arithmetic:

$$\frac{D}{H} \times S = A \qquad \frac{\overset{1}{\cancel{250}} \text{ mg}}{\underset{4}{\cancel{1000}} \text{ mg}} \times 5 \text{ ml} = \frac{5}{4}\overline{)5.0}^{\,1.25}$$

   d.   Answer: Give 1.3 ml IM

   e.   Write on label: Nothing. An ampule must be discarded.

   f.   Storage: No. Discard in a suitable receptacle.

4.   a.   Diluting fluid and number of milliliters: Add 4 ml sterile water for injection

   b.   Solution made and new stock: 222 mg/ml

   c.   Rule and arithmetic:

$$\frac{D}{H} \times S = A \qquad \frac{350 \text{ mg}}{222 \text{ mg}} \times 1 \text{ ml} = \frac{350}{222} \overline{)350.00}^{\,1.57}$$

$$\begin{array}{r} \underline{222} \\ 128\ 0 \\ \underline{111\ 0} \\ 17\ 00 \\ \underline{15\ 54} \\ 1\ 46 \end{array}$$

   d.   Give: 1.6 ml IM

   e.   Write on label: 222 mg/ml date, initials

   f.   Storage: Refrigeration

MENTAL DRILL IN INJECTION FROM POWDER PROBLEMS

Set A

1.   a.   4.6 ml sterile water for injection

   b.   200,000 units/ml

   c.   Give 1.5 ml IM

   d.   200,000 U/ml, date, initials

2.   a.   5 cc sterile water for injection

   b.   100 mg/cc

   c.   Give 2 cc IM

   d.   100 mg/cc, date, initials

3.   a.   2 ml diluent with the vial

   b.   100 mg = 2 ml

   c.   Give entire amount (give 2 ml) IM

   d.   None. Discard empty vial.

4.   a.   4.6 cc sterile water for injection

   b.   200,000 U/ml

   c.   give 2 ml IM

   d.   200,000 U/ml, date, initials

5.   a.   5 ml sterile water for injection

   b.   100 mg/ml

   c. $1\frac{1}{2}$ ml or 1.5 ml IM

   d.   100 mg/ml, date, initials

6.   a.   2.5 ml sterile water for injection. *Note:* Should not be diluted with 5 ml. The answer would be to give 4 ml—this is too much fluid.

   b.   100 mg/ml

   c.   Give 2 ml IM

   d.   None; stock was an ampule. Discard in a suitable receptacle.

7.   a.   1.5 ml sterile water for injection

    b. 500 mg/cc

    c. Give $\frac{1}{2}$ cc or 0.5 cc IM

    d. 500 mg/cc, date, initials

8. a. 3.5 ml sterile water for injection
    b. 75 mg/ml
    c. Give 1.3 ml IM
    d. 75 mg/ml, date, initials

9. a. 1.8 ml of sterile water for injection
    b. 250 mg/ml
    c. Give 1.6 ml IM
    d. 250 mg/ml, date, initials

10. a. 2 ml sterile water for injection
    b. 125 mg/ml
    c. Give 1.2 ml
    d. 125 mg/ml, date, initials

Set B

1. a. 3.0 ml sterile water for injection
    b. 270 mg/ml
    c. Give 0.3 ml IM (3-ml syringe) or 0.33 ml (1-ml precision syringe)
    d. 270 mg/ml, date, initials

2. Two ways are possible: use either one

A	B
a. 4 ml sterile water for injection	5 ml sterile water for injection
b. 1 g/2.5 ml	1 g/3 ml
c. Give 1.3 ml	Give 1.5 ml
d. 1 g/2.5 ml, date, initials	1 g/3 ml, date, initials

3. Two ways are possible: the nurse must assess the patient to determine which is better.

A	B
a. 20 ml sterile water for injection	10 ml sterile water for injection
b. 50,000 U/ml	100,000 U/ml
c. Give 0.8 ml IM	Give 0.4 ml IM
d. 50,000 U/ml, date, initials	100,000 U/ml, date, initials

4. a. 2 ml sterile water for injection
    b. 225 mg/ml
    c. 2 ml IM
    d. 225 mg/ml, date, initials

5. a. 2 ml sterile water for injection
    b. 1 g/2.6 ml
    c. 1.3 ml IM
    d. 1 g/2.6 ml, date, initials

6. a. 3 ml sterile water for injection
    b. 300 mg/ml

   c. Entire amount. Manufacturer says 3.4 ml. Consider two injection sites. Split the dose into two injections of 1.7 ml each.

   d. Nothing! Entire amount has been used. Discard vial in an appropriate receptacle.

7. a. 2 ml sterile water for injection

   b. Table says 227 mg/ml. Really not necessary!

   c. Entire amount in vial; wanted 500 mg, vial has 500 mg.

   d. Nothing. Used entire amount. Discard vial in appropriate receptacle.

8. a. 2 ml sterile water for injection

   b. 400 mg/ml

   c. 1.3 ml IM

   d. 400 mg/ml, date, initials

9. a. 2 ml sterile water for injection

   b. 125 mg/ml

   c. 1.2 ml IM

   d. 125 mg/ml, date, initials

10. Three ways are possible:

A	B	C
a. 23 ml	18 ml	8 ml
b. 200,000 U/ml	250,000 U/ml	500,000 U/ml
c. 1.3 ml IM	1 ml IM	0.5 ml IM
d. 200,000 U/ml, date, initials	250,000 U/ml, date, initials	500,000 U/ml, date, initials

Intravenous Drip Rates and Intermittent Infusions

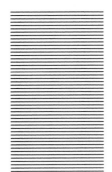

OVERVIEW

Some medications are given intravenously (IV), with the use of sterile technique, to achieve an immediate effect and a high blood level. These drugs, in a powder or liquid form, are diluted and then administered continuously through the primary IV tubing, or through a secondary line attached to the primary IV (Fig. 9-1).

Terms used interchangeably to indicate these lines include

Main IV	Secondary IV
Continuous IV	Intermittent IV
Primary line	Secondary line
Primary IV	Intravenous piggyback (IVPB)

EXAMPLE:

An order for a continuous IV might read
1000 ml D5W IV 8 AM–8 PM

EXAMPLE:

An order for a secondary IV might read
ampicillin 1 g IVPB q6h in 50 ml D5W over 30 minutes

To learn how to prepare these medications and set the drip rate, nurses must first learn about types of IV fluids, IV drip factors, how orders can be written for IVs and IVPBs, and how the nurse calculates the drip rate.

Take the time to study this chapter carefully. Be certain you understand one concept before you move on to the next. Read the terms carefully—ml/hr; μg/min; units/hr; gtt/min can be confusing. After studying this material the following orders for IVs will make sense:

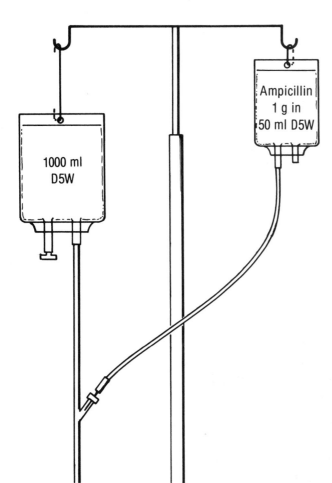

Figure 9-1. *Drawing of a main IV line and an IVPB line. Fluid flows continuously through the main IV line (left) and needle into a patient's vein. At timed intervals medication (right) placed in an intravenous piggyback bag (IVPB) is attached by needle and tubing to the main IV for delivery to the patient.*

EXAMPLE:

Infuse heparin 1200 units/hr via pump

500 ml D5W IVKVO over 24 hr

1 L D5 $\frac{1}{2}$NS with 40 mEq KCl 8 AM–8 PM

Run dopamine drip at 25 μg/min and titrate to maintain diastolic BP > 60.

TYPES OF INTRAVENOUS FLUIDS

A partial listing of IV fluids available at one hospital is shown in Figure 9-2. These fluids are packaged in sterile plastic bags or glass bottles and distributed to the patient care units. The nurse selects the IV fluid needed and prepares the solution. An error in choosing fluid may result in serious fluid and electrolyte imbalance.

Note that one solution is listed as 1000 cc D5%W. This is read as "a thousand cubic centimeters of dextrose five percent in water." Remember 5% means 5 g in 100 ml. Because 1000 ml is ten times 100 ml, this solution contains 50 g of dextrose. The order may be written as 1000 ml D5W.

Another solution is listed as 1000 cc D 5% .9NS. This is read as "1000 cubic centimeters dextrose five percent in nine-tenths normal saline." The order may be written as 1000 ml D5NS

DESCRIPTION	DESCRIPTION
SOLUTIONS	**DINEAL DEXTROSE**
DEXTROSE IN DW	2000 cc D 1.5%
1000 cc D 2½% W GLASS	2000 cc D 4.25%
50 cc D 5% W (PACK OF 4)	**ISOTONIC SODIUM CHLORIDE**
100 cc D 5% W (PACK OF 4)	50 cc 0.9% (PACK OF 4)
250 cc D 5% W	100 cc 0.9% (PACK OF 4)
500 cc D 5% W	250 cc 0.9%
1000 cc D 5% W	500 cc 0.9%
250 cc D 5% W GLASS	1000 cc (IV) 0.9%
500 cc D 10% W	1000 cc 0.9% IRRIGATION
500 cc D 20% W	3000 cc 0.9% CBI
DEXTROSE IN NS	**GENTRAN**
500 cc D 5% W .9 NS	500 cc 6% (70) IN 0.9% NS
1000 cc D 5% W .9 NS	500 cc 10% (40) IN 0.9% NS
500 cc D 5 W .2 SALINE	**LACTATED RINGERS**
250 cc D 5 W .33 SALINE	1000 cc
500 cc D 5 W .33 SALINE	1000 cc WITH 5% DEX
1000 cc D 5 W .33 SALINE	**OSMITROL IN DW**
1000 cc D 10% W .9 NS	500 cc 10%
DEXTROSE IN ½ SALINE	500 cc 20%
500 cc D 2½% W .45 SALINE	**RINGERS (PLAIN)**
1000 cc D 2½% W .45 SALINE	1000 cc
500 cc D 5% W .45 SALINE	
1000 cc D 5% W .45 SALINE	

QUANTITY REQUESTED	UNIT MEASURE	DESCRIPTION	CSS CODE	# ISSUED	QUANTITY REQUESTED	UNIT MEASURE	DESCRIPTION	CSS CODE	# ISSUED
		SOLUTIONS					**DINEAL DEXTROSE**		
		DEXTROSE IN DW				EACH	2000 cc D 1.5%	5B5407	
	EACH	1000 cc D 2½% W GLASS	2A0014			EACH	2000 cc D 4.25%	5B5417	
	EACH	50 cc D 5% W (PACK OF 4)	2B0081P				**ISOTONIC SODIUM CHLORIDE**		
	EACH	100 cc D 5% W (PACK OF 4)	2B0082P			EACH	50 cc 0.9% (PACK OF 4)	2B1301P	
	EACH	250 cc D 5% W	2B0062P			EACH	100 cc 0.9% (PACK OF 4)	2B1302P	
	EACH	500 cc D 5% W	2B0063P			EACH	250 cc 0.9%	2B1322P	
	EACH	1000 cc D 5% W	2B0064			EACH	500 cc 0.9%	2B1323P	
	EACH	250 cc D 5% W GLASS	2A0062			EACH	1000 cc (IV) 0.9%	2B1324	
	EACH	500 cc D 10% W	2B0163P			EACH	1000 cc 0.9% IRRIGATION	2B7124	
	EACH	500 cc D 20% W	2A0213			EACH	3000 cc 0.9% CBI	2B7127	
		DEXTROSE IN NS					**GENTRAN**		
	EACH	500 cc D 5% W .9 NS	2B1063P			EACH	500 cc 6% (70) IN 0.9% NS	2B5013P	
	EACH	1000 cc D 5% W .9 NS	2B1064			EACH	500 cc 10% (40) IN 0.9% NS	2B5043	
	EACH	500 cc D 5 W .2 SALINE	2B1093P				**LACTATED RINGERS**		
	EACH	250 cc D 5 W .33 SALINE	2B1082			EACH	1000 cc	2B2324	
	EACH	500 cc D 5 W .33 SALINE	2B1083P			EACH	1000 cc WITH 5% DEX	2B2074	
	EACH	1000 cc D 5 W .33 SALINE	2B1084				**OSMITROL IN DW**		
	EACH	1000 cc D 10% W .9 NS	2B1164			EACH	500 cc 10%	2D5613P	
		DEXTROSE IN ½ SALINE				EACH	500 cc 20%	2D5433P	
	EACH	500 cc D 2½% W .45 SALINE	2B1023				**RINGERS (PLAIN)**		
	EACH	1000 cc D 2½% W .45 SALINE	2B1024			EACH	1000 cc	2B2304	
	EACH	500 cc D 5% W .45 SALINE	2B1073P						
	EACH	1000 cc D 5% W .45 SALINE	2B1074						

Figure 9-2. *Partial list of IV fluids available at one hospital. (Courtesy of Central Supply Department, St. Vincent Hospital and Medical Center, New York City.)*

or 1000 ml D5S. To make this solution, the manufacturer adds 50 g of dextrose and 154 mEq of sodium chloride to a volume of water that totals 1000 ml.

Normal saline is also known as isotonic sodium chloride or isotonic saline because it has the same osmotic pressure as blood. The prefix *iso* means equal. Normal saline contains 0.9% sodium chloride.

Look further down the list in Figure 9-2. Note 1000 cc D5%W .45 saline. This solution may be ordered as 1000 ml D5 $\frac{1}{2}$ NS because 0.45% is half of 0.9%. If the order read 500 ml D5 $\frac{1}{3}$ NS, the nurse would choose 500 ml D5.33 saline. The stock label may be printed in a different way than the written order. The nurse should *always seek assistance* when in doubt about which solution to use.

Look once more at the list and notice that four solutions have "pack of 4" printed after their name. These are the most common solutions used to dilute medications for IVPB.

50 ml D5W   50 ml D5NS

100 ml D5W   100 ml D5NS

KINDS OF INTRAVENOUS DRIP FACTORS

Intravenous fluids are administered through infusion sets that consist of plastic tubing attached at one end to the IV bag and at the other end to a needle or catheter inserted into a blood vessel, most commonly a vein. The top of the infusion set contains a chamber (Fig. 9-3).

Sets that contain a needle in the chamber are called *microdrip* because the drops are small. To deliver 1 ml of fluid to the patient, 60 drops (gtt) must fall (60 gtt = 1 ml). *All microdrip sets deliver 60 gtt/ml.*

Infusion sets that do not have a needle in the chamber are called *macrodrip.* These sets are not standard. Different manufacturers have a different number of drops per milliliter. Table 9-1 lists examples of macrodrip infusion sets. The package label will state the drops per milliliter (gtt/ml). You need to know this information to calculate the IV drip rates.

The tubing for these sets will include a clamp that the nurse can open or close to regulate the drip rate while using a second-hand on a watch or clock to count the drops per minute.

Use of the Infusion Pump

Many health care institutions use electrical infusion pumps to deliver IV fluid. These are excellent timesaving devices. Some are simple to operate, others are more elaborate. The most basic ones require the nurse to input two pieces of information: the total number of milliliters to be infused and the number of milliliters per hour.

The manufacturer will provide special tubing for the infusion pump or state the type of tubing to be used. The nurse does not need to calculate microdrip or macrodrip.

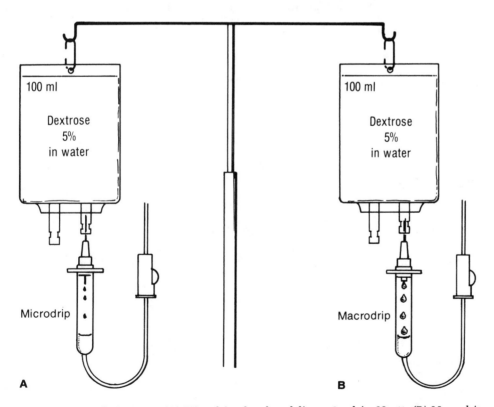

Figure 9-3. Infusion sets. (**A**) *Microdrip chamber delivers 1 ml in 60 gtt.* (**B**) *Macrodrip chamber delivers 1 ml in 10 drips.*

Table 9-1.   Examples of Different Macrodrip Factors

Manufacturer	Drops per Milliliter (gtt/ml)
Travenol	10
Abbott	15
McGaw	15
Cutter	20

EXAMPLE:

Order: 500 ml D5 $\frac{1}{2}$ NS IV; run 50 ml/hr

Available: an infusion pump

The nurse would input on the pump

Total number of milliliters: 500

Milliliters per hour: 50

The pump will deliver 50 ml/hr over 10 hours.

Labeling the Intravenous Fluid

Any IV fluid being administered must be labeled with the following information:

Patient name, room number, and bed location

Date

Physician's order as written

Time for infusion

Rate of flow of IV

Initials of the nurse who prepared the IV

EXAMPLE:

Patient name	John Saxty
Room	1402-1
Date	August 24
Order	500 ml D5 $\frac{1}{2}$ NS IV; run 50 ml/hr
Infusion time	10 AM–10 PM
Rate	50 ml/hr
Nurse	MPB

RULE FOR INTRAVENOUS DRIP RATE

Problems in IV calculations are solved in two steps. Step 1 is used to solve problems requiring an infusion pump and to simplify the arithmetic needed for microdrip and macrodrip. Step 2 will solve micro- and macrodrip problems.

Step 1. $\dfrac{\text{Total number of milliliters ordered}}{\text{number of hours to run}} = \text{number of ml/hr}$

Briefly, $\dfrac{\text{\# ml ordered}}{\text{\# hr to run}} = \text{ml/hr}$

Step 2. $\dfrac{\text{Number of milliliter per hour} \times \text{tubing drip factor}}{\text{number of minutes}} = \text{drops per minute}$

Briefly, $\dfrac{\text{ml/hr} \times \text{TF}}{\text{\# min}} = \text{gtt/min}$

The number of milliliters per hour is obtained in Step 1.

Tubing drip factor (TF) is either microdrip (60 gtt/ml) or macrodrip. Depending on the infusion set, this could be 10 gtt/ml, 15 gtt/ml, or 20 gtt/ml

Number of minutes (# min) is always 60 for this type of problem. The answer to Step 1 is milliliters per hour (ml/hr), but you want drops (gtt) per minute. Because there are 60 minutes in an hour, divide by 60.

Drops per minute (gtt/min) is the drip factor calculated to provide an even flow of a given amount over a specified time.

In the problems requiring calculation in this text, the drip factor will be given to you. In the clinical area, you must read the package label.

Application of the Rule

Three different IV orders and their solutions follow:

> **EXAMPLE:**
>
> Order: 1000 ml Ringer's lactate IV 8 AM–8 PM
>
> Available: An infusion pump
>
> Logic: 8 AM–8 PM is 12 hours for the IV to run. The infusion pump regulates the rate in milliliters per hour. Only Step 1 is necessary.
>
> $\dfrac{\text{\# ml}}{\text{\# hr}} = \text{ml/hr}$

LEARNING AID
Carry out arithmetic one decimal place and round off the answer to the nearest whole number.

$$\frac{1000 \text{ ml}}{12} = \frac{1000}{12} \quad 12\overline{)1000.0} \quad \begin{array}{r} 83.3 \\ \underline{96} \\ 40 \\ \underline{36} \\ 40 \\ \underline{36} \end{array}$$

Label the IV

Set the pump as follows:

Total # ml: 1000

ml/hr: 83

EXAMPLE:

Order: 500 ml D5NS IV 12 N–4 PM

Available: microdrip at 60 gtt/ml; macrodrip at 20 gtt/ml

Logic: The IV will run 4 hours. Since no pump is available, the nurse must choose the drip factor; two steps are necessary. Solve for both drip factors and choose one.

Step 1. $\dfrac{\text{\# ml}}{\text{\# hr}} = \text{ml/hr}$

$\dfrac{500}{4} \quad 4\overline{)500.} \begin{array}{l} 125. \end{array} = 125 \text{ ml/hr}$

Step 2. $\dfrac{\text{ml/hr} \times \text{TF}}{\text{\# min}} = \text{gtt/min}$

Macrodrip

$$\frac{125 \times \overset{1}{\cancel{20}}}{\underset{3}{\cancel{60}}} = \frac{\cancel{125}}{3} \quad 3\overline{)125.0} \begin{array}{r} 41.8 \\ \underline{12} \\ 5 \\ \underline{3} \\ 2\ 0 \end{array}$$

Macrodrip at 42 gtt/min.

Microdrip

$$\frac{125 \times \overset{1}{\cancel{60}}}{\underset{1}{\cancel{60}}} = 125 \text{ gtt/min}$$

Microdrip at 125 gtt/min.

Logic: Answers are macrodrip at 42 gtt/min and microdrip at 125 gtt/min. Choose macrodrip at 42 gtt/min. (See explanation for choosing the infusion set, following this discussion.)

LEARNING AID

1. When the answer is not an even number, carry out arithmetic one decimal place. Round off the answer to the nearest whole number.
2. Note that in Step 2 for microdrip, ml/hr = gtt/min. In other words, when you solve Step 1 you have the microdrip answer in gtt/min. Why? The TF is always 60 and the minutes are always 60. These numbers cancel each other.

Label the IV

Obtain a macrodrip set labeled 20 gtt/ml.

Set drip rate at 42 gtt/min.

EXAMPLE:

Order: 500 ml D5 $\frac{1}{3}$ NS IVKVO for 24°

Available: microdrip at 60 gtt/ml; macrodrip 10 gtt/ml

Logic: Because no pump is available, choose the IV set. This is a two-step problem. The IV will run 24 hr.

Step 1. $\dfrac{\# \text{ ml}}{\# \text{ hr}} = \text{ml/hr}$

$$\frac{500}{24} \quad 24 \overline{)500.0} \begin{array}{r} 20.8 \\ \hline \end{array} = 21 \text{ ml/hr}$$

$$\begin{array}{r} 48 \\ \hline 20\ 0 \\ 19\ 2 \end{array}$$

LEARNING AID

1. Note that the order reads 24°. This abbreviation is used by some physicians to denote hours.
2. Carry out arithmetic one decimal place. Round off the milliliter answer to the nearest whole number.

Step 2. $\dfrac{\text{ml/hr} \times \text{TF}}{\# \text{ min}} = \text{gtt/min}$

Logic: The answer to Step 1 is 21 ml/hr. The number of minutes is 60. Work out the problem for micro- and macrodrip and make a nursing judgment about which tube to use.

Macrodrip

$$21 \times 10 = 21 \quad 6\overline{)21.0} \begin{array}{r} 3.5 \\ \hline \end{array}$$

$$\begin{array}{r} 18 \\ \hline 3\ 0 \\ 3\ 0 \end{array}$$

LEARNING AID

In a two-step IV problem, it is not necessary to show the arithmetic for microdrip because ml/hr = gtt/min.

Macrodrip at 4 gtt/min

Microdrip $\quad \dfrac{21 \times 60}{60} = 21 \text{ gtt/min}$

Logic: 4 gtt/min macrodrip is too slow. Choose microdrip. (See explanation for choosing the infusion set.)

Label the IV

Select a microdrip infusion set

Set the drip rate at 42 gtt/min

Choosing the Infusion Set

Experience will enable you to judge which IV tubing to use. Clinically you will be guided in making a choice. There is no problem when an electric infusion pump is used. The pump will deliver the amount programmed. There are specialized pumps in neonatal and intensive care units that can deliver 1 ml/hr and specialized syringe pumps that can deliver less than 1 ml/hr.

Some guidelines may be helpful when an IV pump is not available.

Use Microdrip When
- The IV is to be administered over a long period
- A small amount of fluid is to be infused
- The macrodrops per minute are too few (Why? IV fluid flows by gravity. Blood flowing in the vein exerts a pressure. If the IV is too slow, blood pressure may force blood into the tube where it clots. The IV will stop.)

Use Macrodrip When
- A large amount of fluid is ordered in a short time
- The microdrips per minute are too many. Counting the drip rate becomes too difficult.

Table 9-2 shows a quick reference chart developed by nurses in a surgical unit for their own use. Look at microdrips per minute (60 gtt = 1 ml). The first heading is *Amount Infused*. Read across—1000 ml, 500 ml, 250 ml, 150 ml. Read down. The heading is *Total Hours for Infusion* —24, 12, 10, 8, 4. When the microdrip rate is 83 gtt/min or more, these nurses use microdrip. Note that in the lower part of the chart, nurses use microdrip when the drip rate is below 10 gtt/min.

Need for Continuous Observation

Many factors may interfere with the drip rate. Do not assume that once an IV is started it will continue to flow at the rate it was set. Check the IV frequently; IVs flow by gravity. As the amount of fluid decreases in the IV bag, pressure changes occur that may affect the rate. The patient's movements may kink the tube and shut off the flow, or they may change the position of the needle or catheter in the vein. The needle may be forced against the side of the blood vessel

Table 9-2.   Quick Reference Chart for IV Drip Factors

Total Hours for Infusion	Amount Infused			
	1000 ml	500 ml	250 ml	150 ml
Microdrops/Minute (60 gtt = 1 ml)				
24	42	21	10	6
12	83/use macro	42	21	12
10	100/use macro	50	25	15
8	125/use macro	63	31	19
4	250/use macro	125/use macro	63	38
Macrodrops/Minute (10 gtt = 1 ml)				
24	7/use micro	Use micro	Use micro	Use micro
12	13	7/use micro	Use micro	Use micro
10	17	8/use micro	Use micro	Use micro
8	21	11	Use micro	Use micro
4	42	21	Use micro	Use micro

Courtesy of the Nursing Department, St. Vincent's Hospital and Medical Center of New York.

changing the flow, or it may be forced out of the vessel allowing fluid to enter the tissues (infiltration).

Infusion pumps have an alarm system that beeps to alert the nurse when the rate cannot be maintained or when the infusion is about to be completed.

CONTINUOUS INTRAVENOUS ADMINISTRATION

When a continuous IV is ordered, the following information will be given:

Type of fluid

Volume to be infused

Time of administration in milliliters per hour (ml/hr) *or* over a number of hours

The order may be written in such a way that no calculation is required.

|| **EXAMPLE:**   250 ml D5W IV; run 25 ml/hr; *pump available*

The order may state milliliters per hour, but an infusion pump is not available; the nurse must decide which tubing should be used.

|| **EXAMPLE:**   1000 ml D5NS; run 100 ml/hr; *no pump available*

The order may be in number of hours and require a choice of IV tubing.

||| **EXAMPLE:**   180 ml D5 $\frac{1}{3}$ NS 12 N–6 PM; *no pump available.*

||| **EXAMPLE:**   1000 ml D5W IV 4 PM–12 mid; *no pump available.*

══════════ PRACTICE EXERCISE 1 ══════════

Calculate the drip factor for the following IV orders given in milliliters per hour or number of hours. Answers may be found at the end of the chapter.

1. Order: 150 ml D5 .33NS IV q8h
    Available: infusion pump

2. Order: 250 cc D5W; run at 25 cc/hr
    Available: infusion pump

3. Order: 1000 ml D5NS; run 100 ml/hr
    Available: macrodrip (20 gtt/ml); microdrip (60 gtt/ml)

(continued)

════════════ PRACTICE EXERCISE 1 *(Continued)* ════════════

4. Order: 180 ml D5 $\frac{1}{3}$ NS 12 N–6 PM

    Available: macrodrip (10 gtt/ml); microdrip (60 gtt/ml)

5. Order: 1000 ml D5 .45S IV 4 PM–12 mid

    Available: macrodrip (15 gtt/ml); microdrip (60 gtt/ml)

MEDICATIONS FOR CONTINUOUS INTRAVENOUS ADMINISTRATION

When a continuous IV order includes a medication, add the medication to the IV and determine the rate of flow. In some institutions, medications are added by the pharmacist; in others, nurses may be required to add the medication.

Ordered Over Several Hours

> *EXAMPLE:*
>
> Order: 1000 ml D5W with 20 mEq KCl IV 10 AM–10 PM
>
> Available: vial of KCl 40 mEq/20 ml; microdrip (60 gtt/min); macrodrip (20 gtt/min)
>
> Logic: $\dfrac{D}{H} \times S = A$ $\quad \dfrac{\overset{1}{\cancel{20}\ \text{mEq}}}{\underset{2}{\cancel{40}\ \text{mEq}}} \times \overset{10}{\cancel{20}}\ \text{ml}$
>
> $\qquad\qquad\qquad\qquad\qquad \dfrac{}{}$
>
> $\qquad\qquad\qquad\qquad 1$
>
> Add 10 ml of KCl to the IV bag.
>
> Use two steps to solve the drip factor.
>
> Choose the tubing. The IV will run 10 hours.
>
> Step 1. $\dfrac{\#\ \text{ml}}{\#\ \text{hr}} = \text{ml/hr}$ $\quad \dfrac{1000}{10} = 100$ ml/hr
>
> Step 2. $\dfrac{\#\ \text{ml/hr} \times \text{TF}}{\#\ \text{min}} = \text{gtt/min}$
>
> For macrodrip: $\dfrac{100 \times \overset{1}{\cancel{20}}}{\underset{3}{\cancel{60}}} = \dfrac{100}{3} = 33$ gtt/min
>
> For microdrip: ml/hr = gtt/min; hence, 100 gtt/min
>
> In this case, choose macrodrip at 33 gtt/min.
>
> Add the KCl to the IV.
>
> Label the IV.

EXAMPLE:

Order: 5 MU penicillin G potassium in 1000 ml D5W IV q8h

Available: macrodrip (10 gtt/ml); microdrip (60 gtt/ml)

Logic: MU means million units. The order is for 5 million U of penicillin G potassium. Penicillin comes in 5 MU vials of powder. Directions say that the drug must be reconstituted with a *minimum* of 100 ml. The order states to add 5 MU to 1000 ml. The order is safe. Use a 10-cc syringe to aseptically remove fluid from the 1000-ml bag of D5W and inject into the powder to make a solution. Withdraw the solution and inject into the bag. You now have 1000 ml D5W with the medication added. The IV will run 8 hours.
Two steps are needed:

Step 1. $\dfrac{\text{\# ml}}{\text{\# hr}} = \text{ml/hr}$ $\dfrac{1000}{8}$ $\dfrac{125}{\overline{)1000.}} = 125 \text{ ml/hr}$

Step 2. $\dfrac{\text{\# ml/hr} \times \text{TF}}{\text{\# min}} = \text{gtt/min}$

Macrodrip: $\dfrac{125 \times 10}{60} = \dfrac{125}{6}$ $\dfrac{20.8}{\overline{)125.0}}$

Microdrip = 125 gtt/min; macrodrip = 21 gtt/min. Choose macrodrip.

Add penicillin 5 MU

Label the IV; set rate at 21 gtt/min macrodrip

Ordered in Milliliters per Hour

Potent medications such as heparin and aminophylline may be added to IVs with the rate ordered in milliliters per hour. It is best to use a pump to deliver these infusions safely. If a pump is not available, a volume control set, such as a Buretrol, should be used (Fig. 9-4).

EXAMPLE:

Order: 10,000 U heparin in 500 ml NS; run at 10 ml/hr

Available: vial of heparin labeled 5000 U/ml; infusion pump

Logic: The vial has 5000 U/ml of heparin. Draw up 2 ml in a syringe; aseptically add this solution to 500 ml NS and label the bag. Because a pump is available, no calculation is necessary. Set the rate at 10 ml/hr.

EXAMPLE:

Order: aminophylline 250 mg in 250 ml D5W IV; run at 50 cc/hr

Available: Ampule of aminophylline labeled 1 g in 10 cc; Buretrol that delivers 60 gtt/ml (microdrip)

Logic: The ampule of aminophylline has 1 g in 10 ml. This is equivalent to 1000 mg in 10 ml. You want 250 mg.

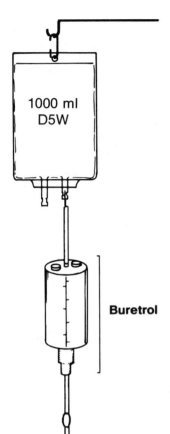

Figure 9-4. *A Buretrol (at bottom) is an IV delivery system with tubing and a chamber that can hold 150 ml delivered as microdrip (1 ml = 60 drops). The top of the Buretrol has a port by means of which a reservoir of fluid can be added. The Buretrol is a volume control because no more than 150 ml can be infused at one time.*

$$\frac{D}{H} \times S = A$$

$$\frac{\overset{1}{\cancel{250}}}{\underset{4}{\cancel{1000}}} \times 10 = \overset{2.5\ ml}{\cancel{10}}\ \underset{4\,\overline{)10.0}}{}$$

Draw up 2.5 ml and inject into 250 ml D5W. You have 250 mg in 250 ml D5W. Label the bag.

You want 50 cc/hr, and you have a Buretrol 60 gtt/ml.

$$\frac{ml/hr \times TF}{60} = \frac{50 \times \cancel{60}}{\cancel{60}} = 50\ gtt/min$$

Actually, since you have a microdrip Buretrol, no calculation is necessary: ml/hr = gtt/min.

Ordered in Units per Hour or Milligrams per Hour

Thus far all the IV problems were solved by determining the milliliters per hour or the drops per minute. Infusion rates can also be calculated when the physician orders the IV to infuse in units per hour (U/hr) or in milligrams per hour (mg/hr). When IVs are ordered in this way, an infusion pump or a control device, such as Buretrol, is necessary.

EXAMPLE:

Order: 20,000 units heparin Na in 500 ml D5W; infusion 1000 U/hr

Available: infusion pump

How will you solve these problems? See them as injections from liquid!

Step 1. Determine the solution made. You will put 20,000 units in 500 ml.

$$\frac{\overset{40}{\cancel{20,000}}\ U}{\cancel{500}\ ml} = 40\ units/ml$$

Step 2. Determine the number of milliliters needed to give the units per hour.

$$\frac{D}{H} \times S = A \qquad \frac{\overset{25}{\cancel{1000}}\ \cancel{units}/hr}{\underset{1}{\cancel{40}\ \cancel{units}}} \times 1\ ml = 25\ ml/hr$$

Logic: If you give 25 ml/hr and each milliliter has 40 units, you will administer 1000 units/hr. Heparin sodium comes as a liquid in a vial labeled 10,000 units/ml.

Add 2 ml of heparin to 500 ml D5W.

Label the IV bag.

Set the infusion pump at 25 ml/hr.

EXAMPLE:

Order: aminophylline 0.5 g in 500 ml D5W; infuse 50 mg/hr via pump

Step 1. Determine the solution made. You have 0.5 g in 500 ml.

$$0.5\ g = 500\ mg$$

$$\frac{\overset{1}{\cancel{500}}\ mg}{\underset{1}{\cancel{500}}\ ml} = 1\ mg/ml$$

Step 2. Actually it is not necessary to calculate. The order calls for 50 mg/hr. The solution is 1 mg/ml. Set the pump for 50 ml/hr. If this is not clear, work it out.

$$\frac{D}{H} \times S = A \qquad \frac{50\ \cancel{mg}/hr}{1\ \cancel{mg}} \times 1\ ml = 50\ ml/hr$$

Aminophylline comes as a liquid in an ampule labeled 1 g in 10 ml.
Add 5 ml aminophylline to 500 ml D5W; label the IV; set pump rate at 50 ml/hr.

Sometimes the order is written in an abbreviated way:

EXAMPLE:

Order: infuse Heparin 1500 U/hr

This IV order is acceptable when the institution has standardized the solution, and it is hospital policy that the drug will be diluted only one way.
A common standard for heparin sodium is 25,000 units in 250 ml D5W.

Step 1. Determine the solution

$$\frac{\overset{100}{\cancel{25,000}}\text{ units}}{\underset{1}{\cancel{250}}\text{ ml}} = 100 \text{ units/ml}$$

Step 2. Determine the number of milliliters needed

$$\frac{D}{H} \times S = A \qquad \frac{1500 \cancel{\text{ U}}/\text{hr}}{100 \cancel{\text{ U}}} \times 1 \text{ ml} = 15 \text{ ml/hr}$$

Heparin sodium comes as a liquid in a vial labeled 5000 units/ml.

Add 5 ml heparin to 250 ml D5W to make 25,000 U/250 ml. Label the IV. Set pump rate at 15 ml/hr.

Ordered in Micrograms per Minute

Nurses in intensive care units care for patients receiving powerful IV drugs that are often ordered in micrograms. These orders differ from any we have yet studied.

EXAMPLE:

Titrate Levophed to maintain arterial mean pressure above 65 and below 95. (*Titrate* means regulate.)

Run dopamine at 2 μg/kg/min IV.

Start dopamine at 400 μg/min IV and titrate to maintain diastole BP > 60 < 75.

Microdrip is used to administer these drugs (60 gtt/ml). Answers to IV problems using microdrip are given in drops per minute (gtt/min). Recall that 1 mg = 1000 μg equivalent. The rule $\frac{D}{H} \times S$ can be used to solve these problems.

EXAMPLE:

Order: start dopamine at 400 μg/min IV and titrate to maintain diastolic BP > 60 < 75

Available: standard dopamine solution of 200 mg in 250 ml D5W. The solution is 200 mg in 250 ml.

Step 1. Change milligrams to micrograms by multiplying by 1000

$$\begin{array}{r} 200 \\ \times\ 1000 \\ \hline 200,000 \text{ μg} \end{array}$$

Step 2. The solution now is

$$\frac{200,000 \text{ μg}}{250 \text{ ml}} \qquad \text{Reduce this large fraction}$$

$$\frac{\overset{800}{\cancel{200,000}}\text{ μg}}{\underset{1}{\cancel{250\text{ ml}}}} = 800 \text{ μg/ml}$$

Step 3. The solution is 800 μg/ml.

Because the IV is administered by microdrip in drops per minute, you can substitute 60 gtt/min for milliliters. The solution is 800 μg/60 gtt/min.

Step 4. Solve using $\dfrac{D}{H} \times S = A$. You desire 400 μg/min.

$$\dfrac{\overset{1}{\cancel{400}\ \mu g}}{\underset{2}{\underset{1}{\cancel{800}\ \mu g}}} \times \overset{30}{\cancel{60}}\ \text{gtt/min} = 30\ \text{gtt/min}$$

Start dopamine at 30 gtt/min and titrate (i.e., regulate the drip) to maintain diastolic BP > 60 and < 75. Label IV.

EXAMPLE:

Order: Aramine 50 mg in 250 ml D5W; titrate to 60 μg/min

Available: vial of Aramine labeled 100 mg in 10 ml. Add 5 ml Aramine to IV. Label: 50 mg in 250 ml D5W.

Step 1. Change milligrams to micrograms

50 mg = 50,000 μg

Step 2. Solution is $\dfrac{\overset{200}{\cancel{50,000}\ \mu g}}{\underset{1}{\cancel{250}\ \text{ml}}} = 200\ \mu$g/ml

Step 3. Substitute 60 gtt/min for the milliliter.

200 μg/60 gtt/min

Step 4. $\dfrac{D}{H} \times S = A$

$$\dfrac{\overset{3}{\cancel{60}\ \cancel{\mu g}}}{\underset{1}{\cancel{200}\ \cancel{\mu g}}} \times \cancel{60}\ \text{gtt/min} = 18\ \text{gtt/min}$$

Label IV.

EXAMPLE:

Order: Levophed 16 μg/min IV

Available: standard solution of 16 mg in 500 cc D5W

Step 1. Change milligrams to micrograms

16 mg = 16,000 μg

Step 2. Reduce solution numbers $\dfrac{\overset{32}{\cancel{16,000}}\ \mu g}{\underset{\cancel{500}}{\cancel{500}}\ ml} = 32\ \mu g/ml$

Step 3. Substitute 60 gtt/min for milliliter. Solution is

32 μg/60 gtt/min

Step 4. $\dfrac{D}{H} \times S = A$ $\dfrac{\overset{1}{\cancel{16}}\ \mu g}{\underset{1}{\cancel{32}}\ \mu g} \times \overset{30}{\cancel{60}}\ gtt/min = 30\ gtt/min$

EXAMPLE:

Order: run Dopamine at 2 μg/kg/min

Available: weight of patient 80 kg; standard dopamine solution of 200 mg/250 ml D5W

Patient weight   80 kg
                 × 2 mg/kg
Order is: 160 μg/min

Step 1. Change milligrams to micrograms in the standard solution

200 mg = 200,000 μg

Step 2. Reduce solution numbers $\dfrac{\overset{800}{\cancel{200,000}}\ \mu g}{\underset{1}{\cancel{250}}\ ml} = 800\ \mu g/min$

Step 3. Substitute 60 gtt/min for milliliters

800 μg/60 gtt/min

Step 4. $\dfrac{D}{H} \times S = A$ $\dfrac{\overset{1}{\cancel{160}}\ \mu g}{\underset{5}{\cancel{800}}\ \mu g} \times \overset{12}{\cancel{60}}\ gtt/min = 12\ gtt/min$

Label the IV.

PRACTICE EXERCISE 2

Solve these problems of medications in continuous IVs ordered in milliliters per hour (ml/hr); number of hours; milligrams per hour (mg/hr); units per hour (U/hr); and micrograms per minute (μg/min). Answers may be found at the end of the chapter.

1. Order: isoproterenol drip IV 3 mcg/min
   Available: standard solution of 1 mg in 250 ml

2. Order: 1500 units heparin qh via pump
Available: institution policy requires standard solution of 25,000 units in 250 ml D5W; vial of heparin 10,000 U/ml

3. Order: 500 ml D5W with 2.5 MU penicillin G sodium IV q12h
Available: vial of powder labeled 20 million units penicillin G sodium. Directions: Add 18 ml NS or DW to make a volume of 1 MU/ml; 500 ml D5W; microdrip tubing

4. Order: aminophylline 1 Gm in 1000 ml D5W IV at 75 ml/hr
Available: infusion pump; vial of aminophylline labeled 1 gram in 10 ml; 1000 ml D5W

MEDICATIONS FOR INTERMITTENT INTRAVENOUS ADMINISTRATION

Some intravenous medications do not have to be administered continuously but only at specific intervals, such as qd, q4h, q6h, q8h. Routinely these drugs are administered piggybacked to the main IV in a small volume of fluid. The route is written *IVPB*, which means intravenous piggyback (see Fig. 9-1).

> ### *EXAMPLE:*
>
> Order: ampicillin sodium 1 g IVPB q6h in 50 ml D5W over 30 minutes
>
> Available: ampicillin sodium 1 g powder; bag of 50 ml D5W; secondary administration IV set (10 gtt/ml). Directions say to dilute the powder in 50 ml D5W and administer over 30–60 minutes. The order specifies the amount of drug, the route, the times of administration, the diluent (type and amount), and the rate of flow.
>
> The rule for solving IVPB drip factors is the same as that for continuous IVs.
>
> $$\frac{\# \text{ ml} \times \text{TF}}{\# \text{ min}} = \text{gtt/min}$$
>
> # ml = 50 ml D5W
>
> TF = 10 gtt/ml
>
> # min. = 30
>
> $$\frac{50 \times \cancel{10}}{\cancel{30}} = \cancel{50} \quad \frac{16.6}{3\,)\overline{50.0}} = 17 \text{ gtt/min}$$
> $$\begin{array}{r} \underline{3} \\ 20 \\ \underline{18} \\ 20 \end{array}$$
>
> You are ready to prepare the IVPB. Because the order is 1 g and the stock is 1 g the preparation is easy. Use a reconstitution device to mix the powder and the diluent. A

reconstitution device is a sterile implement containing two needles that connect the vial and the 50-ml bag. It enables the nurse to dilute the powder and place it in the bag without using a syringe (Fig. 9-5).

With a reconstitution device add 1 g of ampicillin to 50 ml D5W. Label the IVPB.

Drip rate = 17 gtt/min

Label:

   Fred Le Merle

   Room 1006-2

   August 24

   Ampicillin 1 g IVPB q6h in 50 ml D5W over 30 minutes

   12 N–12:30 PM

   Run 17 gtt/min

   RPQ

   Note: the times are q6h: 6 AM–6:30 AM, 12 N–12:30 PM, 6 PM–6:30 PM, 12 M–12:30 AM

Often the doctor will write only the amount of drug and the time interval, relying on the nurse to follow the manufacturer's recommendation for diluent and time to flow. The nurse is then responsible for checking reference materials.

EXAMPLE:

Order: cefonicid sodium 1 g IVPB qd

Available: vial of powder labeled 1 gram (Fig. 9-6); 50-ml bag of sodium chloride; secondary administration set

   The directions on the label state: to reconstitute 1 gram add 50–100 ml of sodium chloride injection. The one factor missing is the amount of time needed to infuse the medication. Some institutions provide guidelines to assist nurses in preparing IVPB infu-

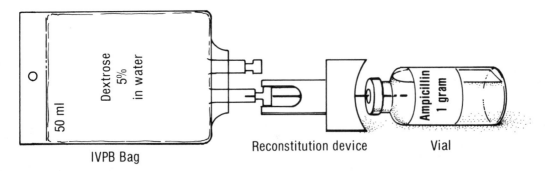

Figure 9-5. *Reconstitution device. The IVPB bag is squeezed forcing fluid into the vial of powder, which is then diluted. The three parts are turned to a vertical position—vial up, IVPB bag down. The IVPB bag is squeezed and released. This creates a negative pressure allowing the diluted medication to flow into the IVPB bag.*

CAUTION—Federal law prohibits dispensing without prescription. U.S. Pat. 4,048,311

NDC 0007-4354-01

Monocid® brand of
sterile cefonicid sodium
(lyophilized)

1 gram equivalent to cefonicid "Piggyback" Vial for Intravenous Admixture

Smith Kline & French Laboratories
Division of SmithKline Beckman Corporation
Philadelphia, PA 19101

Primarily for institutional use.
Usual Adult Dose—1 gram every 24 hours as a single dose. See accompanying literature.

Before reconstitution protect from light and refrigerate (below 8°C.).

Reconstitution
Add 50 to 100 ml. of Sodium Chloride Injection or other intravenous solution listed in accompanying literature. Shake Well. Administer as a single dose with primary intravenous fluids.

Properly reconstituted solutions of 'Monocid' are stable 24 hours at room temperature or 72 hours if refrigerated (5°C.). Slight yellowing does not affect potency.

Each vial contains cefonicid sodium equivalent to 1 gram of cefonicid. Cefonicid sodium contains 85 mg. (3.7 mEq.) sodium per gram of cefonicid activity.

SK&F

Figure 9-6. Label for cefonicid sodium (Monocid). (Courtesy of Smith Kline & French Laboratories.)

sions; one such chart is shown in Table 9-3. Guidelines are determined from package inserts and/or the *Physician's Desk Reference* (PDR).

Note that rates vary on the chart depending upon the dose and volume to be administered and the drug. The higher the dose, the greater the volume of diluent and the longer the rate. Some IVPB medications are painful and require greater dilution. Nursing judgment is required to choose the dilution and the time of infusion when parameters are given.

Use a reconstitution device to add 1 g of cefonicid to 50 ml of sodium chloride injection. Label the IV. Drip rate = 17 gtt/min.

If a reconstitution device is not available, you could use a 10-ml syringe, aseptically withdraw some fluid (3–4 ml) from the IVPB bag, inject into the vial to put the powder into solution, withdraw the fluid containing 1 g, and inject into the IVPB bag. Because you are using the total amount of powder, it is not necessary to be exact in the number of milliliters.

Table 9-3. Pharmacy Guidelines for the Intravenous Administration of Antibiotics by Intermittent Infusion in Adults

Antibiotic (Generic/Trade)	Recommended Volume for Intermittent Infusion/ Infusion Fluid	Infusion Period	Remarks
Acyclovir/Zovirax	100 ml/D5W, NS	1 hr	Use larger volume if concentration exceeds 7 mg/ml
Amikacin/Amikin	100 ml/D5W, NS	1–2 hr	
Amphotericin B/ Fungizone	Dilute to 0.1 mg/ml after reconstitution with 10 ml sterile water/D5W *only*	At least 6 hr	Reconstitute with sterile water for injection without preservatives; Do not administer through filter
Ampicillin/Omnipen, Polycillin-N	50 ml (1 g); 100 ml (2 g)/D5W, NS	15–30 min	Use within 2 hr
Cefazolin/Ancef, Kefzol	50 ml (1 g); 100 ml (2 g)/D5W, NS	15–30 min	
Cefoperazone/ Cefobid	50 ml (1 g); 100 ml (2 g)/D5W, NS	15–30 min	
Cefotaxime/Claforan	50 ml (1 g); 100 ml (2 g)/D5W, NS	15–30 min	
Cefoxitin/Mefoxin	50 ml (1 g); 100 ml (2 g)/D5W, NS	15–30 min	
Cephalothin/Keflin	50 ml (1 g); 100 ml (2 g)/D5W, NS	15–30 min	
Chloramphenicol/ Chloromycetin	50 ml/D5W, NS per g	15–30 min; minimum 20 min/g	
Clindamycin/Cleocin	50 ml (300 mg); 100 ml (600 mg)/D5W, NS	15 min (300 mg) 30 min (600 mg)	
Doxycycline/ Vibramycin	250 ml (100 mg); 500 ml (200 mg)/D5W, NS	At least 1 hr (100 mg) At least 2 hr (200 mg)	

(continued)

Table 9-3. Pharmacy Guidelines for the Intravenous Administration of Antibiotics by Intermittent Infusion in Adults (continued)

Antibiotic (Generic/Trade)	Recommended Volume for Intermittent Infusion/ Infusion Fluid	Infusion Period	Remarks
Erythromycin Lactobionate/ Erythrocin IV	100 ml (500 mg)/NS	20–60 min	Use larger volume if dose is greater than 500 mg; reconstitute with sterile water for injection without preservatives; D5W can be used if buffered with sodium bicarbonate additive
Gentamicin/ Garamycin	100 ml/D5W, NS	30–120 min	
Oxacillin/Bactocill, Prostaphlin	50 ml (1 g); 100 ml (2 g)/D5W, NS	15–30 min	
Penicillin G potassium	50 ml/D5W, NS	30 min (less than 2 million units) 60 min (between 2 and 5 million units) 120 min (more than 5 million units)	
Pentamidine/Pentam 300	250 ml/D5W	At least 1 hr	Reconstitute with sterile water for injection or D5W
Piperacillin/Pipracil	50 ml (2 g); 100 ml (4 g)/D5W, NS	30 min	
Ticarcillin/Ticar	100 ml (3 g)/D5W, NS	30–120 min	
Tobramycin/Nebcin	100 ml/D5W, NS	30–60 min	
Trimethoprim-Sulfamethoxazole/ Bactrim, Septra	One 5-ml vial per 75 ml or 125 ml/D5W	60–90 min	Use within 2 hr if each vial is diluted in 75 ml of D5W; use within 6 hr if each vial is diluted in 125 ml D5W
Vancomycin/ Vancocin, Vancoled	100 ml (500 mg); 250 ml (1 g)/D5W, NS	1 hr (500 mg) 2 hr (1 g)	
Vidarabine/Vira-A	Dilute to 1 mg/2.22 ml (1 L of IV infusion fluid will solubilize a maximum of 450 mg)/D5W, NS	12–24 hr	Shake vial well to obtain a uniform suspension before placing drug in IV container; administer through a 0.22-μm filter

Courtesy of the Pharmacy Department, St. Vincent's Hospital and Medical Center of New York.

====================== **PRACTICE EXERCISE 3** ======================

Calculate the drip factor for the following IVPB orders. Indicate the amount and type of diluent and the minutes to flow. Answers may be found at the end of the chapter.

1. Order: cefazolin (Ancef) 1 g IVPB q6h
    Available: vial of powder labeled 1 g (Fig. 9-7); reconstitution device; secondary administration set
        tubing (1 ml = 10 gtt)
    What diluent and number of milliliters would you choose? Over how many minutes should it flow?

(continued)

Pharmacy Bulk Vials

Add Sterile Water for Injection, Bacteriostatic Water for Injection, or Sodium Chloride Injection according to the table below. SHAKE WELL.

Vial Size	Amount of Diluent	Approximate Concentration	Approximate Available Volume
5 grams	23 ml.	1 gram/5 ml.	26 ml.
	48 ml.	1 gram/10 ml.	51 ml.
10 grams	45 ml.	1 gram/5 ml.	51 ml.
	96 ml.	1 gram/10 ml.	102 ml.

"Piggyback" Vials

Reconstitute with 50 to 100 ml. of Sodium Chloride Injection or other I.V. solution listed under ADMINISTRATION. When adding diluent to vial, allow air to escape by using a small vent needle or by pumping the syringe. SHAKE WELL. Administer with primary I.V. fluids, as a single dose.

ADMINISTRATION

Intramuscular Administration—Reconstitute vials with Sterile Water for Injection according to the dilution table above. Shake well until dissolved. 'Ancef' should be injected into a large muscle mass. Pain on injection is infrequent with 'Ancef'.

Intravenous Administration—Direct (bolus) injection: Following reconstitution according to the above table, further dilute vials with approximately 5 ml. Sterile Water for Injection. Inject the solution slowly over 3 to 5 minutes, directly or through tubing for patients receiving parenteral fluids (see list below).

Intermittent or continuous infusion: Dilute reconstituted 'Ancef' in 50 to 100 ml. of one of the following solutions:

Sodium Chloride Injection, USP
5% or 10% Dextrose Injection, USP
5% Dextrose in Lactated Ringer's Injection, USP
5% Dextrose and 0.9% Sodium Chloride Injection, USP
5% Dextrose and 0.45% Sodium Chloride Injection, USP
5% Dextrose and 0.2% Sodium Chloride Injection, USP

Figure 9-7. *Directions for IVPB dilution of cefazolin sodium (Ancef). (Courtesy of Smith Kline & French Laboratories.)*

Dilution: EACH 5 ML OF SEPTRA I.V. INFUSION SHOULD BE ADDED TO 125 ML OF 5% DEXTROSE IN WATER.

NOTE: **In those instances where fluid restriction is desirable,** each 5 ml may be added to 75 ml of 5% dextrose in water. Under these circumstances the solution should be mixed just prior to use and should be administered within two (2) hours. If upon visual inspection there is cloudiness or evidence of crystallization after mixing, the solution should be discarded and a fresh solution prepared.

DO NOT MIX SEPTRA I.V. INFUSION-5% DEXTROSE IN WATER WITH DRUGS OR SOLUTIONS IN THE SAME CONTAINER.

ADMINISTRATION: The solution should be given by intravenous infusion over a period of 60 to 90 minutes. Rapid infusion or bolus injections must be avoided. Septra I.V. Infusion should not be given intramuscularly.

HOW SUPPLIED: 5 ml ampuls, containing 80 mg trimethoprim (16 mg/ml) and 400 mg sulfamethoxazole (80 mg/ml) for infusion with 5% dextrose in water. Box of 10. (NDC 0081-0856-10)

Figure 9-8. *Directions for IVPB dilution of Septra (trimethoprim and sulfamethoxazole). (Courtesy of Burroughs Wellcome Co.)*

Intermittent intravenous infusion: Kefzol can be administered along with primary intravenous fluid management programs in a volume control set or in a separate, secondary IV bottle. Reconstituted 500 mg or 1 g of Kefzol may be diluted in 50 to 100 mL of one of the following intravenous solutions: 0.9% Sodium Chloride Injection, 5% or 10% Dextrose Injection, 5% Dextrose in Lactated Ringer's Injection, 5% Dextrose and 0.9% Sodium Chloride Injection (also may be used with 5% Dextrose and 0.45% or 0.2% Sodium Chloride Injection), Lactated Ringer's Injection, 5% or 10% Invert Sugar in Sterile Water for Injection, Ringer's Injection, Normosol®-M in D5-W, Inosol® B with Dextrose 5%, or Plasma-Lyte® with 5% Dextrose.

Direct intravenous injection: Dilute the reconstituted 500 mg or 1 g of Kefzol in a minimum of 10 mL of Sterile Water for Injection. Inject solution slowly over 3 to 5 minutes. It may be administered directly into a vein or through the tubing for a patient receiving the above parenteral fluids.

Figure 9-9. *Dilution directions for cefazolin sodium (Kefzol). (Courtesy of Eli Lilly and Co.)*

=============== **PRACTICE EXERCISE 3** *(Continued)* ===============

2. Order: Septra 5 ml in 125 ml of D5W IVPB over 60 minutes
   Available: ampule of Septra labeled 5 ml (Fig. 9-8); 250-ml bag D5W; secondary administration set
        (1 ml = 10 gtt)

3. Order: Kefzol 500 mg IVPB q6h
   Available: vial of powder labeled 500 mg (Fig. 9-9); reconstitution device; secondary administration set
        (1 ml = 10 gtt)

4. Order: kanamycin 1 g IVPB in 400 ml D5W over 100 min
   Available: vial of powder 1 g; reconstitution device (see Fig. 9-5); secondary administration set (1 ml =
        10 gtt)

CHANGING THE INTRAVENOUS DRIP RATE

Setting the drip rate for an IV does not relieve the nurse of the responsibility to check the IV frequently. Many factors can interfere with the flow—kinking of the tube, movement of the client, the effect of gravity, or placement of the needle or catheter. If a discrepancy in flow exists, it may be necessary to recalculate the IV drip.

EXAMPLE:

As you make rounds you check a client's IV. The label reads:

1000 ml D5W IV to run 8 AM–4 PM

The tubing is macrodrip (10 gtt/ml). Rate is set at 20 gtt/min

It is now 1 PM. You note that there is 600 ml left in the IV. Should you change the drip?

Logic: Step 1. Calculate how many milliliters per hour.

$$\frac{1000}{8} = 125 \text{ ml/hr}$$

Step 2. It is now 1 PM. Therefore 5 hours have elapsed since the IV was started.

125 ml/hr
× __5 hr__
625 ml should have been delivered

Step 3. Because there are 600 ml left in the IV, only 400 ml were delivered.

625 ml should have been delivered
__400 ml__ were delivered
225 ml behind

Conclusion: The nurse will have to make a judgment of whether or not to increase the IV drip on the basis of an assessment of the client's status. It may be necessary to consult with the physician.

DETERMINATION OF THE HOURS THAT AN INTRAVENOUS INFUSION WILL RUN

When an IV order reads ml/hr, mg/hr, or units/hr, it is sometimes helpful for the nurse to calculate how long the IV will last so that the next IV can be prepared or new orders written.

EXAMPLE:

Order: 500 ml Ringer's lactate IV; run 75 ml/hr

Divide the number of milliliters by the milliliters per hour

$$
\begin{array}{r}
6.6\ \text{hr} \\
75\ \overline{)500.0} \\
\underline{450} \\
50\ 0
\end{array}
$$

The IV will last approximately 6.6 hr

PRACTICE EXERCISE 4

1. 20,000 units of heparin is added to 500 ml D5W, and the order is to infuse IV at 30 ml/hr. How many hours will the IV run?

SELF-TEST 1

Solve these problems related to intravenous and IVPB drip rates. Aim for a high degree of accuracy. Answers may be found at the end of the chapter. Review material that you find difficult.

1. Order: 1500 ml D5W 8 AM–8 PM
   Available: macrodrip tubing (10 gtt/ml)
   What is the drip rate?

2. Order: 250 ml D5 $\frac{1}{2}$ NS IV KVO (give over 12 hours)
   Available: microdrip tubing
   What is the drip rate?

3. Order: 150 ml D5 $\frac{1}{3}$ NS IV; run 20 ml/hr
   Available: infusion pump
   a. What is the drip rate?
   b. How long will the IV last?

4. Order: heparin 40,000 units in 1000 ml D5W; infuse 800 units/hr
   Available: infusion pump
   What is the drip rate?

(continued)

SELF-TEST 1 (Continued)

5. Order: 1000 ml D5S with 15 mEq KCl IV; run 100 ml/hr
   Available: macrotubing (20 gtt/ml) and microdrip
   a. How many hours will this run?
   b. How many milliliters of KCl will you add to the IV if KCl comes in a vial labeled 40 mEq/20 ml?
   c. What tubing will you use?
   d. What are the gtt/min?

6. Order: nitroglycerin IV at 80 mcg/min
   Available: standard solution of 50 mg in 250 ml D5$\frac{1}{3}$NS
   What are the gtt/min?

SELF-TEST 2

1. Order: aminophylline 1 g in 500 ml D5W IV at 75 ml/hr
   Available: vial of aminophylline 1 g in 10 ml; infusion pump
   a. How many ml of aminophylline should be added to the IV?
   b. How will you set the drip rate?

2. Order: chloramphenicol 2 g in 100 ml D5W IVPB q6h over 40 minutes (see Fig. 9-5)
   Available: 100 ml D5W; vial of chloramphenicol labeled 2 g; reconstitution device; secondary adminis-
         tration set (1 ml = 10 gtt)
   a. What will you do to prepare this IVPB?
   b. What are the gtt/min?

3. Order: dobutamine IV 250 μg/min
   Available: standard IV solution 500 mg in 500 ml D5W
   What are the gtt/min?

4. Order: heparin sodium 800 units/hr IV
   Available: infusion pump; standard solution of 25,000 units in 250 ml D5W
   What is the rate?

5. Order: 500 ml D5 $\frac{1}{2}$ S IV q8h

   Available: microdrip tubing
   What are the gtt/min?

6. Order: bretylium 1 mg/min IV
   Available: standard solution 1 g in 500 ml D5W
   What are the gtt/min?

ANSWERS

PRACTICE EXERCISE 1

1. Logic: This is a continuous IV of 150 ml every 8 hours. There is a pump available. You only need Step 1.

    It will run 8 hr.

    $$\frac{\# \text{ ml}}{\# \text{ hr}} = \text{ml/hr}$$

    $$\begin{array}{r} 18.7 \text{ ml/hr} \\ 8\overline{)150.0} \\ \underline{8} \\ 70 \\ \underline{64} \\ 6\,0 \\ \underline{5\,6} \end{array}$$

    Label the IV. Set the pump as follows:
    Total # ml: 150
    ml/hr: 19

2. Logic: This is a continuous IV. A pump is available. The order states ml/hr. There is no calculation needed. Label the IV. Set the pump as follows:
    Total # ml: 250
    ml/hr: 25

3. Logic: The order gives 100 ml/hr; ml/hr = gtt per minute, so you know the microdrip is 100 gtt/min. Work out the macrodrip factor and choose the tubing. You need Step 2.

    Macrodrip

    Step 2. $\dfrac{\text{ml/hr} \times \text{TF}}{\# \text{ min}} = \text{gtt/min}$

    $$\frac{100 \times \overset{1}{\cancel{20}}}{\underset{3}{\cancel{60}}} = \frac{100}{3} = 33.3$$

    Macrodrip at 33 gtt/min
    Microdrip at 100 gtt/min
    Either drip rate could be used. Choose 33 gtt/min and label the IV.

4. Logic: This is a small volume over several hours; use microdrip. Solve for both macrodrip and microdrip, using two steps.

    Step 1. $\dfrac{\# \text{ ml}}{\# \text{ hr}} = \text{ml/hr}$ $\dfrac{\overset{30}{\cancel{180}}}{\underset{1}{\cancel{6}}} = 30 \text{ ml/hr}$

    Step 2. $\dfrac{\text{ml/hr} \times \text{TF}}{\# \text{ min}} = \text{gtt/min}$

    Microdrip is 30 gtt/min because ml/hr = gtt/min

    Macrodrip

    $$\frac{\overset{5}{\cancel{30}} \times \overset{}{\cancel{10}}}{\underset{1}{\cancel{60}}} = 5 \text{ gtt/min}$$

5. Logic: This is a large volume over several hours; use macrodrip. Solve using two steps and decide.

Step 1. $\dfrac{\# \text{ ml}}{\# \text{ hr}} = \text{ml/hr}$ $\dfrac{\overset{125}{\cancel{1000}}}{\underset{1}{\cancel{8}}} = 125 \text{ ml/hr}$

Step 2. $\dfrac{\text{ml/hr} \times \text{TF}}{\# \text{ min}} = \text{gtt/min}$

You know microdrip will be 125 gtt/min because ml/hr = gtt/min.

Macrodrip

$\dfrac{125 \times \overset{1}{\cancel{15}}}{\underset{4}{\cancel{60}}} = \dfrac{125}{4}$ $\begin{array}{r} 31.2 \\ 4\,\overline{)125.0} \\ \underline{12} \\ 5 \\ \underline{4} \\ 1\,0 \\ \underline{8} \end{array}$

Macrodrip at 31 gtt/min
Microdrip at 125 gtt/min
Use macrodrip
Label the IV. Macrodrip at 31 gtt/min.

PRACTICE EXERCISE 2

1. Logic: You want micrograms per minute. There are four steps. The factor is always microdrip.

Step 1.   Change milligrams to micrograms in the solution.

1 mg = 1000 mcg, hence, you have 1000 mcg in 250 ml

Step 2.   Reduce the number in the solution.

$\dfrac{\overset{4}{\cancel{1000}}\text{ mcg}}{\underset{1}{\cancel{250}}\text{ ml}} = 4 \text{ mcg/ml}$

Step 3.   The TF is microdrip. Change milliliters in the solution to 60 gtt/min. The solution is 4 mcg/60 gtt/min.

Step 4. $\dfrac{D}{H} \times S = A$

$\dfrac{3 \,\cancel{\text{mcg}}}{\underset{1}{\cancel{4}}\,\cancel{\text{mcg}}} \times \overset{15}{\cancel{60}}\text{ gtt/min} = 45 \text{ gtt/min}$

Label the IV: 45 gtt/min.

2. Logic: You are setting up a heparin drip in units per hour. You need two steps. A pump is available.

Step 1.   Determine the solution.

$\dfrac{\overset{100}{\cancel{25,000}}\,\text{U}}{\underset{}{\cancel{250}}\text{ ml}} = 100 \text{ U/ml}$

Step 2.   Determine the milliliters needed.

$$\frac{D}{H} \times S = A \qquad \frac{1500 \text{ U/hr}}{100 \text{ U}} \times 1 \text{ ml} = 15 \text{ ml/hr}$$

The heparin comes in 10,000 U/ml. You want 25,000 U.

$$\frac{D}{H} \times S = A \qquad \frac{\overset{5}{\cancel{25,000}}}{\underset{2}{\cancel{10,000}}} = \frac{5}{2} = 2.5 \text{ ml}$$

Add 2.5 ml heparin to 250 ml D5W to make 25,000 U/250 ml. Label the IV. Set the pump rate at 15 ml/hr.

3.   Logic: This is a continuous IV order with a medication. Add the medication and determine the drip factor. Microdrip tubing is available.

Directions say to add 18 ml NS to 20 MU penicillin to make 1 MU/ml. You want 2.5 MU. Draw up 2.5 ml and add to 500 ml D5W. Label the vial 1 MU/ml and refrigerate. Label the IV bag: 2.5 MU penicillin in 500 ml D5W. You only need one step.

Step 1. $\dfrac{\# \text{ ml}}{\# \text{ hr}} = \text{ml/hr}$

$$500 \quad 12 \overline{)\begin{array}{l} 41.6 = 42 \text{ ml} \\ 500.0 \\ \underline{48} \\ 20 \\ \underline{12} \\ 8\,0 \end{array}}$$

The microdrip is 42 gtt/min because gtt/min = ml/hr.

4.   Logic: This is an IV order in milliliters per hour. Add the medication first and determine the drip rate. An infusion pump is available. You only need to set the pump because the order was written in ml/hr. You want 1 g of aminophylline and it comes as 1 g in 10 ml.

Add 10 ml of aminophylline to 1000 ml D5W and label the IV. Set the pump at 75 ml/hr.

PRACTICE EXERCISE 3

1.   Logic: Directions say to reconstitute 1 g of cefazolin (Ancef) in 50–100 ml of sodium chloride injection or D5W for IVPB. There is no time given. You have a reconstitution device and tubing 10 gtt/ml. Administer over 30 minutes.

Use the reconstitution device to add 1 g of cefazolin to 50 ml D5W. Label the IVPB.

$$\frac{\# \text{ ml} \times \text{TF}}{\# \text{ min}} = \text{gtt/min}$$

$$\frac{50 \times 10}{30} = \frac{50}{3} \quad 3\overline{)\begin{array}{l} 16.6 = 17 \text{ gtt/min} \\ 50.0 \\ \underline{3} \\ 20 \\ \underline{18} \\ 2\,0 \\ \underline{1\,8} \end{array}}$$

Set the rate at 17 gtt/min.

2.   Logic: Directions say that each 5 ml of sulfamethoxazole–trimethoprim (Septra) should be added to 125 ml of D5W and given over 60–90 minutes. Choose 60 minutes.

Because you have a 250-ml bag of D5W, aseptically remove 125 ml. You now have 125 ml D5W in the bag. With a syringe, add 5 ml of Septra to the IV bag. Label the bag.

$$\frac{\# \text{ ml} \times \text{TF}}{60} = \frac{125 \times 10}{60} = \frac{125}{6} \quad \begin{array}{r} 20.8 \\ 6 \overline{\smash{)}125.0} \\ \underline{12} \\ 5\,0 \\ \underline{4\,8} \\ 2 \end{array}$$

Set the rate at 21 gtt/min.

3. Logic: Cefazolin (Kefzol) may be administered IVPB in 50–100 ml D5W or NS. No time for infusion is given. You have a reconstitution device. Use 50 ml D5W. You have tubing (1 ml = 10 gtt). Administer over 30 minutes.

   Use the reconstitution device to add 1 g of cefazolin to 50 ml D5W. Label the bag.

$$\frac{\# \text{ ml} \times \text{TF}}{30} = \text{gtt/min} \qquad \frac{50 \times 10}{30} = \frac{50}{3} = 16.6 \text{ gtt/min}$$

   Set the drip rate at 17 gtt/min.

4. Logic: The order agrees with the literature directions.

   Using the reconstitution device add 1 g of kanamycin to 400 ml D5W. (You will use a 500-ml D5W bag and aseptically remove 100 ml.) Label the bag.

$$\frac{\# \text{ ml} \times \text{TF}}{\# \text{ min}} = \frac{\overset{4}{\cancel{400}} \times 10}{\underset{1}{\cancel{100}}} = 40 \text{ gtt/min}$$

   Set the rate at 40 gtt/min.

PRACTICE EXERCISE 4

1. Logic: There is 500 ml to be administered at 30 ml/hr.

$$\frac{\# \text{ ml}}{\# \text{ hr}} = \frac{500}{30} = \frac{50}{3} \quad \begin{array}{r} 16.6 \\ 3 \overline{\smash{)}50.0} \end{array}$$

   The IV will last about 16.6 hours.

SELF-TEST 1

1. $\dfrac{\# \text{ ml}}{\# \text{ hr}} = \text{ml/hr}$ $\begin{array}{r} \cancel{1500} \quad 125. \\ 12 \overline{\smash{)}1500.} = 125 \text{ ml/hr} \\ \underline{12} \\ 30 \\ \underline{24} \\ 60 \\ \underline{60} \end{array}$

$$\frac{\# \text{ ml/hr} \times \text{TF}}{\# \text{ min}} = \text{gtt/min} \qquad \frac{125 \times 10}{60} = \frac{125}{6} \quad \begin{array}{r} 20.8 \\ 6 \overline{\smash{)}125.0} \\ \underline{12} \\ 5\,0 \\ \underline{4\,8} \end{array}$$

   21 gtt/min

2. $\dfrac{\# \text{ ml}}{\# \text{ hr}} = \text{ml/hr}$ $\begin{array}{r} \cancel{250} \quad 20.8 \\ 12 \overline{\smash{)}250.0} = 21 \text{ ml/hr} \\ \underline{24} \\ 10\,0 \\ \underline{9\,6} \end{array}$

$$\frac{\# \text{ ml/hr} \times \text{TF}}{\# \text{ min}} = \text{gtt/min} \qquad \frac{21 \times \cancel{60}}{\cancel{60}} = 21 \text{ gtt/min}$$

3. $\dfrac{150 \text{ ml}}{20 \text{ ml/hr}} = \dfrac{15}{2} \overline{)15.0}^{\ 7.5 \text{ hr}}$

   a. The drip rate is 20 ml/hr. No math is necessary.

   Set the infusion pump.

   b. The IV will last approximately $7\dfrac{1}{2}$ hours.

4. Step 1. Determine the solution.

$$\frac{40,000 \text{ units}}{1000 \text{ ml}} = 40 \text{ units/ml}$$

Step 2. $\dfrac{D}{H} \times S = A \qquad \dfrac{\overset{20}{800 \text{ units/hr}}}{\underset{1}{40 \text{ units}}} \times 1 \text{ ml} = 20 \text{ ml/hr}$

5. a. $\dfrac{\overset{10}{1000 \text{ ml}}}{\underset{}{100 \text{ ml/hr}}} = 10 \text{ hr}$

   b. $\dfrac{D}{H} \times S = A \qquad \dfrac{15 \text{ mEq}}{\underset{2}{40 \text{ mEq}}} \times \overset{1}{20} \text{ ml} = \dfrac{15}{2} = 7.5 \text{ ml}$

   c. Microdrip at 100 gtt/min or

   macrodrip $\dfrac{100 \times \overset{1}{20}}{\underset{3}{60}} = \dfrac{100}{3} = 33 \text{ gtt/min}$

   Choose macrodrip at 33 gtt/min.

   d. 33 gtt/min

6. Step 1. Change milligrams to micrograms. Solution is 50 mg in 250 ml.

$$50 \text{ mg} = 50,000 \text{ } \mu\text{g}$$

Step 2. Reduce the solution: $\dfrac{\overset{200}{50,000 \text{ } \mu\text{g}}}{\underset{1}{250 \text{ ml}}} = 200 \text{ } \mu\text{g/ml}$

Step 3. Change milliliters to 60 gtt/min. Solution is 200 μg/60 gtt/min.

Step 4. Determine μg/min. $\dfrac{D}{H} \times S = A$

$\dfrac{\overset{4}{80 \text{ } \mu\text{g}}}{\underset{1}{200 \text{ } \mu\text{g}}} \times 60 \text{ gtt/min} = 24 \text{ gtt/min}$

SELF-TEST 2

1. a. You desire 1 g. Aminophylline comes 1 g in 10 ml. Add 10 ml to the IV of 500 ml D5W and label.

   b. You have an infusion pump; there is no math. Set rate at 75 ml/hr.

2. a. Use the reconstitution device to add 2 g to 100 ml D5W. Label the IV.

b. $\dfrac{\overset{25}{\cancel{100}} \times 10}{\underset{1}{\cancel{40}}} = 25$ gtt/min

3. Step 1. Change milligrams to micrograms.

$1 \text{ mg} = 1000 \ \mu g$

Step 2. Solution is $\dfrac{\cancel{500} \text{ mg}}{\cancel{500} \text{ ml}} = 1 \text{ mg/ml} = 1000 \ \mu g/ml$

Step 3. Change milliliters to 60 gtt/min. Hence, 1000 μg/60 gtt/min is the solution, now

Step 4. $\dfrac{D}{H} \times S = A \qquad \dfrac{\overset{1}{\cancel{250}} \ \mu g}{\underset{\underset{1}{\cancel{4}}}{\cancel{1000}} \ \mu g} \times \overset{15}{\cancel{60}} \text{ gtt/min} = 15 \text{ gtt/min}$

4. First, determine the solution: $\dfrac{\overset{100}{\cancel{25{,}000}} \text{ units}}{\cancel{250} \text{ ml}} = 100 \text{ units/ml}$

Second, $\dfrac{D}{H} \times S = A \qquad \dfrac{\overset{8}{\cancel{800}} \ \cancel{\text{units}}/hr}{100 \ \cancel{\text{units}}} \times 1 \text{ ml} = 8 \text{ ml/hr}$

Set the rate on the pump at 8 ml/hr.

5. $\dfrac{\# \text{ ml}}{\# \text{ hr}} = \text{ml/hr} \qquad \begin{array}{r} \cancel{500} \quad 62.5 \\ 8\ )\overline{500.0} \\ \underline{48} \\ 20 \\ \underline{16} \\ 4\,0 \\ \underline{4\,0} \end{array} = 63 \text{ ml/hr}$

Because it is microdrip tubing, there are 63 gtt/min because ml/hr = gtt/min.

6. Order is in milligrams!

Step 1. Determine the solution.

$1 \text{ g} = 1000 \text{ mg; hence,} \dfrac{\overset{2}{\cancel{1000}} \text{ mg}}{\underset{1}{\cancel{500}} \text{ ml}} = 2 \text{ mg/ml}$

Step 2. Change milliliters to 60 gtt/min. Hence, 2 mg/ml = 2 mg/60 gtt/min.

Step 3. $\dfrac{D}{H} \times S = A \qquad \dfrac{1 \ \cancel{\text{mg}}}{\underset{1}{\cancel{2 \ \text{mg}}}} \times \overset{30}{\cancel{60}} \text{ gtt/min} = 30 \text{ gtt/min}$

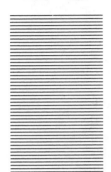

10

Dosage Problems for Infants and Children

In previous chapters we have discussed adult dosages for medications administered orally and parenterally. This chapter considers dosages for infants and children. Because there are wide variations in age, weight, and growth and development within this group, special care must be taken in determining the amount of drug needed to achieve a therapeutic effect.

Before preparing and administering a pediatric order, the nurse determines that the dose is safe for the child. *Safe* means that the amount ordered is not an overdose or an underdose; either may be hazardous. An overdose may produce toxic effects, whereas an underdose may lead to a therapeutic failure. The nurse should check the package insert or another reliable reference.

Manufacturers provide two ways of assessing the safety of a pediatric dose. The more common way is to calculate milligrams per kilograms (mg/kg) of body weight. The second, less used, but more accurate, way is to gauge body surface area (square meters; m^2) by using a scale called a *nomogram*. Additionally, Clark's rule assesses a pediatric dose that is based on the average adult dose and weight. This rule is not as exact as the other two, but it does provide a broad base of comparison for older or less-used drugs that do not have a pediatric dose range listed in the literature.

Keep several equivalents in mind as you begin this chapter.

1 g = 1000 mg

1 kg = 1000 g

1 mg = 1000 μg

1 kg = 2.2 lb

1 tsp = 5 ml

16 oz = 1 lb

Microdrip = 60 gtt/ml

> greater than

< less than

q4° is the abbreviation used for every 4 hours

RULES FOR DETERMINING A SAFE DOSE

Milligrams Per Kilogram

The most common safety check is to multiply milligrams by the child's weight expressed in kilograms. In Table 10-1, the pharmaceutical company gives adult guidelines and pediatric guidelines for methicillin sodium, nafcillin, and oxacillin.

Note that the pediatric dose is given for infants and children weighing less than 40 kg, or 88 lb. When the child is more than that weight, an adult dose is used. For infants and children, methicillin may be given IM 25 mg/kg every 6 hours, but should not be given IV. There is no recommendation for the use of methicillin in neonates.

Nafcillin may be administered IM 25 mg/kg twice daily, and there is a guideline for neonates.

Oxacillin may be given IM or IV 50 mg/kg per day in equal doses every 6 hours for mild to moderate infections, and 100 mg/kg/day IM or IV in equal doses every 4 to 6 hours. Note that the range is 50–100 mg/kg/day. This drug may also be given to premature infants and neonates.

Compare this with Table 10-2, which lists a pediatric dosage guide for cefazolin sodium (Kefzol). The manufacturer gives the child's weight in pounds converted to kilograms. The range is 25 mg/kg/day divided into three or four doses up to 50 mg/kg/day in three or four doses. We are also given the approximate single dose and the amount of fluid to be used for vials of 250-mg and 500-mg powders.

These two tables illustrate the types of information available to the nurse to determine whether or not a dose is safe. How do we use this information?

Step 1. To convert the child's weight from pounds to kilograms:

   a. Divide the number of pounds by 2.2 (2.2 lb = 1 kg). Carry out arithmetic three
       decimal places and round off to two decimal places.

Table 10-1.   Recommended Dosages for Three Parenteral Penicillins

Drug	Adults	Infants and Children < 40 kg (88 lb)	Other Recommendations

Methicillin Sodium	1 gram
	    IM every 4–6 hours
	    IV every 6 hours
		25 mg/kg
		    IM every 6 hours
		    IV not recommended	

Nafcillin	500 mg
	    IM every 4–6 hours
	    IV every 4 hours
	1 gram
	    IM or IV every 4 hours (severe
	        infections)
		25 mg/kg
		    IM twice daily
			Neonates
			    10 mg/kg
			    IM twice daily

Oxacillin	250–500 mg
	    IM or IV every 4–6 hours
	        (mild to moderate infections)
		50 mg/kg/day
		    IM or IV in equally divided doses
		        every 6 hours (mild to
		        moderate infections)	

	1 gram
	    IM or IV every 4–6 hours
	        (severe infections)
		100 mg/kg/day
		    IM or IV in equally divided doses
		        every 4–6 hours (severe
		        infections)
			Premature and neonates
			    25 mg/kg/day
			    IM or IV

Courtesy of Beecham Laboratories.

Table 10-2.   Pediatric Dosage Guide for Cefazolin Sodium (Kefzol)

Weight		25 mg/kg/day Divided Into 3 Doses		25 mg/kg/day Divided Into 4 Doses	
lb	kg	Approximate Single Dose (mg q8h)	Vol. (mL) Needed With Dilution of 125 mg/mL	Approximate Single Dose (mg q6h)	Vol. (mL) Needed With Dilution of 125 mg/mL
10	4.5	40 mg	0.35 mL	30 mg	0.25 mL
20	9	75 mg	0.6 mL	55 mg	0.45 mL
30	13.6	115 mg	0.9 mL	85 mg	0.7 mL
40	18.1	150 mg	1.2 mL	115 mg	0.9 mL
50	22.7	190 mg	1.5 mL	140 mg	1.1 mL

Weight		50 mg/kg/day Divided Into 3 Doses		50 mg/kg/day Divided Into 4 Doses	
lb	kg	Approximate Single Dose (mg q8h)	Vol. (mL) Needed With Dilution of 225 mg/mL	Approximate Single Dose (mg q6h)	Vol. (mL) Needed With Dilution of 225 mg/mL
10	4.5	75 mg	0.35 mL	55 mg	0.25 mL
20	9	150 mg	0.7 mL	110 mg	0.5 mL
30	13.6	225 mg	1 mL	170 mg	0.75 mL
40	18.1	300 mg	1.35 mL	225 mg	1 mL
50	22.7	375 mg	1.7 mL	285 mg	1.25 mL

Courtesy of Smith Kline & French Laboratories.

(continued)

EXAMPLE: 25 lb = _____ kg

$$2.2\overline{)25.0\,000} = 11.36 \text{ kg}$$

$$
\begin{array}{r}
11.363 \\
2.2\,)\,25.0\,000 \\
\underline{22} \\
3\,0 \\
\underline{2\,2} \\
8\,0 \\
\underline{6\,6} \\
1\,40 \\
\underline{1\,32} \\
80
\end{array}
$$

b. Change ounces to a part of a pound by dividing by 16 (16 oz = 1 lb). Carry out arithmetic three places and round off to two places.

EXAMPLE: 24 lb 3 oz = _____ kg

$$\frac{3\ oz}{16\ oz}\,)\,3.000 = 0.19 \text{ lb}$$

$$
\begin{array}{r}
.186 \\
16\ oz\,)\,3.000 \\
\underline{1\,6} \\
1\,40 \\
\underline{1\,28} \\
120 \\
\underline{96}
\end{array}
$$

Hence, 24 lb 3 oz = 24.19 lb. Change this to kilograms.

(continued)

(*continued*)

$$2.2 \overline{)24.1\,900} \quad \frac{10.995}{} = 11 \text{ kg (too close to keep a decimal)}$$

$$\begin{array}{r} 2 \\ \hline 2\ 1\ 9 \\ 1\ 9\ 8 \\ \hline 2\ 10 \\ 1\ 98 \\ \hline 120 \\ \underline{110} \end{array}$$

c. Mentally form an idea of what the kilogram should be as a check. If 2.2 lb = 1 kg, then your answer in kilograms should be a little less than half the number of pounds.

d. You may wish to use a calculator in working out pediatric dosage.

Exercise 1 at the end of this section will test your understanding of these conversions.

Step 2. Identify the dose or the minimum–maximum dose range from the literature.

> **EXAMPLE:**
>
> A child weighing 30 lb has an order for cefazolin (Kefzol) 170 mg IM q6h. Is the dose safe (see Table 10–2)? The range is 25–50 mg/kg/day divided into three or four doses.

Step 3. Multiply the child's weight in kilograms by the range.

30 lb = 13.64 kg

$$\begin{array}{lll} \text{Range} & 25 \text{ mg} & \text{to} & 50 \text{ mg} \\ & \underline{\times\ 13.64 \text{ kg}} & & \underline{\times\ 13.64 \text{ kg}} \\ & 341 \text{ mg/day} & \text{to} & 682 \text{ mg/day} \end{array}$$

Step 4. Compare the ordered amount with the literature to decide if the dose is safe. Order is 170 mg q6h. This means the child receives four doses.

$$\begin{array}{r} 170 \text{ mg} \\ \underline{\times\ 4} \\ 680 \text{ mg} \end{array}$$

The child's order is 680 mg/day. The range is 341–682 mg/day. The order is written within the safe range.

> **EXAMPLE:**
>
> A child weighing 44 lb is ordered nafcillin 0.25 g IM q12h (see Table 10-1). Is the dose safe?
>
> Step 1.   Convert pounds to kilograms
>
> $$2.2 \overline{)44.0} \quad \frac{20.}{} = 20 \text{ kg}$$
> $$\underline{44}$$
>
> Step 2.   Idenitfy the safe dose in the literature (25 mg/kg IM twice a day).
> Step 3.   Multiply the child's weight in kilograms by the safe dose.

(continued)

$$\begin{array}{r} 25 \text{ mg} \\ \underline{\times\ 20 \text{ kg}} \\ 500 \text{ mg/day to be given in two doses} \end{array}$$

Step 4.   Compare the ordered amount with the literature to decide if the dose is safe. Order is 0.25 g IM q12h

$$\begin{array}{r} 0.25 \text{ g} = 250 \text{ mg} \\ \underline{\times\ \ 2 \text{ doses}} \\ 500 \text{ mg} \end{array}$$

The dose is safe. The literature calls for 500 mg/day and the dose is 500 mg/day.

Whenever you determine that the dose ordered is not safe because it is too high or too low, hold the order and consult with the physician who wrote the order. The physician may change the order, explain the reason for the order, or reject your inquiry. If the latter should occur, report your concern to your immediate supervisor.

EXAMPLE:

An 11-lb infant is ordered ampicillin sodium 250 mg IV q6h. Literature states 200 mg/kg/day in divided doses.

1.   Is the dose safe?
2.   If safe, how would you prepare the dose? Ampicillin comes as a powder labeled 500 mg. Directions say to add 1.8 ml sterile water for injection to make a solution of 250 mg/ml. Use within 1 hour.

Step 1. $2.2\overline{)11.0} = 5$ kg

Step 2.   Safe dose is $\begin{array}{r} 200 \text{ mg/kg/day} \\ \underline{\times\ 5 \text{ kg}} \\ 1000 \text{ mg/kg/day} \end{array}$

Step 3.   Infant is receiving 250 mg q6h (i.e., four doses); hence the infant is getting 1000 mg/day.

Step 4.   The dose is safe; the safe dose is 1000 mg/day. Infant is receiving 1000 mg/day.

Step 5.   Dilution and number of milliliters: 1.8 ml sterile water for injection

Solution made and new stock: 250 mg/ml

Rule and arithmetic:

$\dfrac{D}{H} \times S = A$ Not necessary: order is 250 mg, solution is 250 mg/ml.

Prepare 1 ml for IV use.

Storage: No. Directions say to use within 1 hour. Discard the remainder.

=================== EXERCISE 1 ===================

Convert pounds to kilograms. Answers will be found at the end of the chapter.

1. 30 lb   = _____ kg   **4.** 22 lb   = _____ kg

2. 15 lb 5 oz = _____ kg   **5.** 54 lb 8 oz = _____ kg

3. $7\frac{1}{4}$ lb   = _____ kg

=================== SELF-TEST 1 ===================

In these practice problems, determine if the following doses are safe. Answers may be found at the end of the chapter.

1. Order: vancomycin 105 mg IV q8h in D5 $\frac{1}{3}$ NS
   Patient: 1-year-old weighing 15 lb
   Literature: 44 mg/kg in divided doses IV

2. Order: Augmentin 175 mg po q8h
   Patient: child weighing 29 lb
   Literature: 40 mg/kg/day in divided doses

3. Order: Amantadine HCl 35 mg po tid
   Patient: child weighing 35 lb, aged 3 years
   Literature: 4.4–8.8 mg/kg/day po in three divided doses, not to exceed 150 mg/day

4. Order: cefuroxime 210 mg in 50 ml D5 $\frac{1}{3}$ NS q8h
   Patient: infant weighing 4.8 kg
   Literature: 75 mg/kg/day

Body Surface Area

The second method of estimating a safe child's dose is to obtain the child's height in feet, inches, or centimeters; his weight in pounds or kilograms; and, using a scale called a nomogram, determine the body surface area (BSA). Look at Figure 10-1. What is the surface area in square meters (m^2) of a baby 10 inches long and weighing 3 kg? Use a ruler or a straight line to connect 10 inches and 3 kg. The point at which this line intersects the surface area line is the surface area in square meters (0.13 m^2). Body surface area is used most often to calculate doses of cancer drugs for children.

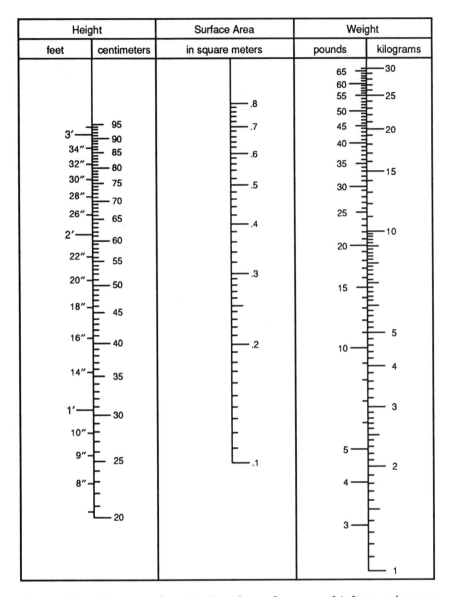

Figure 10-1. *Nomogram for estimating the surface area of infants and young children. To determine the surface area, draw a straight line between the point representing the height on the left vertical scale to the point representing the weight on the right vertical scale. The point at which this line intersects the middle vertical scale represents surface area in* m². *(Courtesy of Abbott Laboratories.)*

RULE FOR CHILD'S DOSE IN SQUARE METERS

When the child's dose is not known, but the adult dose *is* known, this formula can be used.

$$\frac{\text{Child's BSA in m}^2}{1.7 \text{ average adult BSA}} \times \text{adult dose} = \text{child's dose}$$

(continued)

(continued)

EXAMPLE:

An adult dose is 250 mg. What is a safe dose for a child weighing 15 lb with a height of 20 inches? See the nomogram—the BSA of the child is 0.28 m².

Rule: $\dfrac{\text{Child BSA m}^2}{1.7} \times 250 = \text{child's dose}$

$\dfrac{0.28 \text{ m}^2}{1.7} \times 250 = \dfrac{70}{1.7} = 41 \text{ mg}$

EXAMPLE:

An adult dose of a drug is 4 g/day. What would be a safe dose for a child with a BSA of 0.6 m²?

Rule: $\dfrac{0.6 \text{ m}^2}{1.7} \times 4 \text{ g/day} = \dfrac{2.4}{1.7} = 1.4 \text{ g/day}$

SELF-TEST 2

In these practice problems, use body surface area to determine the safe dose. Answers may be found at the end of the chapter.

1. Order: CeeNU (lomustine) 95 mg po q6h
    Available: capsules 5, 10, 40, 100 mg
    Child weighs 55 lb and is 34 inches high.
    Is the dose safe? How would you administer?
    Literature states: 130 mg/m² po q6h

2. Order: etoposide 22 mg IV qd × 4 days
    Available: vial of 20 mg/ml
    Child weighs 20 kg; height 80 cm
    Is the dose safe? What amount would you prepare for administration?
    Literature states: 35 mg/m²/day × 4 days IV to 50 mg/m²/day × 5 days IV

3. Order: acyclovir 165 mg IV q8h over 1 hr in D5$\frac{1}{2}$NS
    Available: vial of 500 mg/10 ml
    Child is 1 year; weighs 55 lb; height is 30 inches
    Is the dose safe? What amount of drug would you prepare?
    Literature states: <12 years IV 250 mg/m² over 1 hr q8h × 1 wk. Make the concentration no greater than 7 mg/ml.

Clark's Rule

This formula can give the nurse a *general idea* of the safety of a child's dose *when the only information available is the average adult dose.* The nurse weighs the child in pounds. The child's dose is based on the comparison of the child's weight with an average adult weight of 150 lb.

Rule: $\dfrac{\text{Child's weight in lb}}{\text{Av adult weight 150 lb}} \times \text{Average adult dose} = \text{child's dose}$

EXAMPLE:

Suppose you knew an average adult dose was 0.4 mg IM. You have an order to give a child 0.25 mg. Is the dose safe? The child weighs 40 lb.

Clark: $\dfrac{40 \text{ lb}}{150 \text{ lb}} \times 0.4 \text{ mg} = \dfrac{16}{150} \overline{)\dfrac{.106}{16.000}} = 0.11 \text{ mg}$

Because the order is over twice the estimated dose when using Clark's rule, check with the physician.

EXAMPLE:

Order: morphine SO_4 4 mg SC q4h prn

Child is 50 lb; age 6 years. Average adult dose is 15 mg SC q4h prn.

By using Clark's rule, decide if this is a safe dose.

$$\dfrac{\overset{1}{\cancel{50 \text{ lb}}}}{\underset{\underset{1}{3}}{\cancel{150 \text{ lb}}}} \times \overset{1}{\cancel{15}} \text{ mg} = 5 \text{ mg}$$

Clark's rule indicates that, in this case, this is a safe dose range because it is less than 5 mg.

═══ SELF-TEST 3 ═══

In these practice problems, use Clark's rule to decide if the following orders are safe doses. Answers will be found at the end of the chapter.

1. Order: phenobarbital 15 mg IM stat
   Baby is 1 year old, weighs 22 lb.
   Usual adult sedative dose is 100 mg.
   Is this a safe dose?

2. Order: Keflin 100 mg IM q6h
   Infant is 4 months old; weighs 25 lb.
   Usual adult dose is 1 g IM q4–6h.
   Is this a safe dose?

(continued)

===================== **SELF-TEST 3** (*Continued*) =====================

3. Order: meperidine HCl 3 mg IM stat
Infant is 4 months old; weighs 10 lb.
Usual adult dose is 50–100 mg IM q4h prn
Is this a safe dose?

========= **DOSAGE CALCULATIONS FOR ORAL ADMINISTRATION** =========

Calculate the following doses. Answers may be found at the end of the chapter. Indicate which rule you used to check the safety of these orders—mg/kg, BSA, or Clark's rule.

1. Order: ethambutal 300 mg po qd
Stock: 100-mg scored tabs
Literature states: 13 years give 15 mg/kg/day
Child is 14 years old and weighs 90 lb.
  a.   Which rule did you use?
  b.   Is the order safe?
  c.   How many tablets would you administer?

2. Order: e1 of ferrous sulfate 200 mg po tid
Stock: bottle of 125 mg/5 ml
Child is 9 years old and weighs 30 kg.
Literature states: children 6–12 years old, 600 mg divided doses tid.
  a.   Is the dose safe?
  b.   How many milliliters would you pour?

3. Order: amoxacillin oral suspension 100 mg po q8h
Stock: bottle of powder labeled unit dose 125 mg; to prepare, add 5 ml water and shake well.
Baby weighs 15 kg.
Literature states: 20–40 mg/kg/day in divided doses
  a.   Is dose safe?
  b.   What would you pour?
  c.   Which rule did you use?

4. Order: Tylenol 80 mg po q4° prn temp 100.9°
Stock: chewable tablets 80 mg
Child is 6 years old; weighs 20.5 kg.
Literature states for child 6–8 years give four tablets. May repeat four or five times daily. Not to exceed five doses in 24 hours.
Is dose safe?

5. Order: Slo-Phyllin 110 mg po q8h
Stock: 160 mg/15 ml
Child is 6 years old; weighs 28 kg.
Literature states: child po 50–100 mg q6h not to exceed 12 mg/kg/24 hour.

    a. Is dose safe?

    b. What would you pour?

    c. Which rule did you use?

6. A 48-lb child who weighs 21.8 kg and has a BSA of 0.84 m^2 is ordered secobarbital 50 mg PO. If the adult dose is 100 mg, is this a safe dose? Which is the *best* rule to follow?

7. Order: vitamin K 5 mg po bid
Stock: 5-mg tablets
Child weighs 65 lb. Suppose there is no statement in the references on pediatric doses. Adult dose is 5–10 mg po daily.
Which rule would you use?
Is this dose safe according to the rule?

8. Order: Lanoxin 0.045 mg po qd
Stock: liquid in a dropper bottle 0.05 mg/l cc
Dose is safe. How much would you prepare?

9. Order: acetaminophen liquid 100 mg po q4h prn. Temp 100.8°
Stock: liquid in a dropper bottle 80 mg/0.8 cc
Dose is safe. How much would you prepare?

10. Order: Slo-Phyllin 35 mg po q4h
Stock: liquid in a bottle labeled 80 mg/15 ml
Dose is safe. How much would you prepare?

═══ DOSAGE CALCULATIONS FOR INJECTIONS FROM LIQUIDS ═══

Calculate these doses. Decide if the dose is safe. Answers may be found at the end of the chapter.

1. Order: Terramycin 150 mg IM q8h
Stock: 100 mg/2-ml ampule; 250 mg/2-ml ampule; 50-mg/ml vial
Child: 10 years old; weighs 60 lb
Literature states: Children above 8 years of age: 15–25 mg/kg body weight up to a maximum of 250 mg per single daily injection. Dose may be divided into 8- to 12-hour intervals.
    a. Is dose safe?
    b. What amount would you prepare?

2. Order: digitoxin 0.02 mg IM qd
Stock: 0.05 mg/ml
Child: 6.8 kg
Literature states: maintenance 0.003 mg/kg qd or 0.75 mg/m^2 qd.
    a. Is dose safe?
    b. What amount would you prepare?

(continued)

‾DOSAGE CALCULATIONS FOR INJECTIONS FROM LIQUIDS (*Continued*) ‾

3. Order: doxycycline hyclate 100 mg po q12h today, then 100 mg po qd
   Stock: syrup labeled 50 mg/ml
   Child: 54 kg
   Literature states: child > 45 kg same as adult. Adult 100 mg q12h first day followed by 100 mg
                    daily.
     a. Is dose safe?
     b. What amount would you prepare?

4. Order: Narcan neonatal 1 mg IV stat; physician to administer
   Stock: ampule 2 mg (2-cc size)
   Infant weighs 2000 g
   Literature states: range 0.5 mg/kg.
     a. Is dose safe?
     b. What amount would you prepare?

5. Order: clindamycin PO_4 90 mg IM q6h
   Stock: 150 mg/ml
   Child: BSA = 0.8 m^2
   Literature states: 350 mg/m^2/day to a maximum of 450 mg/m^2/day for a child.
     a. Is dose safe?
     b. What amount would you prepare?

6. Order: lincomycin 50 mg IM q6h
   Stock: 300 mg/ml
   Literature states: 20 mg/kg/24 hour.
   Child weighs 12 lb 6 oz
     a. Is dose safe?

7. Order: kanamycin 15 mg IM q12h
   Stock: pediatric injection 75 mg/2 ml
   Infant: weighs 4 lb 4 oz
   Literature states: See Table 10-3.

**Table 10-3. Pediatric Dosage Guide
for Kanamycin (Kantrex)***

Weight (lb)	Weight (kg)	Daily Dosage (mg)	Daily Dosage (ml)
2.2	1.00	15.0	0.4
2.8	1.25	18.8	0.5
3.3	1.50	22.5	0.6
3.9	1.75	26.2	0.7
4.4	2.00	30.0	0.8
5.0	2.25	33.8	0.9
5.5	2.50	37.5	1.0
6.0	2.75	41.2	1.1
6.6	3.00	45.0	1.2
7.7	3.50	52.5	1.4
8.8	4.00	60.0	1.6
9.9	4.50	67.5	1.8
11.0	5.00	75.0	2.0

Courtesy of Bristol Laboratories.

a. Is dose safe?

b. What amount would you prepare?

8. Order: diazepam 1 mg IM q3–4h prn

Stock: vial 5 mg/1 ml

Infant 30 days old

Literature states: child < 6 mo IM 1–2.5 mg tid or qid.

a. Is dose safe?

b. How much will you prepare?

9. Order: Mefoxin 250 mg IM q6h

Stock: vial of powder labeled 1 g. Directions: dissolve with 2 ml to make a solution of 400 mg/ml.

Child: 3 years of age; weight 12 kg

Literature states: children 3 months of age and older 80–160 mg/kg of body weight per day divided into four to six equal doses.

a. Is dose safe?

b. How much will you prepare?

10. Order: cefazolin 150 mg IM q8h

Stock: 500-mg vial of powder. Directions say to add 2 ml to make a solution of 225 mg/ml.

Child: 20 lb (9 kg)

Literature states: See Table 10-2.

a. Is dose safe?

b. How much will you prepare?

DOSAGE CALCULATIONS FOR INTRAVENOUS AND INTERMITTENT INTRAVENOUS ADMINISTRATION

Intravenous fluids are administered when the child cannot maintain a normal oral intake or when the child has a fluid and electrolyte imbalance. Intravenous bags of 250 ml or less are used to prevent an accidental fluid overload. In addition, Buretrols are used because they contain chambers that hold no more than 100 to 150 ml at a time. Whenever possible, the IV is set up with an infusion pump to provide another safeguard in administering fluid. In neonatal areas, syringe pumps can deliver very small amounts in syringes, which may range from 1 to 60 ml.

Dosages for IVPB medications are calculated in milligrams per kilogram. The manufacturer will indicate the minimum dilution that is safe. Remember that pediatric nurses give IVPB medications to children who range in weight from the premature infant to a teenager. The IVPB medications must be diluted in differing amounts to meet the fluid restrictions of each age group. A general rule of thumb for IVPB medication dilution is to read the dilution for direct IV or IV push. This is the minimum for safety. As you read the manufacturer's directions for dilution, note the following:

1. *Minimal milligram per milliliter concentration.* The drug must be diluted in at least this amount. A solution that is too concentrated may cause toxic effects.
2. *Minimal milligram per time.* This is the shortest interval over which the drug may be given. If the drug is administered too rapidly, it may cause toxic effects.
3. *Incompatibilities.* Observe the lists of fluids and drugs that must not be administered with the ordered drug.
4. Once the minimum dilution has been met, the drug may be further diluted as necessary.

One last point of great importance: when the entire vial of medication is not used, you must first follow the directions for dilution given by the manufacturer, and then, once the initial dilution is made, withdraw the amount of drug needed and dilute further if necessary.

Many institutions have established guidelines to assist doctors and nurses in pediatric dosage (Table 10-4). If necessary, review Chapter 9 on IV and IVPB medications.

IV AND IVPB DOSAGE PROBLEMS

For the following problems you will be asked how to prepare the intravenous order. Answers will be found at the end of the chapter.

1. Infant weighing 4.3 kg
    Order: IV D5 0.2 NS + 15 mEq KCl/L at 18 cc/hr
    Stock: 250 ml bag D5 0.2 NS; vial of KCl labeled 20 mEq/10 ml; Buretrol; infusion pump
    How would you prepare and administer this IV?

2. Infant weighing 4.3 kg

    Order: ampicillin 100 mg/kg/day = 100 mg in 15 cc D5 $\frac{1}{4}$ NS q6h

    Stock: D5$\frac{1}{4}$ NS; syringe pump (can use a 1-cc syringe to a 60-cc syringe); vial of ampicillin powder labeled 500 mg

    Directions: Add 1.8 ml sterile water for injection to make 250 mg/ml; use within 1 hour (see guidelines in Table 10-4).
    a.   Is this a safe order?
    b.   How should the order be administered?

3. Infant 6.77 kg
    Order: Septra 40 mg (2.5 cc) IV (based on trimethoprim component); bid in 50 ml D5W over 1 hour
    Stock: 250-ml bag D5W; Buretrol; ampule of Septra labeled 5 ml containing trimethoprim 80 mg and sulfamethoxazole 400 mg; infusion pump (see guidelines in Table 10-4)

Table 10-4.   Guidelines for Administration of Selected Intravenous Pediatric Medications

Drug	Maximum Dose	IV Push	IVPB Dilution and Rate
Aminophylline	10 mg/kg/dose for loading; 4–6 mg/kg/dose for loading in neonates	No	Dilute with at least an equal volume of IV fluid. Infuse over 20–30 min
Ampicillin sodium	400 mg/kg/day; 200 mg/kg/day in neonates	Not >100 mg/min	Minimum dilution 1 g/10 ml over 20–30 min (maximum 1 hr)
Gentamicin sulfate	2.5 mg/kg/dose; 2.5 mg/kg/q12h for neonates	No	Concentration not >1 mg/ml over 30–120 min
Isoproterenol	1 µg/kg/min	No	5 ml (1 mg) in 100 ml; infuse at 0.02–0.05 µg/kg/min
Lidocaine hydrochloride	1.5 mg/kg/dose up to 88 µg/kg/min	1 mg/kg over 2 min	20–50 µg/kg/min
Trimethoprim-sulfamethoxazole	20 mg/kg/day; 100 mg/kg/day	No	Minimum dilution is 1 ml in 15 ml D5W over 60–90 min

a. Is this dose safe?

b. How would you prepare the order?

4. 6-year-old weighing 20.5 kg

Order: IV D5 $\frac{1}{3}$ NS + 10 mEq KCl/L at 35 cc/hr (maintenance)

Stock: 1000-ml bag D5 $\frac{1}{3}$ NS; KCl 40 mEq/20 ml; infusion pump; Buretrol (100-ml chamber)

How will you set this up?

5. 18-year-old weighing 73.6 kg

Order: Give bolus of IV aminophylline 50 mg in 50 cc D5W to run in over 30 minutes

Stock: 50-ml bag D5W; infusion pump; vial of aminophylline labeled 250 mg/10 ml (see guidelines in Table 10-4)

a. Is the dose safe?

b. How would you prepare the order?

6. 18-year-old weighing 73.6 kg

Order: gentamicin 75 mg IVPB q8h

Stock: vial of gentamicin 40 mg/ml; secondary infusion set (10 gtt/ml); 100-ml D5W bag; infusion pump

PDR: Adult dose is 3 mg/kg/day q8h, evenly divided. Dilute in 50 to 200 ml with isotonic saline or D5W. Infuse over 30 minutes to 2 hours. Pediatric guidelines state that the concentration should not be greater than 1 mg/ml.

a. Is the dose safe?

b. How will you prepare for IVPB? Dilute in 100 ml and give over 1 hour.

7. Child weighs 20 lb

Order: isoproterenol HCl 1 mg in 100 ml D5W; run 1.8 μg/min

Stock: Vial of isoproterenol 1 mg/5 ml; 100-ml bag D5W; Buretrol (60 gtt/ml); infusion pump (see guidelines in Table 10-4)

a. Does the dilution meet guidelines for pediatric dosage?

b. What is the drip factor?

8. Child weighs 20 lb

Order: lidocaine 100 mg in 250 ml D5W TRA 400 μg/min (TRA is interpreted "to run at")

Stock: 250-ml bag D5W; vial of lidocaine 2% (100 mg/5 ml); (see guidelines in Table 10-4); Buretrol (60 gtt/min); infusion pump

a. Does the dose meet the guidelines for IVPB drip?

b. What is the drip factor?

ASSORTED DOSAGE PROBLEMS

As you develop proficiency in solving pediatric problems, you will be able to calculate many answers without written work. Here is a drill to sharpen your skill. Use a calculator when the solution is not obvious. Answers will be found at the end of the chapter.

(continued)

ASSORTED DOSAGE PROBLEMS (Continued)

1. 10-kg boy with otitis media
   Order: amoxicillin 125 mg po q8h for 10 days
   Stock: bottle labeled amoxicillin 125 mg/5 ml
   Safe range: 20–40 mg/kg/day in divided doses q8h
   Is this dose safe?

2. 9.5-kg girl with febrile seizures
   Order: phenobarbital elixir po 20 mg q12h
   Stock: bottle labeled 20 mg/5 ml
   Safe range: 4–6 mg/kg/day in divided doses q12h
   Is this dose safe?

3. 6-year-old boy weighing 22 kg with asthma
   Order: Proventil elixir 2 mg po q8h
   Stock: bottle labeled 2 mg/5 ml
   Therapeutic dose: The usual starting dosage for children 6 years of age and older is 2 mg (1
   teaspoonful) three or four times a day.

4. 15-year-old boy, 58 kg, with a urinary tract infection
   Order: prophylactic Septra (160 mg TMP/800 mg SMZ) tabs; double-strength 1 tab q12h po
   Stock: tablets labeled Septra Double-Strength
   Therapeutic dose: The usual adult dose in the treatment of urinary tract infection is one Septra DS
   tablet, two Septra tablets, or 4 teaspoonsful (20 ml) Septra Suspension every 12
   hours for 10–14 days.

5. 8-year-old boy, 26 kg, with rheumatic fever
   Order: prophylactic penicillin benzathine 1.2 MU q28d IM
   Stock: vial labeled 600,000 units/ml
   Therapeutic dose: IM 1.2 million units in a single dose q month or 600,000 units q2wk
   a.   Is the dose safe?
   b.   How many milliliters will you administer?

6. 6-year-old girl, 20 kg, with laceration of cheek requiring sutures
   Order: preop medication; Demerol 40 mg; Phenergan 20 mg; Thorazine 20 mg; to be given deep IM
   in a single shot.
   Stock: vials of Demerol HCl 100 mg/ml; Phenergan 50 mg/ml; Thorazine 25 mg/ml
   The dose is safe and no incompatibility will result in combining these drugs in one syringe. What
   amount will you prepare in the syringe?

7. A 17-year-old boy with primary syphilis, weighing 48 kg.
   Order: penicillin G benzathine 2.4 MU IM × 1
   Stock: vial labeled 600,000 units/ml
   Therapeutic dose: literature states IM 50,000 U/kg in a single dose.
   a.   Is the dose safe?
   b.   How many milliliters will you administer?

8. A 3-week-old infant, 4 kg, with fever of unknown origin

   Order: gentamicin 10 mg IV q12h in D5 $\frac{1}{4}$ NS

   Stock: vial labeled Garamycin Pediatric (gentamicin sulfate) 10 mg/ml; syringe pump (ml/hr) (see
   guidelines in Table 10-4).

a. Is this dose safe?

b. How would you prepare this order for administration?

9. A 3-year-old, weight 12 kg, with a reaction to Pen-Vee K

Order: Benadryl 15 mg deep IM q6h

Stock: 50 mg/ml

Therapeutic dose: literature states 5 mg/kg/day in divided doses not to exceed 300 mg/day.

a. Is this dose safe?

b. What amount would you prepare?

10. A 3-year-old with new onset of juvenile and rheumatoid arthritis of knees and ankles; weight 13 kg

Order: aspirin 200 mg q4h po 15–30 minutes after a meal

Stock: tablets 0.2 g

Therapeutic range: literature states 60–90 mg/kg/day; increase at weekly intervals to 80–100 mg/kg/day.

a. Is this dose safe?

ANSWERS

EXERCISE 1

1.
$$2.2\overline{)30.0\,000} = 13.64 \text{ kg}$$

$$\begin{array}{r} 13.636 \\ \hline 2.2)30.0\,000 \\ 22 \\ \hline 8\,0 \\ 6\,6 \\ \hline 1\,4\,0 \\ 1\,3\,2 \\ \hline 80 \\ 66 \\ \hline 140 \end{array}$$

2. $\dfrac{.5 \text{ oz}}{16 \text{ oz}} = 16\overline{)5.000}\ \dfrac{.312}{} = 0.31 \text{ lb}$

Weight is 15.31 lb

Change to kilogram

$$\begin{array}{r} 6.958 \\ \hline 2.2)15.3\,1000 \\ 13\,2 \\ \hline 2\,1\ 1 \\ 1\,9\ 8 \\ \hline 1\ 30 \\ 1\ 10 \\ \hline 200 \\ 176 \end{array} = 6.96 \text{ kg}$$

3. $\dfrac{1}{4} = 0.25 \text{ lb}$

7.25 lb ÷ 2.2

$$\begin{array}{r} 3.295 \\ \hline 2.2)7.2\,500 \\ 6\,6 \\ \hline 6\ 5 \\ 4\ 4 \\ \hline 2\ 10 \\ 1\ 98 \\ \hline 120 \\ 110 \end{array} = 3.3 \text{ kg}$$

4.
$$2.2\overline{)22.0} = 10 \text{ kg}$$

$$\begin{array}{r} 10. \\ \hline 2.2)22.0 \\ 22 \end{array}$$

5. $\dfrac{8 \text{ oz}}{16 \text{ oz}} = \dfrac{1}{2} = 0.5 \text{ lb}$

54.5 lb ÷ 2.2

$$\begin{array}{r} 24.772 \\ \hline 2.2)54.5\,000 \\ 44 \\ \hline 10\ 5 \\ 8\ 8 \\ \hline 1\ 70 \\ 1\ 54 \\ \hline 160 \\ 154 \\ \hline 60 \\ 44 \end{array} = 24.77 \text{ kg}$$

SELF-TEST 1

1. Step 1.   15 lb = _____ kg

$$
\begin{array}{r}
6\,.\,818 \\
2.2_{\!\diagup}\,\overline{)15.\underset{\diagup}{0}\,000}} = 6.82\ \text{kg} \\
\underline{13\ 2}\ \ \ \ \ \ \ \\
1\ 8\ \ 0\ \ \ \ \\
\underline{1\ 7\ \ 6}\ \ \ \ \\
4 0\ \ \\
\underline{2 2}\ \ \\
1 8 0 \\
\underline{1 7 6}
\end{array}
$$

Step 2.
$$
\begin{array}{r}
44\ \text{mg/kg} \\
\times\ 6.82\ \text{kg} \\
\hline
300\ \text{mg/day (calculator)} = \text{safe dose}
\end{array}
$$

Step 3.
$$
\begin{array}{r}
105\ \text{mg} \\
\times\ 3 \\
\hline
315\ \text{mg} = \text{ordered dose}
\end{array}
$$

Step 4.   Order is over the safe dose. Check with the physician.

2. Step 1.   29 lb = 13.18 kg (calculator)

Step 2.
$$
\begin{array}{r}
40\ \text{mg} \\
\times\ 13.18\ \text{kg} \\
\hline
527\ \text{mg (calculator)} = \text{safe dose}
\end{array}
$$

Step 3.
$$
\begin{array}{r}
175\ \text{mg} \\
\times\ 3 \\
\hline
525\ \text{mg} = \text{child's dose}
\end{array}
$$

Step 4.   Order is safe.

3. Step 1.   35 lb = 15.9 kg (calculator)

Step 2.
$$
\begin{array}{rcl}
4.4\ \text{mg} & \text{to} & 8.8\ \text{mg} \\
\times\ 15.9\ \text{kg} & & 15.9\ \text{kg} \\
\hline
70\ \text{mg/day} & & 140\ \text{mg/day} \\
\text{(calculator)} & & \text{(calculator)}
\end{array}
$$

Step 3.
$$
\begin{array}{r}
35\ \text{mg (order)} \\
\times\ 3 \\
\hline
105\ \text{mg (child's dose)}
\end{array}
$$

Step 4.   Dose is safe.

4. Step 1.   Not necessary, 4.8 kg given

Step 2.
$$\begin{array}{r} 4.8 \text{ kg} \\ \times\ 75\ \text{ mg} \\ \hline 360 \text{ mg/day} = \text{safe dose} \end{array}$$

Step 3.
$$\begin{array}{r} 210 \text{ mg} \\ \times\ \ 3 \text{ doses} \\ \hline 630 \text{ mg/day} = \text{child's dose} \end{array}$$

Step 4.   Dose is beyond safe range. Check with the physician.

SELF-TEST 2

1. Weight 55 lb; height 34 in = 0.72 m²
Literature states 130 mg/m² po q6h
130 mg × 0.72 = 93.6 = 94 mg. Order is safe.
Prepare two 40-mg tabs, plus one 10-mg tab, plus one 5-mg tab

2. Weight 20 kg; height 80 cm = 0.62 m²
Literature gives range of 35–50 mg/m²/day
35 × 0.62 = 22 mg   50 × 0.62 = 31 mg
Therefore, for this child a range of 22–31 mg/day is safe.
Dose is safe.

The drug comes 20 mg/ml, so $\dfrac{22}{20} \times 1$ ml = 1.1 ml

3. Weight 55 lb; height 30 in = 0.66 m²
Literature says <12 years 250 mg/m² IV over 1 hour
Therefore, for this child 250 mg × 0.66 = 165 mg.
Dose is safe.

Drug comes 500 mg/10 ml, so $\dfrac{165}{500} \times 10 = \dfrac{165}{50} = 3.3$ ml

Add 3.3 ml to 50 ml D5 $\dfrac{1}{2}$ NS and administer over 1 hour

SELF-TEST 3

1. $\dfrac{22}{150} \times 100$ mg = 14.7 mg.

Dose of 15 mg is safe according to Clark's rule. Use this rule only when there is no literature using BSA or milligrams per kilogram.

2. $\dfrac{25}{150} \times 1000$ mg = 167 mg

Dose of 100 mg is low by Clark's rule. However, this rule is not as exact as use of milligrams per kilogram. Check further.

3. $\dfrac{10}{150} \times 50$ mg = 3.3 mg

Dose of 3 mg is safe according to Clark's rule.

DOSAGE CALCULATIONS FOR ORAL ADMINISTRATION

1. a. Use the rule for milligrams per kilogram.

   Step 1.   Convert pounds to kilograms.

$$2.2\overline{)90.00}\ \begin{array}{r}40.9\\ \hline \end{array} = 41\ kg$$
$$\frac{88}{200}$$

   Step 2.   Identify the safe dose.

   15 mg/kg/day

   Step 3.   Multiply child's weight in kilograms by the safe dose.

$$\begin{array}{r}41\\ \times\ 15\\ \hline 205\\ 41\\ \hline 615\ mg\end{array}$$

   Step 4.   Compare the order with the literature to decide if the dose is safe.

   b. The dose seems to be low. Order is 300 mg/day. Literature indicates it should be in the range of 600 mg.
   c. Check with the physician who wrote the order.
2. a. It was not necessary to use a rule. The literature was clear. Children 6–12 years should receive 600 mg divided into three doses, which equals 200 mg/dose; the ordered dose is safe.

   b. $\dfrac{D}{H} \times S = A \quad \dfrac{200}{125} \times 5 = \dfrac{1000}{125}\ \overline{)1000.}\ 8.0\ ml$

   Give 8 ml

3. a. $\begin{array}{r}20\ mg\\ \times\ 15\ kg\\ \hline 300\ mg/kg\end{array} \quad \begin{array}{r}40\ mg\\ \times\ 15\ kg\\ \hline 600\ mg/kg\end{array}$

   The order is 100 mg × 3 = 300 mg/day. This is safe.

   b. $\dfrac{D}{H} \times S = A \quad \dfrac{100}{125} \times 5 = \dfrac{500}{125}\ \overline{)500.}\ 4.0\ ml$

   c. Milligrams per kilogram rule
4. Tylenol 80 mg seems low. Literature says a child of 6 should receive four chewable tablets. This would be 320 mg (approximately gr v). Check with the physician.
5. a. Literature states dose should not exceed 12 mg/kg/24 hour

   Literature $\begin{array}{r}28\ kg\\ \times\ 12\ mg\\ \hline 336\ mg = safe\ dose\end{array}$ Child $\begin{array}{r}110\ mg\\ \times\ 3\ doses\\ \hline 330\ mg\end{array}$

   Dose is safe

b. $\dfrac{D}{H} \times S = A$ $\dfrac{110}{160} \times 15 = \dfrac{1650}{160} = 10 \text{ ml}$

c. Milligram per kilogram

6. The rule to use is $\dfrac{\text{child's BSA}}{1.7 \text{ adult BSA}} \times \text{adult dose} = \text{child's dose}$

$\dfrac{0.84 \text{ m}^2}{1.7 \text{ m}^2} \times 100 = 49.4 \text{ mg}$ is a safe dose. The ordered 50 mg is safe.

7. Could use Clark's rule $\dfrac{\text{child's lb}}{150} \times \text{adult dose} = \text{child dose}$

$\dfrac{65 \text{ lb}}{150 \text{ lb}} \times 5 \text{ mg} = \dfrac{325}{150} = 2 \text{ mg}.$

The dose is not safe according to Clark's rule.

8. $\dfrac{D}{H} \times S = A$ $\dfrac{0.045 \text{ mg}}{0.05 \text{ mg}} \times 1 \text{ cc} = \dfrac{0.04\!\!\!/\,5}{0.05\!\!\!/} = \dfrac{4.5}{5} = 0.9 \text{ ml}$

9. $\dfrac{D}{H} \times S = A$ $\dfrac{100 \text{ mg}}{80 \text{ mg}} \times 0.8 \text{ cc} = \dfrac{80}{80} = 1 \text{ cc}$

10. $\dfrac{D}{H} \times S = A$ $\dfrac{35 \text{ mg}}{80 \text{ mg}} \times 15 \text{ ml} = \dfrac{525}{80} = 6.6 \text{ ml}$

DOSAGE CALCULATIONS FOR INJECTIONS FROM LIQUIDS

1. a. Step 1.   Determine the kilograms.

$\dfrac{60}{2.2} = 27.27 \text{ kg}$

Step 2.   Determine the safe dose.

Range   15 mg   to   25 mg
            × 27.27 kg   × 27.27 kg
            409 mg/day   to   682 mg/day

Step 3.   Compare safe dose with child's dose.

150 mg
× 3 doses
450 mg/day

Step 4.   Dose is safe.

b. Use 250 mg/1 ml ampule. Other ampules would require 3-ml dose.

$$\dfrac{D}{H} \times S = A \qquad \dfrac{\overset{3}{\cancel{150}} \text{ mg}}{\underset{5}{\cancel{250}} \text{ mg}} \times 2 \text{ ml} = \dfrac{6}{5} \quad 5\overline{)6.0} \;\; 1.2 \text{ ml}$$

Give 1.2 ml IM.

2.   a. $\begin{array}{r} 6.8 \text{ kg} \\ \times\ 0.003 \text{ mg/kg} \\ \hline 0.02 \text{ mg} \end{array}$ This is the safe dose; the order is safe.

    b. $\dfrac{D}{H} \times S = A$ $\dfrac{0.02 \text{ mg}}{0.05 \text{ mg}} = \dfrac{2}{5} = 0.4 \text{ ml}$

3.   a.   According to the literature, this dose is safe.

    b. $\dfrac{D}{H} \times S = A$ $\dfrac{100 \text{ mg}}{50 \text{ mg}} = \times 1 \text{ ml} = 2 \text{ ml}$

4.   a.   Step 1.   Weight in kilograms: 2000 g = 2 kg

          Step 2.   Safe dose: $\begin{array}{r} 0.5 \text{ mg} \\ \times\ 2 \text{ kg} \\ \hline 1.0 \text{ mg} \end{array}$ = safe dose

          Step 3.   Compare neonatal dose with safe dose.

                 Ordered 1 mg   Safe dose = 1 mg

          Step 4.   Order is safe.

    b.   No math necessary. Give 1 ml.

      $\dfrac{1 \text{ mg}}{2 \text{ mg}} \times 2 \text{ ml} = 1 \text{ ml}$

5.   a.   Literature gives range of 350–450 mg/m² per day

       Child's BSA = 0.8 m²

       $\begin{array}{r} 350 \text{ mg} \\ \times\ 0.8 \text{ m}^2 \\ \hline 280 \text{ mg/day} \end{array}$ to $\begin{array}{r} 450 \text{ mg} \\ \times\ 0.8 \text{ m}^2 \\ \hline 360 \text{ mg/day} \end{array}$ is the safe range

       Child is ordered $\begin{array}{r} 90 \text{ mg} \\ \times\ 4 \text{ doses} \\ \hline 360 \text{ mg} \end{array}$ Hence, dose is safe.

    b. $\dfrac{D}{H} \times S = A$ $\dfrac{90 \text{ mg}}{150 \text{ mg}} \times 1 \text{ ml} = \dfrac{9}{15} = 0.6 \text{ ml IM}$

6.   Step 1.   Change pounds to kilograms.

            Change ounces to pounds $\dfrac{6 \text{ oz}}{16 \text{ oz/lb}} = 0.38 \text{ lb}$

            $\dfrac{12.38 \text{ lb}}{2.2} = 5.63 \text{ kg}$

      Step 2.   Determine safe dose.

            $\begin{array}{r} 20 \text{ mg/kg} \\ \times\ 5.63 \text{ kg} \\ \hline 112.6 \text{ mg/day} \end{array}$

Step 3.   Compare safe dose with ordered dose.

Child   50 mg
$\times$ 4 doses
200 mg/day

Step 4.   The dose is excessive according to the literature. Discuss with the physician. Do not prepare the dose.

7.   a.   4 lb 4 oz = 2 kg

Literature says the infant should receive a daily dosage of 30 mg. The order is 15 mg $\times$ 2 = 30 mg. The dose is safe.

b. $\dfrac{D}{H} \times S = A$ $\dfrac{15 \text{ mg}}{75 \text{ mg}} \times 2 \text{ ml} = \dfrac{30}{75} = 0.4 \text{ ml IM}$

8.   a.   The literature states that children under 6 months can receive 1–2.5 mg IM three to four times a day. The individual dose for the infant is 1 mg. This is safe, but the physician wrote q3–4h prn for the time. This would allow six to eight doses per 24 hours. The nurse can give the first dose but should clarify the times with the doctor.

b. $\dfrac{D}{H} \times S = A$ $\dfrac{1 \text{ mg}}{5 \text{ mg}} \times 1 \text{ ml} = 0.2 \text{ ml IM}$

9.   a.   Step 1.   12 kg

Step 2.   Determine safe range.

80 mg   to   160 mg
$\times$ 12 kg $\times$ 12 kg
960 mg/day   to   1920 mg/day

Step 3.   Determine child dose and compare.

250 mg
$\times$ 4 doses
1000 mg/day

Step 4.   Dose is safe.

b. $\dfrac{D}{H} \times S = A$ $\dfrac{250 \text{ mg}}{400 \text{ mg}} \times 1 \text{ ml} = \dfrac{5}{8} = 0.625 = 0.63 \text{ ml}$

10.   a.   Yes, the dose is safe. According to Table 10-2, the range for a 20-lb child is 25–50 mg/kg/day. The child is receiving 150 mg every 8 hours. According to the lower table, this is safe.
   b.   No need to calculate; the chart states 0.7 ml.

Proof: $\dfrac{150 \text{ mg}}{225 \text{ mg}} \times 1 \text{ ml} = 225\overline{)150.00}^{\,.66} = 0.7 \text{ ml}$
135 0
15 00
13 50

IV AND IVPB DOSAGE PROBLEMS

1.   Logic: The order calls for 15 mEq KCl/L, which is 1000 ml. Because you are using 250 ml, which is $\dfrac{1}{4}$ of a liter, determine what $\dfrac{1}{4}$ of 15 is.

$$\begin{array}{r} 3.75 \\ 4\overline{)15.00} \\ \underline{12} \\ 3\,0 \\ \underline{2\,8} \\ 20 \\ \underline{20} \end{array}$$

You need 3.8 mEq of KCl.

KCL comes 20 mEq/10 ml

$$\frac{D}{H} \times S = A \qquad \frac{3.8\ \cancel{mEq}}{20\ \cancel{mEq}} \times 10\ ml = \frac{3.8}{2} = 1.9$$

Add 1.9 ml of KCl to 250 ml D5 0.2 NS. Label the bag. Mix well. Allow 18 ml to flow from the bag into the Buretrol and then to the infusion pump. Set pump to deliver 18 ml/hr.

2. **a.** Logic: Guidelines (see Table 10–4) state that the maximum dose for neonates is 200 mg/kg/day. The physician's order indicates 100 mg/kg/day. The minimum dilution is 1 g/10 ml. This would be 100 mg/1 ml. The order states to give the drug in 15 cc. This is safe. The guidelines state that the drug is to be given over 20–30 minutes (maximum 1 hour). As the order did not indicate the time, choose 1 hour.

b. Dissolve the powder according to the label directions. Add 1.8 ml sterile water to make 250 mg/ml.

$$\frac{D}{H} \times S = A \qquad \frac{\overset{2}{\cancel{100}\ \cancel{mg}}}{\underset{5}{\cancel{250}\ \cancel{mg}}} \times 1\ ml = \frac{2}{5} = 0.4\ ml$$

Remove 0.4 ml from the vial into at least a 20-ml syringe. *Discard the remainder* of the drug because it cannot be stored. Draw up D5 $\frac{1}{4}$ NS into the syringe to reach 15 cc. Set the syringe pump to deliver 15 cc over 1 hour.

3. **a.** Literature lists trimethoprim as 80 mg/5 ml. Order states 40 mg (2.5 cc). This is safe. The maximum pediatric dose is listed as 20 mg/kg per day.

Infant's weight   6.77 kg
$$\underline{\times\ 20\ mg}$$
135.40 mg   is the maximum for this infant

The order is 40 mg twice a day = 80 mg. This is below the maximum dose and is safe.
The minimum dilution is 1 ml of drug in 15 ml D5W over 60–90 minutes. The order is 2.5 ml of drug in 50 ml D5W.

15 ml/fluid
$$\underline{\times\ 2.5\ ml/drug}$$
75
$$\underline{\ \ 30\ \ }$$
37.5 ml   is the minimum safe dilution

There is no problem because 50 ml will result in more dilute solution.

b. Open the ampule. Remove 2.5 ml of Septra. From the reservoir of the bag of D5W allow about 10 ml to flow into the Buretrol. Add the 2.5 ml of Septra. Allow D5W to flow into the Buretrol to complete the volume of 50 ml. Be sure the Septra is evenly dispersed in the Buretrol by rotating the chamber. Label. Set the infusion pump for 50 ml/hr.

4. The order calls for 10 mEq KCl/L. Use 1 L of fluid. First calculate the number of milliliters of KCl needed.

$$\frac{D}{H} \times S = A \qquad \frac{\cancel{10}\ \cancel{mEq}}{\cancel{40}\ \cancel{mEq}} \times \overset{5}{\cancel{20}}\ ml = 5\ ml$$

Add 5 ml KCl to the 1-L bag of D5 $\frac{1}{3}$ NS. Label. Hang bag above Buretrol and attach. Run 35 ml of solution into the Buretrol. Set the infusion pump for 35 ml/hr. Be sure the KCl is evenly distributed in the bag of fluid.

5. a. Because this is an 18-year-old, it is possible to follow directions for an adult dose. The guidelines say 10 mg/kg is the maximum amount for a loading dose. This would be 736 mg for this patient, therefore, 50 mg is a safe dose. The guidelines also say to dilute with at least an equal volume of IV fluid; stock is 50 mg in 50 ml. Finally, directions are to give the IV bolus over 20 to 30 minutes.

 b. First calculate the amount of aminophylline needed.

$$\frac{D}{H} \times S = A \qquad \frac{\overset{1}{\cancel{50\ mg}}}{\underset{\underset{1}{\cancel{5}}}{\cancel{250\ mg}}} \times \overset{2}{\cancel{10}}\ ml = 2\ ml$$

Add 2 ml of drug to 50 ml D5W. Label bag. Infuse over 30 minutes. *Important:* Remember the pump must be set in *ml/hr*. Because you are giving 50 ml over 30 minutes, you must *double* the figures, so set the pump for 100 ml over 1 hour. The pump will deliver the 50 ml in $\frac{1}{2}$ hr.

6. Because the patient is 18 years old, we will follow adult guidelines.

 a. The *PDR* states that 3 mg/kg/day is the adult dose.

73.6 kg	75 mg
$\times$ 3 mg	$\times$ 3 doses
220.8 mg/day is safe	225 mg/day = ordered dose

The order is safe.

 b. The doctor did not order the IV diluent, the amount, or the time. Following the *PDR* directions, dilute the gentamicin in 100 ml D5W and administer IVPB over 1 hour.

$$\frac{D}{H} \times S = A \qquad \frac{\overset{15}{\cancel{75\ mg}}}{\underset{8}{\cancel{40\ mg}}} \times 1\ ml = \begin{array}{r} 1.87 \\ 8\,)\overline{15.00} \\ \underline{8} \\ 7\ 0 \\ \underline{6\ 4} \\ 60 \\ \underline{56} \end{array} = 1.9\ ml$$

Add 1.9 ml of drug to 100 ml D5W and label the bag.

$$\frac{\#\ ml \times TF}{\#\ min} = gtt/min \qquad \frac{100 \times \cancel{10}}{\cancel{60}} = \frac{\cancel{100}}{6} \begin{array}{r} 16.6 \\ )\overline{100.0} \end{array} = 17\ gtt/min$$

Set IVPB drip at 17 gtt/min.

7. The order meets the guidelines in Table 10-4. Add 5 ml of isoproterenol to the 100 ml D5W. Label the bag. You have a solution of 1 mg in 100 ml. Change the milligrams to micrograms.

1 mg = 1000 μg

The solution is 1000 μg in 100 ml. Reduce this number: $\dfrac{1000\ \mu g}{100\ ml} = 10\ \mu g/ml$

You are using a microdrip (60 gtt/ml). Substitute 60 gtt/min for the milliliters. The solution is 10 μg/60 gtt/min.

The order is 1.8 μg/min. Solve

$$\frac{D}{H} \times S = A \qquad \frac{1.8 \,\cancel{\mu g}}{10 \,\cancel{\mu g}} \times 60 \,\text{gtt/min} = \frac{1.8}{\times\ 6}}{10.8} = 11 \text{ gtt/min}$$

Set the drip at 11 gtt/min. Label the IV.

8. a. The guidelines call for 20–50 μg/kg/min. First figure out the child's weight in kilograms.

$$2.2\,\overline{)20.0\,00\text{ lbs}} = 9.1 \text{ kg}$$

$$\begin{array}{r} 9.09 \\ \underline{19\ 8} \\ 200 \\ \underline{198} \end{array}$$

The guidelines list the maximum rate as

$$\begin{array}{r} 50 \text{ μg/kg/min} \\ \times\ 9.1 \text{ kg} \\ \hline 50 \\ 450 \\ \hline 455.0 \text{ μg/kg/min} = \text{maximum safe dose} \end{array}$$

Order is 400 μg/min. Order meets the guidelines.

b. Add 5 ml of lidocaine 2% to 250 ml D5W. Label the bag. The solution is 100 mg in 250 ml. Change the milligrams to micrograms. 1 mg = 1000 μg, so 100 mg = 100,000 μg. The solution is 100,000 μg in 250 ml. Reduce the number:

$$\frac{\cancel{100,000}\,\mu g}{\cancel{250}\text{ ml}} \overset{400}{=} 400 \text{ μg/ml} = \text{solution}$$

You are using a microdrip (60 gtt/ml). Substitute for the milliliters, 60 gtt/min. The solution is now 400 μg/60 gtt/min. This is the order. Set the drip rate at 60 gtt/min. Label the IV.

ASSORTED DOSAGE PROBLEMS

1. Range is

$$\begin{array}{ll} 20 \text{ mg/kg} \quad \text{to} & 40 \text{ mg/kg} \\ \underline{\times 10 \text{ kg}} & \underline{\times 10 \text{ kg}} \\ 200 \text{ mg/day} \quad \text{to} & 400 \text{ mg/day} \end{array}$$

The baby is receiving 125 mg × 3 doses = 375 mg/day. The dosage is safe.

2. Range is

$$\begin{array}{ll} 4 \text{ mg/kg} & 6 \text{ mg/kg} \\ \underline{\times 9.5 \text{ kg}} & \underline{\times 9.5 \text{ kg}} \\ 38.0 \text{ mg/day} \quad \text{to} & 57.0 \text{ mg/day} \end{array}$$

Infant is receiving 20 mg × 2 doses = 40 mg/day. This is within the therapeutic range.

3. No calculation needed. Dose is in the therapeutic range.

4. No calculation necessary. A 15-year-old receives an adult dose. The literature is clear. The dose is safe.

5. No calculation needed. Literature is clear. The dose is safe. Give 2 ml.

6. The amount in the syringe will be 1.6 ml (Demerol 0.4 ml; Phenergan 0.4 ml; Thorazine 0.8 ml).

7. a.   Therapeutic dose

$$
\begin{array}{r}
= 50{,}000 \text{ units} \\
\times\quad 48 \text{ kg} \\
\hline
2{,}400{,}000 = 2.4 \text{ MU. Dose is safe.}
\end{array}
$$

   b.   4 ml

8. a.   Guidelines indicate 2.5 mg/kg q12h is safe; the infant's weight is 4 kg. The 10.0 mg dose is safe.

   b.   Gentamicin pediatric is 10 mg/ml. You need 1 ml. The guidelines state the concentration for IVPB is 1 mg/ml; hence, the volume for the IV will be 10 ml (1 ml drug plus 9 ml diluent). To prepare, draw up 1 ml of drug and 9 ml D5 $\frac{1}{4}$ NS in a syringe. Set the syringe pump to deliver the 10 ml over 30 minutes. (The setting will be 20 ml/hr because the pump is calibrated in milliliters per hour.)

9. a.   The safe dose is 5 mg/kg/day in divided doses. The child's weight is 12 kg; therefore, the therapeutic dose is 60 mg divided. The child is receiving 15 mg × 4 doses daily = 60 mg.

   b. $\dfrac{D}{H} \times S = A \qquad \dfrac{\overset{3}{\cancel{15 \text{ mg}}}}{\underset{10}{\cancel{50 \text{ mg}}}} \times 1 \text{ ml} = \dfrac{3}{10} = 0.3 \text{ ml}$

10.   Safe range is $\qquad$ 60 mg/kg $\quad$ to $\quad$ 90 mg/kg
$\quad$ Child's weight $\qquad \dfrac{\times\ 13 \text{ kg}}{780 \text{ mg/day}}$ $\quad$ to $\quad \dfrac{\times\ 13 \text{ kg}}{1170 \text{ mg/day}}$
$\quad$ Therapeutic range

The child is receiving 200 mg × 6 doses = 1200 mg. This is considered a safe dose. The tablets are not scored and the drug amount will be increased weekly.

11

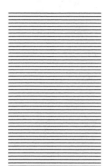

Proficiency Examinations in Dosage

====== TEST 1. ABBREVIATIONS ======

Aim for 90% or better on this test. There are 50 items, each worth 2 points. If you have any difficulty, reread and study Chapter 1, which explains this information. Answers may be found at the end of the chapter.

1. bid _____
2. hs _____
3. prn _____
4. OU _____
5. po _____
6. pr _____
7. SL _____
8. S & S _____
9. tiw _____
10. ml _____
11. q4h _____
12. cc _____
13. SC _____
14. 1 s̈s _____
15. g _____
16. PC _____
17. qd _____
18. stat _____
19. q12h _____
20. tid _____
21. OS _____
22. kg _____
23. ʒ _____
24. qh _____
25. OD _____
26. mEq _____
27. AC _____
28. qid _____
29. mg _____
30. IM _____
31. qod _____
32. BIW _____
33. NGT _____
34. q8h _____
35. L _____
36. mcg _____
37. q6h _____
38. μg _____
39. U _____
40. tsp _____
41. s̈s _____
42. gr _____
43. IV _____
44. mL _____
45. ʒ _____
46. IVPB _____
47. m _____
48. Gm _____
49. q2h _____
50. q3h _____

Your score: _____

TEST 2. EQUIVALENTS

Aim for 90% accuracy or better on this test. There are 50 items each worth 2 points. If you have any difficulty, reread and study Chapter 4, which explains this information. Answers may be found at the end of the chapter.

1. 100 mg = _____ Gm
2. gr $\frac{1}{2}$ = _____ mg
3. ℥ i = _____ cc
4. 1 L = _____ ml
5. gr $\frac{1}{200}$ = _____ mg
6. 325 mg = gr _____
7. 1 tsp = _____ cc
8. 0.4 mg = gr _____
9. gr X = _____ mg
10. 30 mg = gr _____
11. 0.015 g = _____ mg
12. 10 mg = _____ Gm
13. 1 cc = _____ ml
14. gr $\frac{1}{150}$ = _____ mg
15. gr i = _____ gm
16. 0.2 Gm = _____ mg
17. gr xv = _____ Gm

18. 30 mg = _____ g
19. gr III = _____ mg
20. 15 mg = gr _____
21. 500 mg = _____ g
22. gr i = _____ mg
23. 1 oz = _____ ml
24. 1 ml = _____ minims
25. gr $\frac{1}{4}$ = _____ mg
26. 1 tbsp = _____ cc
27. 1 kg = _____ lb
28. 1 g = _____ mg
29. gr i s̈s = _____ Gm
30. 60 mg = _____ g
31. 30 ml = _____ oz
32. 1 minim = _____ gtt
33. gr V = _____ g
34. ℥ ii = _____ ml

35. 1000 mg = _____ Gm
36. gr vii s̈s = _____ gm
37. 0.1 Gm = _____ mg
38. 1 dram = _____ cc
39. 600 mg = gr _____
40. 600 mg = _____ gm
41. 10 mcg = _____ mg
42. 1 L = _____ ml
43. 0.5 μg = _____ mg
44. 0.6 mg = _____ g
45. 250 mcg = _____ mg
46. 1 mg = _____ g
47. 0.125 mg = _____ μg
48. 0.01 mg = _____ mcg
49. 0.001 mg = _____ μg
50. 1 qt = _____ ml

Your score: _____

TEST 3. ORAL CALCULATIONS: SOLIDS AND LIQUIDS

Aim for 90% or better on this test. There are 20 questions, each worth 5 points. Determine the amount to be given. If you have any difficulty, reread Chapter 6, which explains this information. Answers may be found at the end of the chapter.

1. Order: el of potassium chloride 20 mEq po in juice
   Stock: liquid in a bottle labeled 30 mEq/15 ml

2. Order: syrup of tetracycline hydrochloride 80 mg po q6h
   Stock: liquid in a dropper bottle labeled 125 mg/5 ml

3. Order: propranolol 0.02 g po bid
   Stock: scored tablets labeled 10 mg

4. Order: ampicillin sodium 0.5 g po q6h
   Stock: capsules of 250 mg

  5. Order: digoxin 0.5 mg po qd
       Stock: scored tablets of 0.25 mg

  6. Order: Levothroid Susp. 100 mcg qd po
       Stock: liquid in a bottle labeled 0.2 mg/10 ml

  7. Order: hydrochlorothiazide 75 mg po qd
       Stock: scored tablets 50 mg

  8. Order: furosemide 40 mg po qd
       Stock: scored tablets of 80 mg

  9. Order: el digoxin 0.125 mg po
       Stock: liquid in a dropper bottle labeled 500 μg/10 ml

 10. Order: Dilantin Susp 75 mg po tid
       Stock: liquid in a bottle labeled 50 mg/10 ml

 11. Order: diazepam 5 mg po q4h prn
       Stock: scored tablets 2 mg

 12. Order: Synthroid 0.15 mg po qd
       Stock: scored tablets 300 μg

 13. Order: Antabuse 375 mg po today
       Stock: scored tablets 250 mg

 14. Order: ibuprofen 0.6 g po q4h prn
       Stock: Film-coated tablets 300 mg

 15. Order: chlorpheniramine maleate syr 1.5 mg po bid
       Stock: liquid in a bottle 1 mg/8 ml

 16. Order: diphenhydramine maleate syrup 25 mg po q4h while awake
       Stock: liquid labeled 12.5 mg/5 ml

 17. Order: simethicone liq 60 mg po in $\frac{1}{2}$ glass H$_2$O

       Stock: liquid in a dropper bottle labeled 40 mg/0.6 ml

(continued)

═ TEST 3. ORAL CALCULATIONS: SOLIDS AND LIQUIDS (*Continued*) ═

18. Order: chlorothiazide oral susp 0.5 g via NGT po qd
    Stock: liquid labeled 250 mg/5 ml

19. Order: meperidine HCl syrup 150 mg po q4h prn
    Stock: liquid labeled 50 mg/5 ml

20. Order: hydroxyzine syrup 7.5 mg po q6h
    Stock: liquid labeled 10 mg/5 ml

Your score: _____

═══ TEST 4. CALCULATIONS OF INJECTIONS FROM LIQUIDS ═══

Aim for 90% or better on this test. There are 20 questions, each worth 5 points. Determine the amount to be given. If you have any difficulty, reread and study Chapter 7, which explains this information. Answers may be found at the end of the chapter in milliliters to the nearest tenth.

1. Order: Lanoxin 0.25 mg IM qd
    Stock: ampule labeled 0.5 mg/2 ml

2. Order: diphenhydramine hydrochloride 40 mg IM stat
    Stock: ampule labeled 50 mg (2-cc size)

3. Order: morphine sulfate 8 mg SC q4h prn
    Stock: vial labeled 15 mg/ml

4. Order: Demerol Hydrochloride 25 mg IM q4h prn
    Stock: vial labeled 100 mg/ml

5. Order: ascorbic acid 200 mg IM qd
    Stock: ampule labeled 500 mg/2 ml

6. Order: vitamin B_{12} 1500 μg qd IM
    Stock: vial labeled 5000 μg/ml

7. Order: atropine sulfate 0.6 mg SC at 7:30 AM
    Stock: vial labeled 0.4 mg/ml

8. Order: Sodium Amytal 0.1 gm IM stat
    Stock: ampule 200 mg/3 ml

9. Order: hydromorphone HCl 1.5 mg IM q4h prn
    Stock: vial labeled 2 mg/ml

10. Order: penicillin G procaine 600,000 units IM q12h
    Stock: vial labeled 500,000 USP units/ml

11. Order: add nitroglycerin 200 μg to IV stat
    Stock: vial labeled 0.8 mg/ml

12. Order: neostigmine methylsulfate 500 mcg SC
    Stock: ampule labeled 1:4000

13. Order: levorphanol tartrate 3 mg SC
    Stock: vial labeled 2 mg/ml

14. Order: epinephrine 0.4 mg SC stat
    Stock: ampule labeled 1:1000 (2-ml size)

15. Order: magnesium sulfate 500 mg IM
    Stock: ampule labeled 50% (2-ml size)

16. Order: oxymorphone HCl 0.75 mg SC
    Stock: vial labeled 1.5 mg/ml

17. Order: add lidocaine 100 mg to IV stat
    Stock: ampule labeled 20%

18. Order: Lanoxin 0.125 mg IM 10 AM
    Stock: ampule labeled 0.25 mg/2 ml

19. Order: nalbuphine HCl 12 mg IM
    Stock: vial 10 mg/ml

20. Order: add 10 mEq KCl to IV
    Stock: vial 40 mEq/20 ml

Your score: _____

══ TEST 5. CALCULATION OF INJECTIONS FROM POWDERS ══

There are 20 questions each worth 5 points. Aim for 90% or better on this test. If you have any difficulty doing the problems, review and study Chapter 8, which explains this information. Answers may be found at the end of the chapter in milliliters to the nearest tenth.

1. Order: penicillin G potassium 600,000 units IM q8h
   Stock: vial of powder labeled 1 million units (Fig. 11-1)
   Diluting fluid and # ml:

   Solution and new stock:

   Rule and arithmetic:

   Give:

(continued)

Pfizerpen

Approx. Desired Concentration (units/ml)	Approx. Volume (ml) 1,000,000 units	Solvent for Vial of 5,000,000 units	Infusion Only 20,000,000 units
50,000	20.0	. . .	. . .
100,000	10.0	. . .	. . .
250,000	4.0	18.2	75.0
500,000	1.8	8.2	33.0
750,000	. . .	4.8	. . .
1,000,000	. . .	3.2	11.5

(1) Intramuscular Injection: Keep total volume of injection small. The intramuscular route is the preferred route of administration. Solutions containing up to 100,000 units of penicillin per ml of diluent may be used with a minimum of discomfort. Greater concentration of penicillin G per ml is physically possible and may be employed where therapy demands. When large dosages are required, it may be advisable to administer solutions of penicillin by means of continuous intravenous drip.

Buffered Pfizerpen (penicillin G potassium) for Injection is highly water soluble. It may be dissolved in small amounts of Water for Injection, or Sterile Isotonic Sodium Chloride Solution for Parenteral Use. All solutions should be stored in a refrigerator. When refrigerated, penicillin solutions may be stored for seven days without significant loss of potency. Buffered Pfizerpen (penicillin G potassium) for Injection may be given intramuscuiarly or by continuous intravenous drip for dosages of 500,000, 1,000,000, or 5,000,000 units.

Figure 11-1. *Preparation of solution of penicillin G potassium (Pfizerpen). (Courtesy of Roerig–Pfizer Laboratories.)*

⁼ TEST 5. CALCULATION OF INJECTIONS FROM POWDERS *(Continued)* ⁼

Write on label:

Storage:

2. Order: ceftazidime 200 mg IM q8h
Stock: vial of powder labeled 500 mg (Fig. 11-2)
Diluting fluid and # ml:

Solution and new stock:

Rule and arithmetic:

Give:

Write on label:

Storage:

3. Order: carbenicillin disodium 1 g IM q6h
Stock: vial of powder 5 grams (Fig. 11-3)
Diluting fluid and # ml:

Solution and new stock:

Rule and arithmetic:

Give:

Write on label:

Storage:

TAZIDIME® (Ceftazidime, USP, Lilly)

In children, as in adults, the creatinine clearance should be adjusted for body surface area or lean body mass and the dosing frequency should be reduced in cases of renal insufficiency.

In patients undergoing hemodialysis, a loading dose of 1 g of Tazidime is recommended, followed by 1 g after each hemodialysis period.

Tazidime can also be used in patients undergoing intraperitoneal dialysis (IPD) and continuous ambulatory peritoneal dialysis (CAPD). In such patients, a loading dose of 1 g of Tazidime may be given, followed by 500 mg every 24 hours. In addition to intravenous use, Tazidime can be incorporated in dialysis fluid at a concentration of 250 mg/2 L of dialysis fluid.

NOTE: Tazidime should generally be continued for 2 days after the signs and symptoms of infection have disappeared; however, in complicated infections, longer therapy may be required.

Administration—Tazidime may be given intravenously or by deep intramuscular injection into a large muscle mass (such as the upper outer quadrant of the gluteus maximus or lateral part of the thigh).

Intramuscular Administration—For intramuscular administration, Tazidime should be reconstituted with 1 of the following diluents: Sterile Water for Injection, Bacteriostatic Water for Injection, or 0.5% or 1.0% Lidocaine Hydrochloride Injection. Refer to Table 5.

Intravenous Administration—The IV route is preferable for patients with bacterial septicemia, bacterial meningitis, peritonitis, or other severe or life-threatening infections. It is also preferable for patients who may be poor risks because of lowered resistance resulting from such debilitating conditions as malnutrition, trauma, surgery, diabetes, heart failure, or malignancy, particularly if shock is present or impending.

For direct intermittent intravenous administration, reconstitute Tazidime with Sterile Water for Injection (see Table 5). Slowly inject the solution directly into the vein over a period of 3 to 5 minutes or give through the tubing of an administration set while the patient is also receiving 1 of the compatible intravenous fluids (see Compatibility and Stability).

For intravenous infusion, reconstitute the 1-g or 2-g piggyback (100-mL) vial with 50 or 100 mL Sterile Water for Injection or 1 of the compatible intravenous fluids listed in the Compatibility and Stability section. Alternatively, reconstitute the 500-mg, 1-g, or 2-g vial, and add an appropriate quantity of the resulting solution to an IV container with 1 of the compatible intravenous fluids.

Intermittent intravenous infusion with a Y-type administration set can be accomplished with compatible solutions. However, during infusion of a solution containing ceftazidime, it is desirable to discontinue the other solution.

ADD-Vantage® vials are to be used only with Abbott ADD-Vantage diluent bags according to the printed tray card instructions included in each Traypak of vials.

ADD-Vantage vials that have been joined to Abbott ADD-Vantage bags of diluent and activated to dissolve the drug are stable for 24 hours at room temperature. Joined Vials which have not been activated may be used within a 14-day period; this period corresponds to that for use of Abbott ADD-Vantage containers following removal of the outer packaging (overwrap).

Freezing solutions of Tazidime in the ADD-Vantage system is not recommended.

Table 5. Preparation of Solutions of Tazidime

	Amount of Diluent to Be Added (mL)	Approximate Available Volume (mL)	Approximate Ceftazidime Concentration (mg/mL)
Intramuscular			
500 mg, Vial No. 7230	1.5	1.8	280
1 g, Vial No. 7231	3.0	3.6	280
Intravenous			
500 mg, Vial No. 7230	5	5.3	100
1 g, Vial No. 7231	5 or 10	5.6 or 10.6	180 or 100
2 g, Vial No. 7234	10	11.2	180
Piggyback (100 mL)			
1 g, Vial No. 7238	50* or 100*	50 or 100	20 or 10
2 g, Vial No. 7239	50* or 100*	50 or 100	40 or 20

COMPATIBILITY AND STABILITY

Intramuscular: Vials of Tazidime, when reconstituted as directed with Sterile Water for Injection, Bacteriostatic Water for Injection, or 0.5% or 1% Lidocaine Hydrochloride Injection, maintain satisfactory potency for 24 hours at room temperature or for 10 days under refrigeration. Solutions in Sterile Water for Injection that are frozen immediately after reconstitution in the original container are stable for 3 months when stored at −20°C. Once thawed, solutions should not be refrozen. Thawed solutions may be stored for up to 24 hours at room temperature or for 4 days in a refrigerator.

Figure 11-2. Preparation of solution of ceftazidime (Tazidime). (Courtesy of Eli Lilly and Co.)

For Intramuscular Use: The 2 g vial should be reconstituted with 4.0 ml of Sterile Water for Injection, 0.5% Lidocaine Hydrochloride (without epinephrine), or Bacteriostatic Water containing 0.9% benzyl alcohol. (Preparations containing benzyl alcohol should not be used in neonates.) In order to facilitate reconstitution up to 7.2 ml of diluent can be used.

Amount of Diluent to be Added to the 2 g Vial	Volume to be Withdrawn for a 1 g Dose
4.0 ml	2.5 ml
5.0 ml	3.0 ml
7.2 ml	4.0 ml

The 5 g vial should be reconstituted with 7.0 ml of Sterile Water for Injection, 0.5% Lidocaine Hydrochloride (without epinephrine), or Bacteriostatic Water containing 0.9% benzyl alcohol. (Preparations containing benzyl alcohol should not be used in neonates.) In order to facilitate reconstitution, up to 17 ml of diluent can be used.

Amount of Diluent to be Added to the 5 g Vial	Volume to be Withdrawn for a 1 g Dose
7.0 ml	2.0 ml
9.5 ml	2.5 ml
12.0 ml	3.0 ml
17.0 ml	4.0 ml

After reconstitution, no significant loss of potency occurs for up to 24 hours at room temperature, and for 72 hours if refrigerated. Any of these unused solutions should be discarded.

Figure 11-3. Preparation of solution of carbenicillin disodium. (Courtesy of Roerig–Pfizer Laboratories.)

4. Order: ampicillin sodium 400 mg IM q8h

Stock: vial of powder labeled 500 mg (Fig. 11-4)

Diluting fluid and # ml:

Solution and new stock:

(continued)

Intramuscular Use: 125 mg vial: Add 1 ml Sterile Water for Injection, USP, or Bacteriostatic Water for Injection, USP (TUBEX® Sterile Cartridge-Needle Unit) to give a final concentration of 125 mg per ml. For fractional doses, withdraw the ampicillin sodium solution as follows:

Dose	Withdraw
25 mg	0.2 ml
50 mg	0.4 ml
75 mg	0.6 ml
100 mg	0.8 ml
125 mg	1 ml

250 mg vial: Add 0.9 ml Sterile Water for Injection, USP, or Bacteriostatic Water for Injection, USP (TUBEX) to give a final concentration of 250 mg/ml. For fractional doses, withdraw the ampicillin sodium solution as follows:

Dose	Withdraw
125 mg	0.5 ml
150 mg	0.6 ml
175 mg	0.7 ml
200 mg	0.8 ml
225 mg	0.9 ml
250 mg	1 ml

For dilution of 500-mg, 1-gram, and 2-gram vials, dissolve contents of a vial with the amount of Sterile water for Injection, USP, or Bacteriostatic Water for Injection, USP, listed in the table below:

Label Claim	Recommended Amount of Diluent	Withdrawable Volume	Concentration in mg/ml
500 mg	1.8 ml	2.0 ml	250 mg
1.0 gram	3.4 ml	4.0 ml	250 mg
2.0 gram	6.8 ml	8.0 ml	250 mg

While the 1-gram and 2-gram vials are primarily for intravenous use, they may be administered intramuscularly when the 250-mg or 500-mg vials are unavailable. In such instances, dissolve in 3.4 or 6.8 ml Sterile Water for Injection, USP, or Bacteriostatic Water for Injection, USP, to give a final concentration of 250 mg/ml
The above solutions must be used within one hour after reconstitution.

Figure 11-4. *Reconstitution directions for ampicillin sodium. (Courtesy of Wyeth-Ayerst Laboratories, Philadelphia, PA.)*

¯ TEST 5. CALCULATION OF INJECTIONS FROM POWDERS (*Continued*) ¯

Rule and arithmetic:

Give:

Write on label:

Storage:

5. Order: ampicillin sodium 300 mg IM q8h
Stock: vial of 500 mg powder (Fig. 11-5)
Diluting fluid and # ml:

Solution and new stock:

Rule and arithmetic:

Give:

Write on label:

Storage:

6. Order: cefazolin sodium 0.33 g IM q8h
Stock: vial of powder labeled 1 gram (Fig. 11-6)
Diluting fluid and # ml:

Solution and new stock:

Label Claim	Recommended Amount of Diluent	Withdrawable Volume	Concentration in mg/ml
500 mg	1.8 ml	2.0 ml	250 mg
1.0 gram	3.4 ml	4.0 ml	250 mg
2.0 gram	6.8 ml	8.0 ml	250 mg

While the 1-gram and 2-gram vials are primarily for intravenous use, they may be administered intramuscularly when the 250-mg or 500-mg vials are unavailable. In such instances, dissolve in 3.4 or 6.8 ml Sterile Water for Injection, USP, or Bacteriostatic Water for Injection, USP, to give a final concentration of 250 mg/ml

The above solutions must be used within one hour after reconstitution.

Figure 11-5. *Preparation of solution of ampicillin sodium (Omnipen). (Courtesy of Wyeth–Ayerst Laboratories, Philadelphia, PA.)*

Vial Size	Diluent to Be Added	Approximate Available Volume	Approximate Average Concentration
250 mg	2 ml	2 ml	125 mg/ml
500 mg	2 ml	2.2 ml	225 mg/ml
1 g*	2.5 ml	3 ml	330 mg/ml

* The 1-g vial should be reconstituted only with Sterile Water for Injection or Bacteriostatic Water for Injection.

STABILITY
Reconstituted Kefzol (cefazolin sodium, Lilly) and dilutions of Kefzol in the recommended intravenous fluids are stable for 24 hours at room temperature and for 96 hours stored under refrigeration (5°C).

Figure 11-6. *Dilution table for cefazolin sodium (Kefzol). (Courtesy of Eli Lilly and Co.)*

Rule and arithmetic:

Give:

Write on label:

Storage:

7. Order: cefoperazone 0.5 g IM q12h
   Stock: 1-g vial of powder (Fig. 11-7)
   Diluting fluid and # ml:

   Solution and new stock:

   Rule and arithmetic:

   Give:

   Write on label:

   Storage:

(continued)

RECONSTITUTION

The following solutions may be used for the initial reconstitution of CEFOBID sterile powder:

Table 1. Solutions for Initial Reconstitution

5% Dextrose Injection (USP)	0.9% Sodium Chloride Injection (USP)
5% Dextrose and 0.9% Sodium Chloride Injection (USP)	Normosol* M and Dextrose Injection
5% Dextrose and 0.2% Sodium Chloride Injection (USP)	Normosol* R
10% Dextrose Injection (USP)	Sterile Water for Injection*
Bacteriostatic Water for Injection [Benzyl Alcohol or Parabens] (USP)*†	

*Not to be used as a vehicle for intravenous infusion
†Preparations containing Benzyl Alcohol should not be used in neonates.

Preparation for Intramuscular Injection

Any suitable solution listed above may be used to prepare CEFOBID sterile powder for intramuscular injection. When concentrations of 250 mg/ml or more are to be administered, a lidocaine solution should be used. These solutions should be prepared using a combination of Sterile Water for Injection and 2% Lidocaine Hydrochloride Injection (USP) that approximates a 0.5% Lidocaine Hydrochloride Solution. A two-step dilution process as follows is recommended: First, add the required amount of Sterile Water for Injection and agitate until CEFOBID powder is completely dissolved. Second, add the required amount of 2% lidocaine and mix.

	Final Cefoperazone Concentration	Step 1 Volume of Sterile Water	Step 2 Volume of 2% Lidocaine	Withdrawable Volume*†
1 g vial	333 mg/ml	2.0 ml	0.6 ml	3 ml
	250 mg/ml	2.8 ml	1.0 ml	4 ml
2 g vial	333 mg/ml	3.8 ml	1.2 ml	6 ml
	250 mg/ml	5.4 ml	1.8 ml	8 ml

When a diluent other than Lidocaine HCl Injection (USP) is used reconstitute as follows:

	Cefoperazone Concentration	Volume of Diluent to be Added	Withdrawable Volume*
1 g vial	333 mg/ml	2.6 ml	3 ml
	250 mg/ml	3.8 ml	4 ml
2 g vial	333 mg/ml	5.0 ml	6 ml
	250 mg/ml	7.2 ml	8 ml

*There is sufficient excess present to allow for withdrawal of the stated volume.
†Final lidocaine concentration will approximate that obtained if a 0.5% Lidocaine Hydrochloride Solution is used as diluent

Figure 11-7. *Dilution directions for cefoperazone sodium (Cefobid). (Courtesy of Roerig–Pfizer Laboratories.)*

RECONSTITUTION

Preparation of Parenteral Solution

Parenteral drug products should be SHAKEN WELL when reconstituted, and inspected visually for particulate matter prior to administration. If particulate matter is evident in reconstituted fluids, the drug solutions should be discarded. When reconstituted or diluted according to the instructions below, Ancef (sterile cefazolin sodium, SK&F) is stable for 24 hours at room temperature or for 96 hours if stored under refrigeration. Reconstituted solutions may range in color from pale yellow to yellow without a change in potency.

Single-Dose Vials

For I.M. injection, I.V. direct (bolus) injection, or I.V. infusion, reconstitute with Sterile Water for Injection according to the following table. SHAKE WELL.

Vial Size	Amount of Diluent	Approximate Concentration	Approximate Available Volume
250 mg.	2.0 ml.	125 mg./ml.	2.0 ml.
500 mg.	2.0 ml.	225 mg./ml.	2.2 ml.
1 gram	2.5 ml.	330 mg./ml.	3.0 ml.

Figure 11-8. *Dilution table for cefazolin sodium (Ancef). (Courtesy of Smith Kline & French Laboratories.)*

⁼ TEST 5. CALCULATION OF INJECTIONS FROM POWDERS (*Continued*) ⁼

8. Order: cefazolin sodium 300 mg IM q8h

Stock: vial of powder labeled 1 gram (Fig. 11-8)

Diluting fluid and # ml:

Solution and new stock:

Rule and arithmetic:

Give:

Write on label:

Storage:

9. Order: Mefoxitin 300 mg IM q4h

Stock: vial of powder 1 gram (Fig. 11-9)

Diluting fluid and # ml:

Solution and new stock:

	Table 3 — Preparation of Solution		
Strength	Amount of Diluent to be Added (mL)+ +	Approximate Withdrawable Volume (mL)	Approximate Average Concentration (mg/mL)
1 gram Vial	2 (Intramuscular)	2.5	400
2 gram Vial	4 (Intramuscular)	5	400
1 gram Vial	10 (IV)	10.5	95
2 gram Vial	10 or 20 (IV)	11.1 or 21.0	180 or 95
1 gram Infusion Bottle	50 or 100 (IV)	50 or 100	20 or 10
2 gram Infusion Bottle	50 or 100 (IV)	50 or 100	40 or 20
10 gram Bulk	43 or 93 (IV)	49 or 98.5	200 or 100

+ +Shake to dissolve and let stand until clear.

Intramuscular
MEFOXIN, as constituted with Sterile Water for Injection, Bacteriostatic Water for Injection, or 0.5 percent or 1 percent lidocaine hydrochloride solution (without epinephrine), maintains satisfactory potency for 24 hours at room temperature, for one week under refrigeration (below 5°C), and for at least 30 weeks in the frozen state.

Figure 11-9. *Directions to reconstitute Mefoxitin (cefoxitin sodium). (Courtesy of Merck Sharp & Dohme.)*

Rule and arithmetic:

Give:

Write on label:

Storage:

10. Order: Claforan 200 mg IM q6h
    Stock: vial of powder labeled 1 gram (Fig. 11-10)
    Diluting fluid and # ml:

    Solution and new stock:

    Rule and arithmetic:

    Give:

    Write on label:

    Storage:

11. Order: cephradine 108 mg IM q8h
    Stock: vial of 250 mg of powder (Fig. 11-11)
    Diluting fluid and # ml:

    Solution and new stock:

    Rule and arithmetic:

    Give:

(*continued*)

PREPARATION OF CLAFORAN STERILE

Claforan for IM or IV administration should be reconstituted as follows:

Strength	Diluent (mL)	Withdrawable Volume (mL)	Approximate Concentration (mg/mL)
1g vial (IM)*	3	3.4	300
2g vial (IM)*	5	6.0	330
1g vial (IV)*	10	10.4	95
2g vial (IV)*	10	11.0	180
1g infusion	50-100	50-100	20-10
2g infusion	50-100	50-100	40-20
10g bottle	47	52.0	200
10g bottle	97	102.0	100

(*) in conventional vials

Shake to dissolve; inspect for particulate matter and discoloration prior to use. Solutions of Claforan range from very pale yellow to light amber, depending on concentration, diluent used, and length and condition of storage.

For Intramuscular use: Reconstitute VIALS with Sterile Water for Injection or Bacteriostatic Water for Injection as described above.

COMPATIBILITY AND STABILITY

Solutions of Claforan Sterile reconstituted as described above (**Preparation of Claforan Sterile**) maintain satisfactory potency for 24 hours at room temperature (at or below 22°C), 10 days under refrigeration (at or below 5°C), and for at least 13 weeks frozen.

Figure 11-10. Preparation of cefotaxime sodium (Claforan) solution. (Courtesy of Hoechst–Roussel Pharmaceuticals, Inc.)

VELOSEF FOR INJECTION
(Cephradine for Injection USP)

IM DILUTION TABLE

Vial Size	Volume of Diluent	Approximate Available Volume	Approximate Available Concentration
250 mg	1.2 mL	1.2 mL	208 mg/mL
500 mg	2.0 mL	2.2 mL	227 mg/mL
1 g	4.0 mL	4.5 mL	222 mg/mL

For I.M. Use.—Aseptically add Sterile Water for Injection or Bacteriostatic Water for Injection (containing 0.9% [w/v] benzyl alcohol, or 0.12% methylparaben and 0.014% propylparaben) according to the following table [i.e., the table entitled "IM Dilution Table" below].

Intramuscular solutions should be used within two hours at room temperature; if stored in the refrigerator at 5° C., solutions retain full potency for 24 hours. Constituted solutions may vary in color from light straw to yellow; however, this does not affect the potency.

Figure 11-11. IM dilution table for Velosef (cephradine for injection). (Package insert used by permission of E. R. Squibb & Sons, Inc., copyright owner.)

⁻ TEST 5. CALCULATION OF INJECTIONS FROM POWDERS (*Continued*) ⁻

Write on label:

Storage:

12. Order: oxacillin sodium 100 mg IM q6h
     Stock: vial of powder 250 mg (Fig. 11-12)
             Diluting fluid and # ml:

     Solution and new stock:

> *For intramuscular injection:* To obtain a solution containing 250 mg of drug in 1.5 ml of solution, add 1.1 ml of sterile water for injection to the 250 mg vial. The solution will be stable in the refrigerator for 5 days and at room temperature for 24 hours.

Figure 11-12. *Hypothetical directions for reconstitution of oxacillin sodium.*

Rule and arithmetic:

Give:

Write on label:

Storage:

13. Order: Streptomycin sulfate 0.15 g q6h IM
     Stock: vial of powder labeled 1 gram (Fig. 11-13)
             Diluting fluid and # ml:

Solution and new stock:

Rule and arithmetic:

Give:

Write on label:

Storage:

14. Order: penicillin G potassium 120,000 units q4h IM
     Stock: vial of powder 1 million units (see Fig. 11-1)
             Diluting fluid and # ml:

Solution and new stock:

Rule and arithmetic:

(continued)

> The dry powder is dissolved by adding Water for Injection, USP or Sodium Chloride Injection, USP in an amount to yield the desired concentration as indicated in the following table:
>
> | Approx. Conc. (mg/ml) | Volume (ml) of Solvent | |
> | --- | --- | --- |
> | | 1 g Vial | 5 g Vial |
> | 200 | 4.2 | — |
> | 250 | 3.2 | — |
> | 400 | 1.8 | 9.0 |
>
> Sterile reconstituted solutions should be protected from light and may be stored at room temperature for four weeks without significant loss of potency.

Figure 11-13. *Reconstitution directions for streptomycin sulfate. (Courtesy of Roerig–Pfizer Laboratories.)*

ˉ TEST 5. CALCULATION OF INJECTIONS FROM POWDERS (*Continued*) ˉ

Give:

Write on label:

Storage:

15. Order: ampicillin sodium 0.25 g IM q6h
Stock: vial of powder labeled 250 mg (Fig. 11-14)
Diluting fluid and # ml:

Solution and new stock:

Rule and arithmetic:

Give:

Write on label:

Storage:

16. Order: cefoxitin 100 mg IM q12h
Stock: vial of powder 1 gram (see Fig. 11-9)
Diluting fluid and # ml:

Solution and new stock:

Rule and arithmetic:

Give:

Write on label:

Storage:

17. Order: cefazolin 150 mg IM q12h
Stock: vial of powder 250 mg (see Fig. 11-6)
Diluting fluid and # ml:

Solution and new stock:

250 mg vial: Add 0.9 ml Sterile Water for Injection, USP, or Bacteriostatic Water for Injection, USP (TUBEX) to give a final concentration of 250 mg/ml. For fractional doses, withdraw the ampicillin sodium solution as follows:

Dose	Withdraw
125 mg	0.5 ml
150 mg	0.6 ml
175 mg	0.7 ml
200 mg	0.8 ml
225 mg	0.9 ml
250 mg	1 ml

Figure 11-14. *Reconstitution directions for ampicillin sodium (Omnipen). (Courtesy of Wyeth–Ayerst Laboratories, Philadelphia, PA.)*

Rule and arithmetic:

Give:

Write on label:

Storage:

18. Order: ticarcillin 0.2 g q4h IM
Stock: vial of powder labeled 1 g (Fig. 11-15)
Diluting fluid and # ml:

Solution and new stock:

Rule and arithmetic:

Give:

Write on label:

Storage:

19. Order: cefotaxime sodium 0.5 g IM q8h
Stock: vial of powder labeled 2 grams (see Fig. 11-10)
Diluting fluid and # ml:

Solution and new stock:

Rule and arithmetic:

Give:

Write on label:

Storage:

20. Order: penicillin G potassium 800,000 units IM q8h
Stock: vial of powder labeled 5 million units (Fig. 11-16)
Diluting fluid and # ml:

(continued)

DIRECTIONS FOR USE
—1 Gm, 3 Gm and 6 Gm Standard Vials—
INTRAMUSCULAR USE: (Concentration of approximately 385 mg/ml).
For initial reconstitution use Sterile Water for Injection, U.S.P., Sodium Chloride Injection, U.S.P. or 1% Lidocaine Hydrochloride solution* (without epinephrine).
Each gram of Ticarcillin should be reconstituted with 2 ml of Sterile Water for Injection, U.S.P., Sodium Chloride Injection, U.S.P. or 1% Lidocaine Hydrochloride solution* (without epinephrine) and **used promptly.** Each 2.6 ml of the resulting solution will then contain 1 Gm of Ticarcillin.
*[For full product information, refer to manufacturer's package insert for Lidocaine Hydrochloride.]
As with all intramuscular preparations, TICAR (Ticarcillin Disodium) should be injected well within the body of a relatively large muscle, using usual techniques and precautions.

Figure 11-15. Directions for the use of ticarcillin disodium (Ticar). (Courtesy of Beecham Laboratories.)

Preparation of Solutions

Solutions of penicillin should be prepared as follows: Loosen powder. Hold vial horizontally and rotate it while *slowly* directing the stream of diluent against the wall of the vial. Shake vial vigorously after all the diluent has been added. Depending on the route of administration, use Sterile Water for Injection USP, isotonic Sodium Chloride Injection USP, or Dextrose Injection USP. NOTE: Penicillins are rapidly inactivated in the presence of carbohydrate solutions at alkaline pH.

RECONSTITUTION: 1,000,000 u vial—add 9.6 ml, 4.6 ml, or 3.6 ml diluent to provide 100,000 u, 200,000 u, or 250,000 u per ml, respectively: 5,000,000 u vial—add 23 ml, 18 ml, 8 ml, or 3 ml diluent to provide 200,000 u, 250,000 u, 500,000 u, or 1,000,000 u per ml, respectively. *For IV infusion only:* 10,000,000 u vial—add 15.5 ml or 5.4 ml diluent to provide 500,000 u or 1,000,000 u per ml,

respectively: 20,000,000 u vial—add 31.6 ml diluent to provide 500,000 u per ml.

HOW SUPPLIED

Penicillin G Potassium for Injection USP is available in vials providing 1, 5, 10 and 20 million u of crystalline penicillin G potassium.

Storage

The dry powder is relatively stable and may be stored at room temperature without significant loss of potency. Sterile solutions may be kept in the refrigerator one week without significant loss of potency. Solutions prepared for intravenous infusion are stable at room temperature for at least 24 hours.

Figure 11-16.   Preparation of solution of penicillin G potassium. (Package insert used by permission of E. R. Squibb & Sons, Inc., copyright owner.)

͟ TEST 5. CALCULATION OF INJECTIONS FROM POWDERS (*Continued*) ͟

Solution and new stock:

Rule and arithmetic:

Give:

Write on label:

Storage:

Your score: _____

͟ TEST 6. CALCULATION OF IVPB AND IV DRIP FACTORS ͟

Aim for 90% or better on this test. There are 20 questions each worth 5 points. If you have any difficulty doing these problems, review and study Chapter 9, which explains this information. Answers may be found at the end of this chapter.

1.   Order: aqueous penicillin G 1 MU in 100 ml D5W IVPB q6h over 40 minutes (macrodrip tubing at 10 gtt/ml)

   Stock: vial labeled 5 million units of powder. Directions say to inject 18 ml of sterile water for injection to yield 20 ml of solution. Reconstituted solution is stable for 1 week.

   a.   How would you prepare the penicillin?

   b.   What solution will you make?

   c.   What amount of penicillin solution should be placed into the bag of 100 ml D5W?

   d.   What is the drip factor for the IVPB?

2. You have a 250-ml bag of D5W to which has been added 25,000 units of Liquaemin Sodium. You have an order to give the patient 1200 units IV per hour using an infusion pump.
   a.   What should be the drip rate in cubic centimeters per hour (cc/hr)?

   b.   How many hours will this IV run?

3. 1000 ml of an IV solution is to infuse at 100 ml/hr. If the infusion starts at 8 AM, at what time will it be completed?

4. Order: Gentamicin 60 mg IVPB in 50 ml D5W over 30 minutes using macrodrip (20 gtt/cc).
   Stock: vial of gentamicin 40 mg/ml; 50-ml bag of D5W. Order is correct.
   a.   How many ml of gentamicin will you add to the 50-ml bag of D5W?

   b.   What is the drip factor for the IVPB?

5. Calculate the drip factor for 1500 ml D5 $\frac{1}{2}$ NS to run 12 hours by macrodrip (10 gtt/ml).

6. Intralipid, 500 ml q6h, is ordered for a patient together with an IV that is infusing at 80 ml/hr. Calculate the 24-hour parenteral intake.

7. Order: 1000 ml D5W with 20 mEq KCl and 500 mg Vit C at 60 ml/hr. No infusion pump is available.
   a.   Approximately how many hours will the IV run?

   b.   Which tubing will you choose—macrodrip at 10 gtt/ml or microdrip at 60 gtt/ml?

   c.   What are the drops per minute (gtt/min) for the tubing that you chose?

8. Order: 1000 ml D5NS; run 150 ml/hr IV
   Stock: IV bag of 1000 ml D5NS
   a.   Approximately how many hours will the IV run?

   b.   Which tubing will you choose—macrodrip at 10 gtt/ml or microdrip at 60 gtt/ml?

   c.   What will be the drip rate?

9. Order: 100 ml Ringer's solution 12 noon–6 PM IV
   a.   What size tubing will you use?

   b.   What are the gtt/min?

(continued)

⊏ TEST 6. CALCULATION OF IVPB AND IV DRIP FACTORS (*Continued*) ⊐

10. Order: 150 ml NS IV over 3 hours
    Stock: bag of 250 ml normal saline for IV and macrotubing 15 gtt/ml; microtubing (60 gtt/ml)
    a.   What would you do to obtain 150 ml NS?

    b.   What IV tubing would you use?

    c.   What are the gtt/min?

11. Order: Liquaemin Sodium 1500 units/hr IV
    Stock: standardized solution of Liquaemin 100 units/ml. An infusion pump is available. What
             should be the setting on the infusion pump?

12. Order: 500 ml D5W IVKVO. Solve for 24 hours. An infusion pump is available. What should be the
             setting on the infusion pump?

13. Order: cefazolin sodium 1 g IVPB q8h × 3 doses
    Stock: Kefzol (cefazolin sodium) 1 g powder and IVPB tubing (10 gtt/ml) (Fig. 11-17)
    a.   The doctor did not order the fluid for dilution, the amount to be used, or the time for
         infusion. What do the reconstitution directions state?

    b.   State the amount and type of IV fluid you will use and the time for infusion you will use.

    c.   What are the gtt/min?

14. Order: aminophylline 250 mg in 250 ml D5W to run 8 hours IV. Tubing is microdrip. What are the
             gtt/min?

15. Order: Isuprel 2 mg in 250 ml D5W IV; titrate at 4 µg/min
    Stock: ampule of Isuprel labeled 1 mg in 5 ml; microdrip tubing
    a.   How much Isuprel will you add to the IV?

    b.   What will be the gtt/min?

Intermittent <u>intravenous infusion</u>: Kefzol can be administered along with primary intravenous fluid management programs in a volume control set or in a separate, secondary IV bottle. Reconstituted 500 mg or 1 g of Kefzol may be diluted in 50 to 100 mL of one of the following intravenous solutions: 0.9% Sodium Chloride Injection, 5% or 10% Dextrose Injection, 5% Dextrose in Lactated Ringer's Injection, 5% Dextrose and 0.9% Sodium Chloride Injection (also may be used with 5% Dextrose and 0.45% or 0.2% Sodium Chloride Injection), Lactated Ringer's Injection, 5% or 10% Invert Sugar in Sterile Water for Injection, Ringer's Injection, Normosol®-M in D5-W, Inosol® B with Dextrose 5%, or Plasma-Lyte® with 5% Dextrose.
<u>Direct intravenous injection</u>: Dilute the reconstituted 500 mg or 1 g of Kefzol in a minimum of 10 mL of Sterile Water for Injection. Inject solution slowly over 3 to 5 minutes. It may be administered directly into a vein or through the tubing for a patient receiving the above parenteral fluids.

Figure 11-17. Reconstitution directions for cefazolin sodium (Kefzol). (Courtesy of Eli Lilly & Co.)

16. A patient is receiving an IV at the rate of 125 ml/h. The doctor orders cefoxitin 1 g in 75 ml D5W q6h. Calculate the 24-hour parenteral intake.

17. Order: 1000 ml D5 $\frac{1}{2}$ NS to run at 90 ml/hr; infusion pump available

    a. What will be the pump setting?

    b. Approximately how long will the IV run?

18. Order: Aramine 50 mg IV in 250 ml D5W; titrate to 60 μg/min
    Stock: vial of Aramine 100 mg in 10 ml; microtubing

    a. How much Aramine would you add to the IV?

    b. What will be the gtt/min?

19. A doctor orders 500 ml of aminophylline 0.5 g to infuse at 50 ml/hr. How many milligrams will the patient receive each hour?

20. Order: ampicillin sodium 0.5 g in 50 ml D5W IVPB q6h; tubing is macrodrip (10 gtt/ml) (Fig. 11-18)

    a. According to the dilution directions, is the order correct?

    b. What will be the gtt/min if the infusion is given over 20 minutes?

Your score: _____

FOR ADMINISTRATION BY INTRAVENOUS DRIP
Stability studies on ampicillin sodium in various intravenous solutions indicate the drug will lose less than 10% activity at room temperature (70° F) for the time periods and concentrations stated:

IV Solution	Concentrations	Stability Periods
Sterile Water for Injection	Up to 30 mg/mL	8 hours
Isotonic Sodium Chloride	Up to 30 mg/mL	8 hours
M/6 Sodium Lactate Solution	Up to 30 mg/mL	8 hours
5% Dextrose in Water	Up to 20 mg/mL	2 hours
5% Dextrose in 0.45% Sodium Chloride	Up to 2 mg/mL	4 hours
10% Invert Sugar	Up to 2 mg/mL	4 hours
Lactated Ringer's Solution	Up to 30 mg/mL	8 hours

If the solutions below are stored under refrigeration, they will remain stable for the time periods indicated:

PIGGYBACK UNITS (for Intravenous Drip Use)—Use Sterile Water for Injection or Isotonic Sodium Chloride
500-MG BOTTLE:
Add a minimum of 50 mL water or saline, and shake well. If lower concentrations are desired, the solution could be further diluted with up to a total of 100 mL of diluent.

Diluent Amount	Solution Concentration
50 mL	10 mg/mL
100 mL	5 mg/mL

ONE-GRAM BOTTLE:
Add a minimum of 49 mL water or saline, and shake well. If lower concentrations are desired, the solution could be further diluted with up to a total of 99 mL of diluent.

Diluent Amount	Solution Concentration
49 mL	20 mg/mL
99 mL	10 mg/mL

Figure 11-18. *Reconstitution directions for ampicillin sodium IVPB. (Courtesy of Wyeth Laboratories, Philadelphia, PA.)*

TEST 7. CALCULATION OF DOSAGE FOR INFANTS AND CHILDREN

Questions for this test are presented in two parts. Part I deals with calculations. Part II asks you to determine whether the dosages ordered are within a therapeutic range. Calculations are not required.

Part I

In this exercise 10 problems in dosage calculation are presented. Each problem is worth 5 points. Decide if the order is within the therapeutic range. If safe, calculate the dose. Aim for 100% accuracy. If you have any difficulty, reread and study Chapter 10. Answers will be found at the end of the chapter.

1. Order: Tylenol 80 mg po q4° prn temp 100.9°
   Stock: liquid labeled 165 mg/5 ml
   Weight: 8.4 kg
   Literature recommends 10 mg/kg

2. Order: tobramycin 40 mg IVPB D5 $\frac{1}{3}$ NS 50 cc q8h

   Stock: vial labeled 80 mg/2 ml
   Weight: 19 kg; aged 6
   Literature recommends
   a. 6–7.5 mg/kg/day in three or four equally divided doses
   b. Volume of diluent 50–100 ml. Use 50 ml.
   c. Infuse over 20–60 minutes. Use 60 minutes.

3. Order: Augmentin 40 mg/kg/day = 175 mg po q8°
   Stock: oral suspension 125 mg/5 ml
   Weight: 4.3 kg; aged 3
   Literature recommends 40 mg/kg/day in divided doses every 8 hours

4. Order: IV D5 $\frac{1}{3}$ NS + 70 mEq KCl/L at 35 cc maintenance

   Available: 500-ml bag D5 $\frac{1}{3}$ NS; KCl 40 mEq/20 ml; infusion pump (ml/hr)

5. Order: Proventil Syrup 2 mg po q8°
   Stock: liquid labeled 2 mg per 5 ml
   Weight: 41.6 lb
   Literature recommends 0.1 mg/kg three times a day, not to exceed 2 mg three times a day

6. Order: Septra (trimethoprim) (2.5 cc) IV bid in 50 cc D5W over 1 hr
   Stock: 5-ml ampule labeled 80 mg trimethoprim and 400 mg sulfamethoxazole
   Weight: 6.77 kg
   Literature recommends the total daily dose is 15–20 mg/kg based on the trimethoprim component in three to four equally divided doses or 8–10 mg/kg based on the trimethoprim component in two to

four equally divided doses. Each 5 ml of Septra should be added to 125 ml of suitable solution over 60 to 90 minutes.

7. Order: Slo-Phylline 125 mg po q8h
   Stock: liquid labeled 80 mg/15 ml
   Weight: 18.9 kg; aged 6
   Literature recommends 5-mg/kg loading dose and 4 mg/kg q6h. If dose needs to be adjusted for children ages 1–9 do not exceed 24 mg/kg/day.

8. Order: IV D5 0.20 NS + KCl 15 mEq/L at 18 cc/hr
   Available: 250-ml bag of D5 0.02 NS; infusion pump (ml/hr); KCl 20 mEq/40 ml

9. Order: vancomycin 100 mg IVPB q8° in 50 ml D5 $\frac{1}{3}$ NS over 1 hour

   Available: vial labeled 500 mg powder; IV bag of 250 ml D5 $\frac{1}{3}$ NS; infusion pump (ml/hr)

   Weight: 6.8 kg
   Literature recommends total daily dose is 44 mg/kg/day in divided doses; give over 30–60 minutes. Vancomycin directions: Dilute 500 mg with 10 ml sterile water for injection. Further dilution is required. After dilution, vials may be stored in the refrigerator up to 14 days. (*Note:* There is no displacement with vancomycin, so 500 mg = 10 ml.)

10. Order: cefuroxime 75 mg/kg/day = 210 mg in 50 cc D5 $\frac{1}{3}$ NS q8h IVPB

    Available: 750-mg vial of powder; infusion pump (ml/hr)
    Weight: 8.4 kg
    Literature recommends 50–100 mg/kg/day in equally divided doses every 6–8 hours. Dilute 750 mg IV initially with 10 ml sterile water for injection to provide 90 mg/ml. Further dilute with 50–100 ml of acceptable solution and administer over 30–60 minutes. Remaining solution can be stored in refrigerator for 48 hours.

Your score Part I _____

Part II

In this exercise 10 problems are presented. Determine if the dosages ordered are within the therapeutic range for children and infants according to the weight and body surface area. Aim for 100% accuracy. If you have any difficulty, reread and study Chapter 10. Answers may be found at the end of the chapter. Each problem is worth 5 points.

1. An infant with a severe infection caused by *Escherichia coli* weighs 2000 g. Carbenicillin sodium 200 mg IM stat is ordered and then 150 mg IM q6h. The literature states that infants over 2000 g should receive an initial dose of 100 mg/kg and subsequent doses of 75 mg/kg/6 hr (300 mg/kg/day).
   a. What rule will you use to check the safety of this dose?
   b. Is this dose safe? Explain.

(continued)

⊏ TEST 7. CALCULATION OF DOSAGE FOR INFANTS AND CHILDREN ⊐
(Continued)

2. A 32-lb child with an anaerobic septicemia is ordered carbenicillin 1.5 g IVPB q6h. Literature states that 400–500 mg/kg/day should be given IV in divided doses or by continuous drip.
   a. What rule will you use to check the safety of this dose?
   b. Is this dose safe? Explain.

3. A 40-lb child with a postoperative infection is ordered to receive cefazolin sodium 150 mg IM q8h (Fig. 11-19). Is this a safe dose? Explain.

4. A baby weighing 10 lb is ordered cefazolin sodium 55 mg IM q6h. (see Fig. 11-19). Is this a safe dose? Explain.

5. A 6-lb baby of normal height has a BSA of 0.2 m². If an adult dose of atropine sulfate is 0.4 mg IM, what would be a safe dose for this baby?

6. A child weighing 15.4 lb has a respiratory infection and is ordered ampicillin sodium 100 mg IM q6h. Literature states that 25–50 mg/kg/day q6h in equal doses is safe. Is this dose safe for the child? Explain.

7. A baby weighing 5 lb 10 oz is ordered ampicillin sodium 150 mg po q8h. Literature states that 25–50 mg/kg q6h in divided doses is safe. Is this dose safe? Explain.

8. If an adult dose of a drug is 10 mg,
   a. What would be a safe dose for a child weighing 30 lbs?
   b. Which rule did you use to reach an answer?

KEFZOL® (Cefazolin Sodium, USP, Lilly)

TABLE 5. PEDIATRIC DOSAGE GUIDE

Weight		25 mg/kg/Day Divided into 3 Doses		25 mg/kg/Day Divided into 4 Doses	
lb	kg	Approximate Single Dose (mg q8h)	Vol (mL) Needed with Dilution of 125 mg/mL	Approximate Single Dose (mg q6h)	Vol (mL) Needed with Dilution of 125 mg/mL
10	4.5	40 mg	0.35 mL	30 mg	0.25 mL
20	9	75 mg	0.6 mL	55 mg	0.45 mL
30	13.6	115 mg	0.9 mL	85 mg	0.7 mL
40	18.1	150 mg	1.2 mL	115 mg	0.9 mL
50	22.7	190 mg	1.5 mL	140 mg	1.1 mL

Weight		50 mg/kg/Day Divided into 3 Doses		50 mg/kg/Day Divided into 4 Doses	
lb	kg	Approximate Single Dose (mg q8h)	Vol (mL) Needed with Dilution of 225 mg/mL	Approximate Single Dose (mg q6h)	Vol (mL) Needed with Dilution of 225 mg/mL
10	4.5	75 mg	0.35 mL	55 mg	0.25 mL
20	9	150 mg	0.7 mL	110 mg	0.5 mL
30	13.6	225 mg	1 mL	170 mg	0.75 mL
40	18.1	300 mg	1.35 mL	225 mg	1 mL
50	22.7	375 mg	1.7 mL	285 mg	1.25 mL

In children with mild to moderate renal impairment (creatinine clearance of 70 to 40 mL/min), 60% of the normal daily dose given in divided doses every 12 hours should be sufficient. In children with moderate impairment (creatinine clearance of 40 to 20 mL/min), 25% of the normal daily dose given in divided doses every 12 hours should be sufficient. In children with severe impairment (creatinine clearance of 20 to 5 mL/min), 10% of the normal daily dose given every 24 hours should be adequate. All dosage recommendations apply after an initial loading dose.

Figure 11-19. Pediatric dosage guide of cefazolin sodium (Kefzol) (Courtesy of Eli Lilly & Co.)

9. The BSA of a child is 1.3 m^2. If an adult dose of a drug is 50 mg,
    a. What would be a safe dose for this child?
    b. Which rule did you use to reach an answer?

10. A child weighing 40 lb, of normal height, is ordered phenytoin sodium 50 mg po tid. Literature states that the safe dose for this child is 5 mg/kg/day. Is this dose safe? Explain.

Your score Part II _____

TEST 8. ASSORTED DOSAGE PROBLEMS: I

Twenty problems are presented. Aim for 100% accuracy! If you have any difficulty review the relevant material in the beginning chapters. Each problem is worth 5 points. For injection answers using a 3-ml syringe, carry out arithmetic two decimal places and report to the nearest tenth. For the 1-ml precision syringe, carry out arithmetic three decimal places and report to the nearest hundredth. Answers will be found at the end of the chapter.

1. Order: digoxin 0.125 mg po qd
    Stock: bottle of liquid labeled 0.5 mg per 20 ml

2. Order: Levothroid 100 µg qd po
    Stock: scored tablets 0.2 mg

3. Order: Meperidine HCl 35 mg IM stat
    Stock: vial labeled 100 mg/ml. Use 1-ml precision syringe.

4. Order: 1500 ml D5W IVKVO (solve for 24 hr); include drip factor in gtt/min and type of tubing: macrodrip 15 gtt/ml or microdrip 60 gtt/ml

5. Order: heparin 25,000 units in 250 ml D5W IV. Infuse 1500 units/hour. Infusion pump is available.

6. Order: pediatric digitoxin 0.07 mg po qd
    Stock: dropper bottle labeled 0.25 mg/cc

7. Order: add KCl 1.5 mEq to IV stat
    Stock: vial labeled 2 mEq per ml. Use a 3-ml syringe.

(continued)

TEST 8. ASSORTED DOSAGE PROBLEMS: I (*Continued*)

8. Order: penicillin G potassium 150,000 units IM
   Stock: vial of powder labeled 1 million units
   Directions for reconstitution: Add 3.6 ml sterile water for injection to make a concentration of
   200,000 units/ml. Store in refrigerator. Use a 3-ml syringe.

9. Order: ampicillin sodium 2 g in 50 ml D5W IVPB over 30 minutes q6h. What is the gtt/min?
   Macrodrip 10 gtt/ml

10. Order: 1000 ml D5NS with 500 mg vitamin C; run 80 ml/hr. An infusion pump is available.
    a. How would you set the drip rate?
    b. How many hours will this IV run?

11. Order: ascorbic acid 150 mg IM q8h
    Stock: ampule labeled 500 mg/2 ml. Use a 3-ml syringe.

12. Order: tobramycin 0.6 gm IM q6h
    Stock: vial of liquid labeled 300 mg/ml. Use a 3-ml syringe.

13. Order: Lanoxin 0.125 mg qd po
    Stock: scored tablets 0.25 mg

14. Order: cephalexin 0.5 g IM q4h
    Stock: vial of powder labeled 1 gram
    Directions for reconstitution: Add 4 ml sterile water for injection. Made as directed, 500 mg = 2.2 ml.
    Store in refrigerator.

15. Order: quinidine sulfate susp. 200 mg po tid
    Stock: bottle of liquid labeled 0.1 gm = 5 ml

16. Order: 500 ml D5W IV from 8 AM–8 PM; macrodrip (10 gtt/ml); microdrip (60 gtt/ml)
    a. What type of tubing should be used?
    b. What is the gtt/min?

17. Order: el Dimetane 12 mg po q4h prn
    Stock: bottle of liquid labeled 4 mg/5 ml

18. Order: oxytetracycline 0.5 g po q6h
    Stock: capsules labeled 250 mg

19. Order: cefoxitin 0.6 g IM q6h
    Stock: vial of powder labeled 2 grams
    Directions for reconstitution: Add 6.8 ml of sterile water for injection to make a solution of 250
    mg/ml. Entire contents should be withdrawn.

20. Order: NPH insulin units 20 qd SC at 7:30 AM
    Stock: vial of insulin labeled NPH units 100/ml. An insulin syringe marked U 100 is available.

Your score: _____

═══════ TEST 9. ASSORTED DOSAGE PROBLEMS: II ═══════

Twenty problems are presented. Aim for 100% accuracy! If you have any difficulty, review the relevant material in the beginning chapters. Each problem is worth 5 points. Answers will be found at the end of the chapter.

1. Order: potassium chloride elixir 30 mcg po
   Stock: bottle of liquid labeled 40 mcg = 30 ml

2. Order: codeine phosphate 0.06 Gm po
   Stock: tablets of 30 mg and 15 mg. How would you prepare this dose?

3. Order: digoxin 0.25 mg po
   Stock: tablets labeled 0.125 mg

4. Order: 500 ml D5W IV over 6 hours
       a. Which tubing would you use—macrodrip (10 gtt/ml) or microdrip (60 gtt/ml)?
       b. What is the drip rate?

5. Order: cefoxitin 0.4 g IM q6h
   Stock: vial of powder labeled 1 gram
   Directions: Add 2 ml of sterile water for injection to make a solution of 400 mg/ml; stable in the
   refrigerator.

6. Order: Lanoxin 0.125 mg po qd
   Stock: bottle of liquid labeled digoxin 0.5 mg/20 ml

(continued)

═══ TEST 9. ASSORTED DOSAGE PROBLEMS: II (*Continued*) ═══

7. Order: 250 ml Ringer's solution IV at 50 ml/hr
   Stock: infusion pump; bag of IV fluid labeled 250 ml Ringer's solution
       a. How many hours will this IV run?
       b. How should the drip factor be set on the pump?

8. Order: Liquaemin Sodium 50,000 units in 500 ml D5W IV; infuse 1500 units per hour
   Stock: vial of Liquaemin Sodium labeled 10,000 units/ml; bag of IV fluid labeled 500 ml D5W;
           infusion pump is available.
       a. How much Liquaemin Sodium will be added to the IV?
       b. How many hours will this IV run?
       c. How should the drip factor be set on the pump?

9. Order: propranolol 0.02 Gm po q6h
   Stock: scored tablets 0.01 Gm

10. Order: Dilaudid 1.5 mg IM stat
    Stock: vial labeled 2 mg/ml. Use a 3-ml syringe.

11. Order: ampicillin sodium 0.5 g IM q6h
    Stock: vial of powder labeled 1 g
    Directions: Give reconstituted drug within 1 hour because potency may decrease significantly after
            this time. The 1-g vial may be diluted in two ways: add 7.4 ml sterile water for injection
            to make 125 mg/ml, or add 3.4 ml sterile water for injection to make 250 mg/ml.
        a. Which dilution will you use?
        b. How many milliliters will you give the patient?

12. Order: Humulin insulin 7 units SC stat
    Stock: vial of Humulin insulin labeled U 100/ml; U 100 regular insulin syringe (2 units = 1 line); U
            100 low-dose insulin syringe (1 unit = 1 line)
        a. Which syringe should be used?
        b. Explain how you would prepare the dose.

13. Order: start dopamine drip at 200 μg/min and titrate to maintain BP
    Stock: standardized hospital solution of 200 mg in 250 ml D5W
    What is the drip factor?

14. Order: nystatin susp. 300,000 U po qid S & S
    Stock: bottle of liquid labeled 100,000 units/5 ml

15.　Order: erythromycin lactobionate 1 g IVPB in 200 ml NS q6h; administer over 60 min.
　　Stock: vial of powder 1 g; reconstitution device; 250-ml bag of normal saline; IVPB tubing (10 gtt/ml)
　　What is the gtt/min?

16.　Order: diphenhydramine syrup 25 mg po q4h prn
　　Stock: liquid in a bottle labeled 12.5 mg/5 ml

17.　Order: nalbuphine HCl 15 mg IM q4h prn
　　Stock: vial of liquid labeled 20 mg/ml. Use a 3-ml syringe.

18.　Order: keep IV open with 500 ml D5 $\frac{1}{2}$ NS for 24 hours

　　Stock: bag of IV fluid D5 $\frac{1}{2}$ NS

　　a.　What tubing would you use—microdrip or macrodrip (10 gtt/ml)?
　　b.　What are the gtt/min?

19.　Order: kanamycin 500 mg IVPB in 200 ml D5W q8h × 3 days
　　Stock: vial of powder 500 mg; reconstitution device; IV bag of D5W labeled 250 ml. Literature states
　　to administer this amount over 50 minutes.
　　What are the gtt/min?

20.　Order: epinephrine 0.5 mg SC stat
　　Stock: ampule labeled 1:1000 (2-ml size)

Your score: _____

═══ TEST 10. MENTAL DRILL FOR ASSORTED DOSAGE PROBLEMS ═══

*Twenty problems are presented in this set. Each problem is worth 5 points. Aim for 100% accuracy! It is
only necessary to write the answer. If the arithmetic is not obvious, by all means work it out on paper.*

1.　Order: atropine sulfate 0.6 mg SC
　　Stock: vial of liquid labeled 0.4 mg/cc

2.　Order: infuse heparin sodium 1,200 U/hr. An infusion pump is available. What solution will you
　　make? How will you set the flow on the pump?

(continued)

══ TEST 10. MENTAL DRILL FOR ASSORTED DOSAGE PROBLEMS ══
(*Continued*)

3. Order: el potassium chloride 20 mEq po bid
   Stock: bottle of liquid labeled 30 mEq/15 ml

4. Order: Synthroid 0.3 mg po qd
   Stock: scored tablets labeled 150 μg

5. Order: morphine sulfate 10 mg SC stat
   Stock: vial labeled 15 mg/ml. Use a 1-ml precision syringe.

6. Order: cefoxitin 0.6 g IM q6h
   Stock: 1 g powder in a vial
   Directions: Add 2 ml sterile water for injection to make a solution of 400 mg/ml. Stable in the
   refrigerator.

7. Order: 1000 ml D5S with 20 mEq KCl IV; run 150 ml/hr; macrodrip tubing 10 gtt/ml
   What is the drip factor?

8. Order: Thorazine 50 mg IM stat
   Stock: vial of liquid labeled 0.1 gm/2 ml

9. Order: digoxin 0.5 mg po qd
   Stock: scored tablets 0.25 mg

10. Order: Pen-Vee 400,000 units po
    Stock: bottle of liquid labeled 300,000 units/5 cc

11. Order: oxacillin sodium 0.25 g q6h IM
    Stock: vial of powder labeled 1 gram
    Directions: Add 5.7 ml sterile water for injection to make a solution of 250 mg/1.5 ml; stable in the
    refrigerator.

12. Order: el phenobarbital 25 mg po q6h
    Stock: liquid in a bottle labeled 10 mg/4 ml

13. Order: 500 ml D5W to run 8 AM–8 PM
What tubing will you use?
What is the drip rate?

14. Order: Dimetane 6 mg po bid
Stock: scored tablets of 4 mg

15. Order: aq. penicillin G potassium 400,000 units IM q6h
Stock: vial of powder labeled 1 million units
Directions: Add 3.6 ml of sterile water for injection to make a solution of 250,000 units/cc

16. Order: haloperidol 2 mg IM stat
Stock: vial of liquid labeled 5 mg/ml

17. Order: Bactrim 80 mg IVPB in 125 ml D5W q6h; run over 1 hr
Stock: 80-mg vial of liquid in 5 ml labeled Bactrim; 150-ml bag of D5W
What is the drip factor?

18. 1000 ml of an IV is infusing at 100 ml/hr. If it is 10 AM when the infusion starts, at what hour will it be completed?

19. Order: kanamycin 1 g in 200 ml D5W IVPB over 2 hours
Stock: vial of kanamycin 1 g powder; reconstitution device; 250-ml bag of D5W; IVPB tubing macrodrip 20 gtt/ml
What is the drip factor?

20. Order: nafcillin 0.5 g IM q6h
Stock: 2-gram vial of powder
Directions: Add 6.6 ml sterile water for injection to make a concentration of 250 mg/ml; stable in the
refrigerator.

Your score: _____

ANSWERS

TEST 1. ABBREVIATIONS

1. Twice a day
2. Hour of sleep
3. When necessary
4. Both eyes
5. By mouth
6. By rectum
7. Sublingually
8. Swish and swallow
9. Three times a week
10. Milliliter
11. Every 4 hours
12. Cubic centimeters
13. Subcutaneously
14. One and a half
15. Gram
16. After meals
17. Every day
18. Immediately
19. Every 12 hours
20. Three times a day
21. Left eye
22. Kilogram
23. Dram
24. Every hour
25. Right eye
26. Milliequivalent
27. Before meals
28. Four times a day
29. Milligram
30. Intramuscularly
31. Every other day
32. Twice a week
33. Nasogastric tube
34. Every 8 hours
35. Liter
36. Microgram
37. Every 6 hours
38. Microgram
39. Unit
40. Teaspoon
41. A half
42. Grain
43. Intravenously
44. Milliliter
45. Ounce
46. Intravenous piggyback
47. Minim
48. Gram
49. Every 2 hours
50. Every 3 hours

TEST 2. EQUIVALENTS

1. 0.1
2. 30
3. 30
4. 1000
5. 0.3
6. v
7. 5
8. $\dfrac{1}{150}$
9. 600
10. $\dfrac{1}{2}$
11. 15
12. 0.01
13. 1
14. 0.4
15. 0.06
16. 200
17. 1
18. 0.03
19. 200
20. $\dfrac{1}{4}$
21. 0.5
22. 60
23. 30
24. 16
25. 15
26. 15
27. 2.2
28. 1000
29. 0.1
30. 0.06
31. 1
32. 1
33. 0.3
34. 8
35. 1
36. 0.5
37. 100
38. 4
39. x
40. 0.6
41. 0.01
42. 1000
43. 0.0005
44. 0.0006
45. 0.25
46. 0.001
47. 125
48. 10
49. 1
50. 1000

TEST 3. ORAL CALCULATIONS: SOLIDS AND LIQUIDS

1. $\dfrac{20\ \text{mEq}}{30\ \text{mEq}} \times \overset{5}{15}\ \text{ml} = 10\ \text{ml}$

2. $\dfrac{80\ \text{mg}}{125\ \text{mg}} \times 5\ \text{ml} = \dfrac{80}{25} = \dfrac{16}{5} = 5\overline{)16.0}\;^{3.2} = 3.2\ \text{ml}$

   If you do not have a dropper bottle, you could use a syringe without the needle to obtain the dose.

3. 0.02 g = 20 mg

   $\dfrac{20\ \text{mg}}{10\ \text{mg}} \times 1\ \text{tab} = 2\ \text{tablets}$

4. 0.5 g = 500 mg

   $\dfrac{500\ \text{mg}}{250\ \text{mg}} \times 1\ \text{cap} = 2\ \text{capsules}$

5.
$$\frac{0.50 \text{ mg}}{0.25 \text{ mg}} \times 1 \text{ tab} = 2 \text{ tablets}$$
(2 over 0.50, 1 under 0.25)

6. 100 mcg = 0.1 mg
$$\frac{0.1 \text{ mg}}{0.2 \text{ mg}} \times 10 \text{ ml} = 5 \text{ ml}$$
(5 over 10)

7.
$$\frac{75 \text{ mg}}{50 \text{ mg}} \times 1 \text{ tab} = \frac{3}{2} \overline{)3.0}^{1.5} = 1.5 \text{ tablets}$$
(3 over 75, 2 under 50)

8.
$$\frac{40 \text{ mg}}{80 \text{ mg}} \times 1 \text{ tab} = \frac{1}{2} \text{ tablet}$$
(1 over 40, 2 under 80)

9. 0.125 mg = 125 μg
$$\frac{125 \text{ μg}}{500 \text{ μg}} \times 10 \text{ ml} = \frac{5}{2} \overline{)5.0}^{2.5} = 2.5 \text{ ml}$$
(1 over 125, 4 under 500, 5 over 10, 2 under 4)

10.
$$\frac{75 \text{ mg}}{50 \text{ mg}} \times 10 \text{ ml} = 15 \text{ ml}$$
(3 over 75, 2 under 50, 5 over 10, 1 under 2)

11.
$$\frac{5 \text{ mg}}{2 \text{ mg}} \times 1 \text{ tab} = \frac{5}{2} \overline{)5.0}^{2.5} = 2\frac{1}{2} \text{ tablets}$$

12. 0.15 mg = 150 μg
$$\frac{150 \text{ μg}}{300 \text{ μg}} \times 1 \text{ tab} = \frac{1}{2} \text{ tablet}$$
(1 over 150, 2 under 300)

13.
$$\frac{375 \text{ mg}}{250 \text{ mg}} \times 1 \text{ tab} = \frac{3}{2} \overline{)3.0}^{1.5} = 1\frac{1}{2} \text{ tablets}$$
(3 over 375, 2 under 250)

14. 0.6 g = 600 mg
$$\frac{600 \text{ mg}}{300 \text{ mg}} \times 1 \text{ tab} = 2 \text{ tablets}$$
(2 over 600, 1 under 300)

15.
$$\frac{15 \text{ mg}}{10 \text{ mg}} \times 8 \text{ ml} = 12 \text{ ml; pour 3 drams!}$$
(3 over 15, 4 over 8, 2 under 10, 1 under 2)

16.
$$\frac{25.0 \text{ mg}}{12.5 \text{ mg}} \times 5 \text{ ml} = 10 \text{ ml}$$
(2 over 25.0, 1 under 12.5)

17.
$$\frac{60 \text{ mg}}{40 \text{ mg}} \times 0.6 \text{ ml} = \frac{1.8}{2} = 0.9 \text{ ml}$$
(3 over 60, 2 under 40)

18. 0.5 g = 500 mg
$$\frac{500 \text{ mg}}{250 \text{ mg}} \times 5 \text{ ml} = 10 \text{ ml}$$
(2 over 500, 1 under 250)

19.
$$\frac{150 \text{ mg}}{50 \text{ mg}} \times 5 \text{ ml} = 15 \text{ ml}$$
(3 over 150, 1 under 50)

20.
$$\frac{7.5 \text{ mg}}{10.0 \text{ mg}} \times 5 \text{ ml} = \frac{15}{4} \overline{)15.00}^{3.75} = 3.8 \text{ ml}$$
(3 over 7.5, 4 under 10.0)

If you do not have a dropper, use a syringe minus the needle to get the dose.

TEST 4. CALCULATIONS OF INJECTIONS FROM LIQUIDS

1.
$$\frac{0.25 \text{ mg}}{0.50 \text{ mg}} \times 2 \text{ ml} = 1 \text{ ml}$$
(1 over 0.25, 2 under 0.50, 1 over 2, 1 under)

2.
$$\frac{40 \text{ mg}}{50 \text{ mg}} \times 2 \text{ cc} = \frac{8}{5} \overline{)8.0}^{1.6} = 1.6 \text{ ml}$$

3.
$$\frac{8 \text{ mg}}{15 \text{ mg}} \times 1 \text{ ml} = \frac{8}{15} \overline{)8.00}^{.53} = 0.5 \text{ ml}$$
$$\underline{7\ 5}$$
$$50$$
$$\underline{45}$$

4. $\dfrac{\cancel{25}\ \cancel{mg}}{\cancel{100}\ \cancel{mg}} \times 1\ ml = \dfrac{1}{4}\overset{.25}{\overline{)1.00}} = 0.3\ ml$

    You could use the 1-ml precision syringe (0.25 ml).

5. $\dfrac{\cancel{200}\ \cancel{mg}}{\cancel{500}\ \cancel{mg}} \times 2\ ml = \dfrac{4}{5}\overset{.8}{\overline{)4.0}} = 0.8\ ml$

6. $\dfrac{\cancel{1500}\ \cancel{\mu g}}{\cancel{5000}\ \cancel{\mu g}} \times 1\ ml = \dfrac{3}{10}\overset{.3}{\overline{)3.0}} = 0.3\ ml$

7. $\dfrac{\cancel{0.6}\ \cancel{mg}}{\cancel{0.4}\ \cancel{mg}} \times 1\ ml = \dfrac{3}{2}\overset{1.5}{\overline{)3.0}} = 1.5\ ml$

8. $0.1\ gm = 100\ mg$

    $\dfrac{\cancel{100}\ \cancel{mg}}{\cancel{200}\ \cancel{mg}} \times 3\ ml = \dfrac{3}{2}\overset{1.5}{\overline{)3.0}} = 1.5\ ml$

9. $\dfrac{\cancel{15}\ \cancel{mg}}{\cancel{20}\ \cancel{mg}} \times 1\ ml = \dfrac{3}{4}\overset{.75}{\overline{)3.00}} = 0.8\ ml$

    You could use a 1-ml precision syringe (0.75 ml).

10. $\dfrac{\cancel{600,000\ units}}{\cancel{500,000\ units}} \times 1\ ml = \dfrac{6}{5}\overset{1.2}{\overline{)6.0}} = 1.2\ ml$

11. $200\ \mu g = 0.2\ mg$

    $\dfrac{\cancel{0.2}\ \cancel{mg}}{\cancel{0.8}\ \cancel{mg}} \times 1\ ml = \dfrac{1}{4}\overset{.25}{\overline{)1.00}} = 0.3\ ml$

    You could use a precision syringe (0.25 ml).

12. 1:4000 means 1 g in 4000 ml

    1 g = 1000 mg

    500 mcg = 0.5 mg

13. $\dfrac{3\ \cancel{mg}}{2\ \cancel{mg}} \times 1\ ml = \dfrac{3}{2}\overset{1.5}{\overline{)3.0}} = 1.5\ ml$

14. 1:1000 means 1 g = 1000 ml

    1 g = 1000 mg

    $\dfrac{0.4\ \cancel{mg}}{\cancel{1000}\ \cancel{mg}} \times \cancel{1000}\ ml = 0.4\ ml$

15. 50% means 50 g in 100 ml

    500 mg = 0.5 g

    $\dfrac{0.5\ \cancel{g}}{\cancel{50}\ \cancel{g}} \times \overset{2}{\cancel{100}}\ ml = 1.0\ ml$

16. $\dfrac{\cancel{0.75}\ \cancel{mg}}{\cancel{1.50}\ \cancel{mg}} \times 1\ ml = \dfrac{1}{2}\ ml\ or\ 0.5\ ml$

17. 20% means 20 g in 100 ml

    100 mg = 0.1 g

    $\dfrac{0.1\ \cancel{g}}{\cancel{20}\ \cancel{g}} \times \overset{5}{\cancel{100}}\ ml = 0.5\ ml$

18. $\dfrac{\cancel{0.125}\ \cancel{mg}}{\cancel{0.250}\ \cancel{mg}} \times \overset{1}{\cancel{2}}\ ml = 1\ ml$

19. $\dfrac{\cancel{12}\ \cancel{mg}}{\cancel{10}\ \cancel{mg}} \times 1\ ml = \dfrac{6}{5}\overset{1.2}{\overline{)6.0}} = 1.2\ ml$

20. $\dfrac{\cancel{10}\ \cancel{mEq}}{\cancel{40}\ \cancel{mEq}} \times \overset{5}{\cancel{20}}\ ml = 5\ ml$

TEST 5. CALCULATION OF INJECTIONS FROM POWDERS

1. 1.8 ml sterile water for injection
    500,000 units/ml

    $\dfrac{D}{H} \times S = A$ $\dfrac{\cancel{600,000}\ \cancel{U}}{\cancel{500,000}\ \cancel{U}} \times 1\ ml = \dfrac{6}{5}\overset{1.2}{\overline{)6.0}}$

1.2 ml IM
500,000 units/ml; date; initials
Refrigerator

2. 1.5 ml sterile water for injection
280 mg/ml

$$\frac{D}{H} \times S = A \qquad \frac{\cancel{280}\ \cancel{mg}}{\cancel{280}\ \cancel{mg}} \times 1\ ml = \cancel{5} \ \ \frac{.71}{7\,)5.00}$$

$$\frac{4\ 9}{10}$$
$$\frac{\ \ \ 7}{}$$

0.7 ml IM
280 mg/ml; date; initials
Refrigerator

3. 7 ml sterile water for injection
1 g/2.0 ml
Not necessary. Order is 1 g
2 ml IM
1 g/ml; date; initials
Refrigerator

4. 1.8 ml sterile water for injection
250 mg/ml

$$\frac{D}{H} \times S = A \qquad \frac{\overset{8}{\cancel{400\ mg}}}{\underset{5}{\cancel{250\ mg}}} \times 1\ ml = \cancel{8} \ \ \frac{1.6}{5\,)8.0}$$

1.6 ml IM
Nothing. Note that the solution cannot be stored. Must be used within 1 hour.
No. *Discard the vial in an appropriate receptacle.*

5. 1.8 ml sterile water for injection
250 mg/ml

$$\frac{D}{H} \times S = A \qquad \frac{\overset{3}{\cancel{300\ mg}}}{\underset{5}{\cancel{250\ mg}}} \times 1\ ml = \cancel{6} \ \ \frac{1.2}{5\,)6.0}$$

1.2 ml IM
Nothing! Discard the vial. Directions say solution must be used within 1 hour.
No. *Discard the vial in an appropriate receptacle.*

6. 2.5 ml sterile water for injection
330 mg/ml

$$\frac{D}{H} \times S = A \qquad \text{Not necessary.}$$
0.33 g is 330 mg

1 ml IM
330 mg/ml; date; initials
Refrigerator

7. 2.8 ml sterile water for injection; 1 ml 2% lidocaine
250 mg/ml

$$\frac{D}{H} \times S = A \qquad 0.5\ g = 500\ mg$$

$$\frac{\overset{2}{\cancel{500\ mg}}}{\underset{1}{\cancel{250\ mg}}} \times 1\ ml = 2\ ml$$

2 ml IM
250 mg/ml; date; initials
Refrigerator

8. 2.5 ml sterile water for injection
330 mg/ml

$$\frac{D}{H} \times S = A \qquad \frac{\cancel{300\ mg}}{\cancel{330\ mg}} \times 1\ ml = \frac{\cancel{30}}{33}$$

$$\begin{array}{r} .90 \\ 33\overline{)30.00} \\ \underline{29\ 7} \\ 30 \end{array}$$

0.9 ml IM
330 mg/ml; date; initials
Refrigerator

9. 2 ml sterile water for injection
400 mg/ml

$$\frac{D}{H} \times S = A \qquad \frac{\cancel{300\ mg}}{\cancel{400\ mg}} \times 1\ ml = \frac{\cancel{3}}{4}$$

$$\begin{array}{r} .75 \\ 4\overline{)3.00} \\ \underline{2\ 8} \\ 20 \\ \underline{20} \end{array}$$

0.8 ml IM
400 mg/ml; date; initials
Refrigerator

10. 3 ml sterile water for injection
300 mg/ml

$$\frac{D}{H} \times S = A \qquad \frac{\cancel{200\ mg}}{\cancel{300\ mg}} \times 1\ ml = \frac{\cancel{2}}{3}$$

$$\begin{array}{r} .66 \\ 3\overline{)2.00} \\ \underline{1\ 8} \\ 20 \\ \underline{18} \end{array}$$

0.7 ml IM
300 mg/ml; date; initials
Refrigerator

11. 1.2 ml sterile water for injection
208 mg/ml

$$\frac{D}{H} \times S = A \qquad \frac{108\ mg}{208\ mg} \times 1\ ml = \frac{\cancel{108}}{208}$$

$$\begin{array}{r} .51 \\ 208\overline{)108.00} \\ \underline{104\ 0} \\ 4\ 00 \\ \underline{2\ 08} \end{array}$$

0.5 ml IM
208 mg/ml; date; initials
Refrigerator

12.   1.1 ml sterile water for injection
          250 mg/1.5 ml

$$\frac{D}{H} \times S = A \qquad \frac{\overset{2}{\cancel{100}\text{ mg}}}{\underset{5}{\cancel{250}\text{ mg}}} \times 1.5\text{ ml} = \frac{\cancel{3.0}}{5} \quad 5\overline{)3.0}^{\,.6}$$
$$\qquad\qquad\qquad\qquad\qquad\qquad\qquad\qquad\quad \underline{3\ 0}$$

0.6 ml IM
250 mg/1.5 ml; date; initials
Refrigerator

13.   Best to use 4.2 ml sterile water for injection because it is the most dilute
          200 mg/ml
          0.15 g = 150 mg

$$\frac{D}{H} \times S = A \qquad \frac{\overset{3}{\cancel{150}\text{ mg}}}{\underset{4}{\cancel{200}\text{ mg}}} \times 1\text{ ml} = \frac{\cancel{3}}{4} \quad 4\overline{)3.00}^{\,.75}$$
$$\qquad\qquad\qquad\qquad\qquad\qquad\qquad\qquad\quad \underline{2\ 8}$$
$$\qquad\qquad\qquad\qquad\qquad\qquad\qquad\qquad\qquad\ 20$$
$$\qquad\qquad\qquad\qquad\qquad\qquad\qquad\qquad\qquad\underline{20}$$

0.8 ml IM
200 mg/ml; date; initials
Room temperature

14.   Closest is 10 ml sterile water for injection
          100,000 units/ml

$$\frac{D}{H} \times S = A \qquad \frac{\overset{6}{\cancel{120,000}\text{ units}}}{\underset{5}{\cancel{100,000}\text{ units}}} \times 1\cdot\text{ml} = \frac{\cancel{6}}{5} \quad 5\overline{)6.0}^{\,1.2}$$

1.2 ml IM
100,000 units/ml; date; initials
Refrigerator

15.   0.9 ml sterile water for injection
          250 mg/ml
          Not necessary. Order is 250 mg.
          Entire amount in the vial (250 mg in 1 ml) in solution
          Nothing
          None. Discard vial in a proper receptacle.

16.   2 ml sterile water for injection
          400 mg/ml

$$\frac{D}{H} \times S = A \qquad \frac{\cancel{100}\text{ mg}}{\cancel{400}\text{ mg}} = \frac{1}{4} \quad 4\overline{)1.00}^{\,.25} = 0.3\text{ ml}$$

0.3 ml IM
400 mg/ml; date; initials
Refrigerator

17.   2 ml sterile water for injection. (It is the first listed.)
          125 mg/ml

$$\frac{D}{H} \times S = A \qquad \frac{\overset{6}{\cancel{150}\text{ mg}}}{\underset{5}{\cancel{125}\text{ mg}}} \times 1\text{ ml} = \frac{\cancel{6}}{5} \quad 5\overline{)6.0}^{\,1.2}$$

1.2 ml IM
125 mg/ml; date; initials
Refrigerator

18. 2 ml sterile water for injection
1 g = 2.6 ml

$\dfrac{D}{H} \times S = A$
1 g = 1000 mg
0.2 g = 200 mg

$$\dfrac{\overset{1}{\cancel{200\ \text{mg}}}}{\underset{5}{\cancel{1000\ \text{mg}}}} \times 2.6\ \text{ml} = \dfrac{\overset{.52}{\cancel{2.6}}}{5} \quad 5\overline{)2.60}$$
$$\underline{2\ 5}$$
$$10$$

0.5 ml IM
1 g = 2.6 ml; date; initials
Not given. Check package insert.

19. 5 ml sterile water for injection
330 mg/ml

$\dfrac{D}{H} \times S = A$ 0.5 g = 500 mg

$$\dfrac{500\ \cancel{\text{mg}}}{330\ \cancel{\text{mg}}} \times 1\ \text{ml} = \dfrac{50}{33} \quad 33\overline{)50.00}^{\,1.51}$$
$$\underline{33}$$
$$17\ 0$$
$$\underline{16\ 5}$$
$$50$$
$$\underline{33}$$

1.5 ml IM
330 mg/ml; date; initials
Refrigerator

20. 8 ml sterile water for injection
500,000 units/ml

$\dfrac{D}{H} \times S = A$ $\dfrac{\cancel{800,000\ \text{u}}}{\cancel{500,000\ \text{u}}} \times 1\ \text{ml} = \dfrac{8}{5} \quad 5\overline{)8.0}^{\,1.6}$

1.6 ml IM
500,000 units/ml; date; initials
Refrigerator
Note that you could have diluted the powder with 3 ml to yield a solution of 1 million units/ml. You would then have administered 0.8 ml IM.

TEST 6. CALCULATION OF IVPB AND IV DRIP FACTORS

1. a. Add 18 ml of sterile water for injection to the vial of 5 million units (5 MU).
   b. Solution is 5 MU/20 ml

   c. You want 1 MU so $\dfrac{D}{H} \times S = A$ $\dfrac{1\ \cancel{\text{MU}}}{\cancel{5\ \text{MU}}} \times \overset{4}{\cancel{20}}\ \text{ml} = 4\ \text{ml}$

   d. $\dfrac{\#\ \text{ml} \times \text{TF}}{\#\ \text{min}} = \text{gtt/min}$ $\dfrac{\overset{25}{\cancel{100}}\ \text{ml} \times \cancel{10}}{\underset{1}{\cancel{40}}} = 25\ \text{gtt/min}$

2. a. Logic: You have $\dfrac{\overset{100}{\cancel{25,000}}\ \text{units of drug}}{\underset{1}{\cancel{250}}\ \text{ml bag}} = 100\ \text{units/ml}$

The solution is 100 units/ml. The order calls for

$$\frac{1200 \text{ units/hr}}{100 \text{ units/ml}} = 12 \text{ ml/hr}$$

The drip rate is 12 cc/hr. Set the infusion pump for 12 ml/hr.

b. If you deliver 12 ml/hr and the IV bag contains 250 ml, then

$$\frac{250}{12} \quad 12\overline{)250.0}^{\,20.8} = \text{approximately 21 hours.}$$

$$\begin{array}{r} 24 \\ \hline 10\ 0 \\ 9\ 6 \\ \hline 4 \end{array}$$

3. Logic: 1000 ml is infusing at 100 ml/hr, so the IV will take

$$\frac{\overset{10}{\cancel{1000}}}{\underset{1}{\cancel{100}}} = 10 \text{ hours to complete.}$$

If it starts at 8 AM, it should finish 10 hours later at 6 PM.

4. a. $\dfrac{D}{H} \times S = A$ $\quad \dfrac{\overset{3}{\cancel{60}\text{ mg}}}{\underset{2}{\cancel{40}\text{ mg}}} \times 1 \text{ ml} = \dfrac{3}{2} \quad 2\overline{)3.0}^{\,1.5 \text{ ml}}$

b. $\dfrac{\text{\# ml} \times \text{TF}}{\text{\# min}} = \text{gtt/min}$ $\quad \dfrac{50 \text{ ml} \times \cancel{20}}{\cancel{30}} = \dfrac{100}{3} \quad 3\overline{)100.00}^{\,33.3} = 33 \text{ gtt/min}$

5. Step 1. $\dfrac{\text{\# ml}}{\text{\# hr}} = \text{ml/hr}$ $\quad \dfrac{\cancel{1500}}{12} \quad 12\overline{)1500.}^{\,125.} = 125 \text{ ml/hr}$

$$\begin{array}{r} 12 \\ \hline 30 \\ 24 \\ \hline 60 \\ 60 \\ \hline \end{array}$$

Step 2. $\dfrac{\text{\# ml/hr} \times \text{TF}}{60} = \text{gtt/min}$ $\quad \dfrac{125}{\cancel{60}} \times \cancel{10} = \dfrac{\cancel{125}}{6} \quad 6\overline{)125.0}^{\,20.8} = 21 \text{ gtt/min}$

$$\begin{array}{r} 12 \\ \hline 5\ 0 \\ 4\ 8 \\ \hline \end{array}$$

6. Logic: Intralipid 500 ml q6h means the patient is receiving 500 ml four times every 24 hours.

$$\begin{array}{r} 500 \\ \times\ \ 4 \\ \hline 2000 \text{ ml} \end{array}$$

The IV is infusing 80 ml/hr. There are 24 hr in a day so

$$\begin{array}{r} 24 \\ \times 80 \\ \hline 1920 \end{array}$$

Adding these we have   2000 ml
                         + 1920 ml
                          3920 ml

7. a. You have 1000 ml running at 60 ml/hr; therefore,

$$60 \overline{)1000.0} = \text{approximately } 16\frac{1}{2} \text{ hours}$$

$$\begin{array}{r} 16.6 \\ 60 \overline{)1000.0} \\ \underline{60} \\ 400 \\ \underline{360} \\ 400 \end{array}$$

b. Logic: If you want 60 ml/hr and use microdrip tubing, the drip factor will be 60 gtt/min:

$$\frac{\#\ ml \times TF}{60} = \frac{60 \times \cancel{60}}{\cancel{60}} = 60 \text{ gtt/min}$$

If you use macrodrip you have $\dfrac{\cancel{60} \times 10}{\cancel{60}} = 10$ gtt/min

Because the IV will run over 16 hours, choose *microdrip tubing.*

c. The drip factor will be 60 gtt/min.
Note: It is not incorrect to choose the macrodrip at 10 gtt/min. However, because the IV will run so many hours, a good flow might help to keep the IV running.

8. a. You have 1000 ml running at 150 ml/hr; therefore,

$$\frac{\cancel{1000}}{\cancel{15}} = \frac{\cancel{20}}{3} \quad 3\overline{)20.0} = \text{approximately } 6\frac{1}{2} \text{ hours}$$

$$\begin{array}{r} 6.6 \\ 3 \overline{)20.0} \\ \underline{18} \\ 2\ 0 \\ \underline{1\ 8} \end{array}$$

b. Given: macrodrip = 25 gtt/min   microdrip = 150 gtt/min

$$\frac{\#\ ml \times TF}{60} \quad \frac{150 \times 10}{60} = 25 \qquad \frac{150 \times \cancel{60}}{\cancel{60}} = 150$$

You would choose macrodrip tubing.

c. 25 gtt/min

9. a. Because the amount is small and will run over 6 hours, choose *microdrip tubing.*

b. Step 1. $\dfrac{\#\ ml}{hr} = ml/hr = \dfrac{\cancel{100}}{6} \quad 6\overline{)100.0} = 17$ ml/hr

$$\begin{array}{r} 16.6 \\ 6 \overline{)100.0} \\ \underline{6} \\ 40 \\ \underline{36} \\ 40 \\ \underline{36} \end{array}$$

Step 2. $\dfrac{\#\ ml/hr \times TF}{60} = \dfrac{17 \times \cancel{60}}{\cancel{60}} = 17$ gtt/min

10. a. Because the stock bag is 250 ml NS, you would aseptically allow 100 ml to run off. This will leave 150 ml NS.

    b. *Microdrip,* because:

Step 1. $\dfrac{\#\ ml}{\#\ hr} = ml/hr$ $\dfrac{\overset{50}{\cancel{150}\ ml}}{\cancel{3}\ hr} = 50\ ml/hr$

Step 2. $\dfrac{\#\ ml/hr \times TF}{60} = gtt/min$

With microdrip the # ml/hr = gtt/min; hence, microdrip would be 50 gtt/min. Proof: $\dfrac{50 \times \cancel{60}}{\cancel{60}}$

= 50 gtt/min

Macrodrip would be $\dfrac{50 \times \overset{1}{\cancel{15}}}{\underset{4}{\cancel{60}}} = \dfrac{\cancel{50}}{4} \overset{12.5}{\overline{)50.0}} = 13\ gtt/min$

$$\begin{array}{r} 4 \\ \hline 10 \\ 8 \\ \hline 2\,0 \\ 2\,0 \\ \hline \end{array}$$

  c. 50 gtt/min

    Note: It would not be incorrect to choose the macrodrip. However, 50 gtt/min provides a better flow.

11. 15 ml/hr

    Logic: You have to give 1500 units/hr and have a solution of 100 units/ml;

    therefore, $\dfrac{1500\ \cancel{units}/hr}{100\ \cancel{units}/ml} = 15\ ml/hr$

12. 21 ml/hr

    Logic: Step 1. $\dfrac{\#\ ml}{\#\ hr} = ml/hr$

$$\dfrac{500\ ml}{24\ hr} \overset{20.8}{\overline{)500.0}} = 21\ ml/hr$$

$$\begin{array}{r} 48 \\ \hline 20\ 0 \\ 19\ 2 \\ \hline \end{array}$$

        Step 2.   Not necessary; you have an infusion pump that delivers milliliters per hour.

13. a. The reconstitution directions state that you can use 50 ml–100 ml of several solutions to dilute the powder, and it can be given along with the primary IV or as a secondary IV (IVPB).

        No time for the IVPB is given; however, a direct IV push can be given over 3–5 minutes. It is safe to use a longer period. A rule of thumb is to give 50 ml over 30 minutes.

    b. 1 g of cefazolin sodium dissolved in 50 ml D5W, given over 30 minutes.

    c. $\dfrac{\#\ ml \times TF}{30} = gtt/min$ $\dfrac{50 \times 10}{30} = \dfrac{\cancel{50}}{3} \overset{16.6}{\overline{)50.0}} = 17\ gtt/min$

$$\begin{array}{r} 3 \\ \hline 20 \\ 18 \\ \hline 20 \\ 18 \\ \hline \end{array}$$

14.   31 gtt/min

Step 1. $\dfrac{\#\ ml}{\#\ hr} = ml/hr$

$$\begin{array}{r} 31.3 \\ 8\,\overline{)250.0} \\ \underline{24} \\ 10 \\ \underline{8} \\ 20 \end{array}$$

The IV will run 31 ml/hr

Step 2.   You are using microdrip (60 gtt/ml); ml/hr = gtt/min

Proof: $\dfrac{\#\ ml \times TF}{60} = \dfrac{31 \times 60}{60} = 31\ gtt/min$

15.   a.   Use two ampules of Isuprel 1 mg in 5 ml; therefore, add 10 ml to the IV.
      b.   30 gtt/min
Logic: You have 2 mg in 250 ml; 2 mg = 2000 μg.
         Therefore, you have 2000 μg in 250 ml. Reduce this solution:

$$\dfrac{\overset{8}{\cancel{2000}}\ \mu g}{\underset{1}{\cancel{250}}\ ml} = \dfrac{8}{1}$$

Therefore, the solution is 8 μg/1 ml. The tubing is microdrip (60 gtt/ml). Substitute for 8 μg/1 ml, 8 μg/60 gtt/min
You want 4 μg/min

$$\dfrac{D}{H} \times S = A \qquad \dfrac{\overset{1}{\cancel{4}}\ \cancel{\mu g}}{\underset{\underset{1}{\cancel{2}}}{\cancel{8}\ \cancel{\mu g}}} \times \overset{30}{\cancel{60}}\ gtt/min = 30\ gtt/min$$

16.   3300 ml
Logic: The patient gets 125 ml/hr and there are 24 hours in a day; hence,

$$\begin{array}{r} 125 \\ \times\ 24 \\ \hline 500 \\ 250 \\ \hline 3000\ ml \end{array}$$

The patient gets 75 ml q6h and, therefore, is receiving 75 ml four times in 24 hours

so $\begin{array}{r} 75 \\ \times\ 4 \\ \hline 300 \end{array}$

$$\begin{array}{r} 3000\ ml \\ +\ 300\ ml \\ \hline 3300\ ml \end{array}$$

17.   a.   90 ml/hr

b. $\dfrac{\text{total \# ml}}{\text{ml/hr}} = \text{hr}$ $\begin{array}{r} 11.1 \\ 90\,)\overline{1000.0} \\ \underline{90} \\ 100 \\ \underline{90} \\ 100 \end{array}$

Approximately 11 hours

18. a. 5 ml

$\dfrac{D}{H} \times S = A$ $\dfrac{\overset{1}{\cancel{50\ mg}}}{\underset{\underset{1}{\cancel{2}}}{\cancel{100\ mg}}} \times \overset{5}{\cancel{10}}\,ml = 5\ ml$

b. 18 gtt/min

Logic: The order calls for titrating the IV to 60 μg/min.

Have 50 mg in 250 ml

50 mg = 50,000 μg

Have 50,000 μg in 250 ml

Reduce these numbers:

$\dfrac{\overset{200}{\cancel{50,000}}\ \mu g}{\underset{1}{\cancel{250}}\ ml} = \dfrac{200\ \mu g}{1\ ml}$

Tubing is microtubing and delivers 60 gtt/ml

Substitute for 200 μg/1 ml:

200 μg/60 gtt/min

The order calls for titrating to 60 μg/min

$\dfrac{D}{H} \times S = A$ $\dfrac{\overset{}{\cancel{60}\ \mu g}}{\underset{1}{\cancel{200}\ \mu g}} \times \overset{3}{\cancel{60}} = 18\ gtt/min$

19. 50 mg

Logic: Have 0.5 g in 500 ml. Substitute milligrams for grams: 0.5 g = 500 mg. The solution is 500 mg in 500 ml. Reducing this means 1 mg in 1 ml. As the patient is receiving 50 ml/hr, he is receiving 50 mg of aminophylline per hour.

20. a. Yes

b. $\dfrac{\text{\# ml} \times \text{TF}}{20} = \dfrac{\overset{25}{\cancel{50}} \times \cancel{10}}{\underset{1}{\cancel{20}}} = 25\ gtt/min$

TEST 7. PART I: CALCULATION OF DOSAGES FOR INFANTS AND CHILDREN

1. Literature recommends 10 mg/kg

$\begin{array}{r} \times\ wt\ \underline{8.4\ kg} \\ 40 \\ \underline{80} \\ 84.0\ mg\ \text{recommended dose} \end{array}$

Order of 80 mg is in the therapeutic range

$$\frac{D}{H} \times S = A \qquad \frac{\overset{1}{\cancel{80\ mg}}}{\underset{33}{\cancel{165\ mg}}} \times \cancel{5}\ ml = \frac{80}{33} \quad \overset{2.42}{33)\overline{80.}}$$

$$\begin{array}{r} \underline{66} \\ 140 \\ \underline{132} \\ 80 \end{array}$$

Dose is 2.4 ml if needed.

2. Literature recommends 6 mg/kg/day   to   7.5 mg/kg/day

$$\times\ wt\ \underline{19\ kg} \qquad\qquad \times\ wt\ \underline{19\ kg}$$
$$\begin{array}{r} 54 \\ \underline{6} \\ 1\overline{14}\ mg/day \end{array} \quad to \quad \begin{array}{r} 675 \\ \underline{75} \\ 142.5\ mg/day \end{array}$$

The order of 40 mg $\times$ three doses per day (120 mg) is in the therapeutic range.

$$\frac{D}{H} \times S = A \qquad \frac{\overset{1}{\cancel{40\ mg}}}{\underset{2}{\cancel{80\ mg}}} \times \overset{1}{\cancel{2}}\ ml = 1\ ml$$
$$\underset{1}{\cancel{2}}$$

Statement: Use a Buretrol and run in 50 ml D5 $\frac{1}{3}$ NS; add 1 ml tobramycin; infuse over 1 hour. Set pump for 50 ml/hr; label IV.

3. Literature recommends 40 mg/kg/day in divided doses

$$\times\ wt\ \underline{4.3\ kg}$$
$$\begin{array}{r} 120 \\ \underline{160} \\ 172.0\ mg/day \end{array}$$

Order of 175 mg $\times$ three doses/day = 525 mg/day
Dose is excessive. Check with physician.

4. Available IV fluid is 500 ml. Must give half of 70 mEq KCl = 35 mEq

$$\frac{D}{H} \times S = A \qquad \frac{\overset{7}{\cancel{35\ mEq}}}{\underset{8}{\cancel{40\ mEq}}} \times 20\ ml = \frac{\overset{140}{\cancel{140}}}{8} \quad \overset{17.5}{8)\overline{140.0}}$$

$$\begin{array}{r} \underline{8} \\ 60 \\ \underline{56} \\ 40 \end{array}$$

Add 17.5 ml KCl to IV bag and label IV.
No IV calculation necessary. Set pump for 500 ml total IV and rate at 35 ml/hr.

5. Literature recommends 0.1 mg/kg three times a day not to exceed 2 mg three times a day.

41.6 lb = 18.9 kg

18.9 kg $\times$ 0.1 mg = 1.89 mg (approximately 2 mg.)

Order of 2 mg three times a day is the upper therapeutic range. No calculation necessary. Stock comes in 2 mg/5 ml. Give 5 ml.

6. Order is bid. Literature recommends 8 mg/kg to 10 mg/kg in two divided doses based on trimethoprim.

```
        8 mg/kg   to        10 mg/kg
×  wt  6.77 kg          ×  wt  6.77 kg
       54.16 mg   to        67.7 mg
```

Order calls for 2.5 cc. Because trimethoprim is 80 mg in 5 cc, half of that is 40 mg. Twice a day = 80 mg, which is above the therapeutic range of 54–68 mg. The order calls for 50 cc. The literature indicates that 2.5 cc of the drug should be diluted in 62.5 ml. Check with the physician.

7. Literature recommends 4 mg/kg/q6h   75.6 mg
```
             ×  wt 18.9 kg          ×      4 doses
                   75.6 mg q6h      302.4 mg
```

Literature further says that if dose is adjusted for children ages 1–9, do not exceed 24 mg/kg/day.

```
           24 mg               Order is    125 mg
×  wt     18.9 kg                       ×      3 doses
          216                             375 mg
          192
           24
          453.6 mg/kg maximum
```

Order is within the therapeutic range.

$$\frac{D}{H} \times S = A \qquad \frac{\overset{25}{\cancel{125}\ mg}}{\underset{16}{\cancel{80}\ mg}} \times 15\ ml = \frac{\overset{23.43}{\cancel{375}}}{16} \underset{\begin{array}{r}32 \\ \hline 55 \\ 48 \\ \hline 70 \\ 64 \\ \hline 60\end{array}}{)\overline{375.00}}$$

Pour 23.4 cc

8. Available IV fluid is 250 ml. The order is 15 mEq/L; take $\frac{1}{4}$ of 15 mEq. Because you are taking only $\frac{1}{4}$ of a liter (250 ml) you must reduce the milliequivalents.

```
        3.75 mEq
   4 )15.00
      12
       30
       28
       20
       20
```

$$\frac{D}{H} \times S = A \qquad \frac{3.75\ \cancel{mEq}}{\underset{1}{\cancel{20}\ mEq}} \times \overset{2}{\cancel{40}}\ ml = \begin{array}{r}3.75 \\ \times\ \ 2 \\ \hline 7.50\end{array}$$

Add 7.5 ml of KCl to IV bag and label IV.

No calculation is necessary. Set pump for 250 ml total and rate at 18 ml/hr.

9. a. Literature recommends 44 mg/kg/day in divided doses
```
              ×  wt  6.8 kg
                   352
                   264
                   299.2 mg/day
```

$$\begin{array}{r} 100 \text{ mg} \\ \underline{\times\ 3 \text{ doses}} \\ 300 \text{ mg} = \text{order} \end{array}$$

Order is within therapeutic range.

b. Diluting fluid and # ml: 10 ml sterile water for injection
    Solution made and new stock: 500 mg/10 ml (vancomycin does not have displacement)
    Rule and arithmetic:

$$\frac{D}{H} \times S = A \qquad \frac{\overset{1}{\cancel{100}} \text{ mg}}{\underset{\underset{1}{\cancel{5}}}{\cancel{500}} \text{ mg}} \times \overset{2}{\cancel{10}} \text{ ml} = 2 \text{ ml}$$

Label on vial: 500 mg/10 ml; date; initials
Storage: refrigerator

c. Use a Buretrol and run in 50 ml D5 $\frac{1}{3}$ NS.

Add 2 ml vancomycin. Label IV.
No calculation necessary. Set pump at 50 ml/hr.

10. Literature recommends:

$$\begin{array}{cc} 50 \text{ mg/kg/day} \quad \text{to} & 100 \text{ mg/kg/day} \\ \times \text{ wt } \underline{\quad 8.4 \text{ kg}} & \times \text{ wt } \underline{\quad 8.4 \text{ kg}} \\ 420.0 \text{ mg/kg} & 840. \text{ mg/kg} \end{array}$$

Order is 210 mg × 3 doses = 630 mg/day.
Order is within the therapeutic range.
Diluting fluid and # ml: 10 ml sterile water for injection
Solution and new stock: 90 mg/ml
Rule and arithmetic:

$$\frac{D}{H} \times S = A \qquad \frac{\cancel{210} \text{ mg}}{\cancel{90} \text{ mg}} \times 1 \text{ ml} = \frac{\overset{21}{\cancel{21}}}{9} \quad \begin{array}{r} 2.33 \\ 9\overline{)21.00} \\ \underline{18} \\ 30 \\ \underline{27} \\ 30 \\ \underline{27} \end{array}$$

Answer: 2.33 ml
Label: 90 mg/ml; date; initials
Storage: refrigerator

Use a Buretrol and run in 50 cc D5 $\frac{1}{3}$ NS

Add 2.33 ml cefuroxime. Label IV. Run in over 60 minutes.
No calculation necessary. Set pump at 50 ml/hr.

TEST 7. PART II: CALCULATIONS OF DOSAGE FOR INFANTS AND CHILDREN

1. The infant weighs 2000 g. To convert this to kilograms, use the equivalent 1000 g = 1 kg. The infant weighs 2 kg. Compare the literature with the order to decide if the dose is safe.

Literature	Order	Nursing Judgment
Initial dose 100 mg/kg (100 mg × 2 = 200 mg)	200 mg IM	Follows guideline
Subsequent doses 75 mg/kg/q6h (75 mg × 2 = 150 mg) q6h = 4 doses 150 mg × 4 = 600 mg)	150 mg IM q6h (q6h = 4 doses) 150 mg × 4 = 600 mg	Follows guideline
Maximum daily dose 300 mg/kg/day (300 mg × 2 kg = 600 mg)	150 mg q6h q6h = 4 doses 150 × 4 = 600 mg	Follows guideline

    a. Milligrams per kilogram rule

    b. The dose is safe. The order complies exactly with the literature.

2. The child weighs 32 lb. Convert this to kilograms using the equivalent 2.2 lb = 1 kg

```
            1 4 . 5 4
   2.2 )32.0 00
        22
        100
         88
        120
        110
         100
          88
          12
```

The child weighs 14.54 kg

The literature gives a range of 400–500 mg/kg/day

The range for this child will be

```
   14.54 kg              14.54 kg
   × 400 mg        to    × 500 mg
5816.00 mg = 5.8 g  to  7270.00 mg = 7.3 g
```

The range for this child is approximately 5.8–7.3 g in divided doses.

The child receives 1.5 g four times in 24 hours:

```
 1.5 g
 × 4
 6.0 g in 24 hours, which is within the range
```

    a. Milligrams per kilogram rule

    b. Yes, the dose is safe.

3. The child weighs 40 lbs. Figure 11-19 indicates that the range for this child is 25–50 mg/kg divided into three or four daily doses. The figure also tells us that 40 lb = 18.1 kg. Determine the range.

```
 18.1 kg           18.1 kg
 × 25 mg     to    × 50 mg
  905              906.0 mg
 362
 452.5 mg
```

The safe range is approximately 450–900 mg.

The child is receiving 150 × 3 doses = 450 mg daily.

The dose is safe.

4. The range of dosage is 25–50 mg/kg/day divided into three or four doses.

The baby weighs 10 lb. The table shows that this is 4.5 kg. Determine the safe range:

$$
\begin{array}{cc}
25 \text{ mg} & 50 \text{ mg} \\
\underline{\times 4.5 \text{ kg}} \quad \text{to} \quad & \underline{\times 4.5 \text{ kg}} \\
125 & 250 \\
\underline{100} & \underline{200} \\
112.5 & 225.0
\end{array}
$$

The safe range is approximately 110–225 mg daily in divided doses.
The baby is receiving 55 mg in four doses daily:

$$
\begin{array}{c}
55 \text{ mg} \\
\underline{\times 4 \text{ doses}} \\
220 \text{ mg}
\end{array}
$$

The dose is within the safe range.

5. Use the BSA rule:

$$\frac{m^2}{1.7 \text{ m}^2} \times \text{average adult dose} = \text{child dose}$$

$$\frac{0.2 \text{ m}^2}{1.7 \text{ m}^2} \times 0.4 \text{ mg} = \begin{array}{c} 0.2 \\ \underline{\times 0.4} \\ 0.08 \end{array} = \begin{array}{r} 0.047 \\ 1.7\,\overline{)0.0800} \\ \underline{68} \\ 120 \\ \underline{119} \end{array}$$

The dose is 0.05 mg.
Change this to micrograms.
0.05 mg = 50 μg is a safe dose for this baby.

6. Change 15.4 lb to kilograms dividing by 2.2

$$
\begin{array}{r}
7. \\
2.2\,\overline{)15.4} \\
\underline{15.4}
\end{array}
$$

The child weighs 7 kg. The literature states the safe range as 25–50 mg/kg/day in divided doses. Determine what the range is.

$$
\begin{array}{cc}
25 \text{ mg} \quad \text{to} & 50 \text{ mg} \\
\underline{\times 7 \text{ kg}} & \underline{\times 7 \text{ kg}} \\
175 \text{ mg} \quad \text{to} & 380 \text{ mg}
\end{array}
$$

The safe range is 175–380 mg in divided doses. The child is receiving 100 mg × 4 doses daily = 400 mg. The order is above the range. The nurse should check the prescription with the physician who wrote the order.

7. The baby weighs 5 lb 10 oz.
First determine what part of a pound is 10 oz. There are 16 oz in a pound;

$$
\text{hence, } \frac{10}{16}\,\begin{array}{r} .62 \\ \overline{)10.00} \\ \underline{9\;6} \\ 40 \end{array}
$$

The baby weighs 5.6 lb.
Convert this to kilograms. Divide by 2.2.

$$
\begin{array}{r}
2.54 \\
2.2\,\overline{)5.6\,00} \\
\underline{4\;4} \\
1\;2\;0 \\
\underline{1\;1\;0} \\
1\;00 \\
\underline{88} \\
12
\end{array}
$$

The baby weighs 2.54 kg.
The literature states the safe dose is 25–50 mg/kg/q6h in divided doses. Determine the range.

$$\begin{array}{r} 2.54 \text{ kg} \\ \times\ 25 \text{ mg} \\ \hline 1270 \\ 508 \quad\ \\ \hline 63.50 \end{array} \quad \text{to} \quad \begin{array}{r} 2.54 \text{ kg} \\ \times\ 50 \text{ mg} \\ \hline 127.00 \text{ mg} \end{array}$$

The safe range is approximately 60–125 mg $\times$ 4 doses daily, i.e., 240–500 mg.
The baby is receiving 150 mg $\times$ 3 doses daily = 450 mg.
The dose is safe.

8.   Use Clark's rule:

$$\frac{\text{Child's wt in lb}}{150 \text{ lb}} \times \text{adult dose} = \text{child's dose}$$

$$\frac{\overset{1}{\cancel{30 \text{ lb}}}}{\underset{\underset{1}{\cancel{5}}}{\cancel{150 \text{ lb}}}} \times \overset{2}{\cancel{10}} \text{ mg} = 2 \text{ mg}$$

9.   a. $\dfrac{\text{Child's BSA}}{1.7 \text{ m}^2} \times \text{adult dose} = \text{child's dose}$

$$\frac{1.3 \text{ m}^2}{1.7 \text{ m}^2} \times 50 \text{ mg} = \frac{\cancel{65}}{1.7} \quad \begin{array}{r} 3\,8\,.\,2 \\ 1.7\overline{)65.0\ 0} \\ \underline{51\ \ } \\ 14\,0 \\ \underline{13\,6} \\ 40 \end{array} = 38 \text{ mg}$$

   b.   Use the BSA rule.

10.   Change 40 lb to kilograms. Divide by 2.2:

$$2.2\overline{)40.0\ 00} \quad \begin{array}{r} 1\,8\,.\,18 \\ \underline{22\ \ \ } \\ 18\,0 \\ \underline{17\,6} \\ 40 \\ \underline{22} \\ 180 \\ \underline{176} \end{array}$$

The child's weight is

$$\begin{array}{r} 18.18 \text{ kg} \\ \times\ \ \ 5 \text{ mg} \\ \hline 90.90 \end{array}$$

The safe dose is approximately 90 mg/day.
The child is ordered 50 mg $\times$ 3 doses/day = 150 mg.
The dose is beyond the guideline. Check with the physician who wrote the order.

TEST 8. ASSORTED DOSAGE PROBLEMS: I

1. $\dfrac{D}{H} \times S = A$ $\dfrac{0.\overset{5}{\cancel{125}}\ \text{mg}}{0.\underset{20}{\underset{1}{\cancel{500}}}\ \text{mg}} \times \overset{1}{\cancel{20}}\ \text{ml} = 5\ \text{ml}$

2. $\dfrac{D}{H} \times S = A$ $0.2\ \text{mg} = 200\ \mu g$

$$\frac{\overset{1}{\cancel{100}}\ \mu g}{\underset{2}{\cancel{200}}\ \cancel{\mu g}} \times \text{tab} = \frac{1}{2}\ \text{tablet}$$

3. $\dfrac{D}{H} \times S = A$ $\dfrac{\overset{7}{\cancel{35}}\ \cancel{\text{mg}}}{\underset{20}{\cancel{100}}\ \cancel{\text{mg}}} \times 1\ \text{ml} = \overset{.35}{20\overline{\smash{)}7.00}} = 0.35\ \text{ml}$

$$\begin{array}{r} \underline{6\ 0}\ \ \\ 1\ 00 \\ \underline{1\ 00} \end{array}$$

4. Step 1. $\dfrac{\#\ \text{ml}}{\#\ \text{hr}} = \text{ml/hr}$ $\cancel{1500}\ \ \overset{62.5}{24\overline{\smash{)}1500.0}} = 63\ \text{ml/hr}$

$$\begin{array}{r} \underline{144}\ \ \\ 60 \\ \underline{48}\ \\ 120 \\ \underline{120} \end{array}$$

Step 2. $\dfrac{\#\ \text{ml/hr} \times TF}{\#\ \text{min}} = \text{gtt/min}$

Macrodrip (15 gtt/ml)

$$\frac{63 \times \overset{1}{\cancel{15}}}{\underset{4}{\cancel{60}}} = \overset{}{\cancel{63}}\ \frac{15.6}{4\overline{\smash{)}63.0}} = 16\ \text{gtt/min}$$

Microdrip

Remember ml/hr = gtt/min, hence, microdrip is 63 gtt/min.

Proof: $\dfrac{63 \times \cancel{60}}{\cancel{60}} = 63\ \text{gtt/min}$

Use microdrip.

5. Logic: You have $\dfrac{\overset{100}{\cancel{25,000}}\ \text{units}}{\underset{1}{\cancel{250}}\ \text{ml bag}}$ of drug = 100 units/ml

The solution is 100 units/ml. The order calls for 1500 units/hr.

$$\frac{D}{H} = \frac{150\cancel{0}\ \cancel{\text{units}}/\text{hr}}{10\cancel{0}\ \cancel{\text{units}}/\text{ml}} = 15\ \text{ml/hr}$$

Set the infusion pump at 15 ml/hr.

6. $\dfrac{D}{H} \times S = A$ $\quad \dfrac{0.07 \text{ mg}}{0.25 \text{ mg}} \times 1 \text{ cc} = \dfrac{.28}{25 \overline{)7.00}} = 0.28 \text{ cc} = 0.28 \text{ ml}$

$$\begin{array}{r} 5\ 0 \\ \hline 2\ 00 \\ 2\ 00 \end{array}$$

7. $\dfrac{D}{H} \times S = A$ $\quad \dfrac{\overset{3}{1.5} \text{ mEq}}{\underset{4}{2.0} \text{ mEq}} \times 1 \text{ ml} = \dfrac{.75}{4 \overline{)3.00}} = 0.8 \text{ ml}$

8. Diluent and # ml: 3.6 ml sterile water for injection
Solution made and new stock: 200,000 units/ml
Rule and arithmetic:

$\dfrac{D}{H} \times S = A$ $\quad \dfrac{\overset{3}{\cancel{150,000 \text{ units}}}}{\underset{4}{\cancel{200,000 \text{ units}}}} \times 1 \text{ ml} = \dfrac{3}{4} \dfrac{.75}{\overline{)3.00}} = 0.75 \text{ ml}$

Give: 0.8 ml IM
Label: 200,000 units/ml; date; initials
Storage: Information not provided. Check the label on the package insert.

9. $\dfrac{\text{\# ml} \times \text{TF}}{\text{\# min}} = \text{gtt/min}$ $\quad \dfrac{50 \times \cancel{10}}{\underset{3}{\cancel{30}}} = \dfrac{50}{3} \dfrac{16.6}{\overline{)50.0}} = 17 \text{ gtt/min}$

$$\begin{array}{r} 3 \\ \hline 20 \\ 18 \\ \hline 20 \\ 18 \end{array}$$

10. a. You have an infusion pump; no calculation is necessary. Set the pump at 80 ml/hr.

b. $\dfrac{\overset{25}{\cancel{1000 \text{ ml}}}}{\underset{2}{\cancel{80 \text{ ml/hr}}}} = \dfrac{25}{2} \dfrac{12.5}{\overline{)25.0}} = \text{approximately } 12\dfrac{1}{2} \text{ hours}$

11. $\dfrac{D}{H} \times S = A$ $\quad \dfrac{\overset{3}{\cancel{150} \text{ mg}}}{\underset{\underset{5}{\cancel{10}}}{\cancel{500} \text{ mg}}} \times \overset{1}{\cancel{2}} \text{ ml} \quad \dfrac{3}{5} \dfrac{.6}{\overline{)3.0}} = 0.6 \text{ ml}$

12. $\dfrac{D}{H} \times S = A$ $\quad 0.6 \text{ gm} = 600 \text{ mg}.$

$\dfrac{\overset{2}{\cancel{600} \text{ mg}}}{\underset{1}{\cancel{300} \text{ mg}}} \times 1 \text{ ml} = 2 \text{ ml}$

13. $\dfrac{D}{H} \times S = A$ $\quad \dfrac{\overset{1}{0.125 \text{ mg}}}{\underset{2}{0.250 \text{ mg}}} = \dfrac{1}{2} \text{ tablet}$

14. Diluent and # ml: 4 ml sterile water for injection
Solution made and new stock: 500 mg = 2.2 ml. Label, date.
Rule and arithmetic: 0.5 g = 500 mg; no calculation needed
Give: 2.2 ml IM. Refrigerate remainder.

15. $\dfrac{D}{H} \times S = A$ 0.1 gm = 100 mg

$$\frac{200 \text{ mg}}{100 \text{ mg}} \times 5 \text{ ml} = 10 \text{ ml}$$

16. Step 1. $\dfrac{\# \text{ ml}}{\# \text{ hr}} = \text{ml/hr}$ $12\overline{)500.0}\;\dfrac{41.6}{} = 42$ ml/hr

$$\begin{array}{r} 48 \\ \hline 20 \\ 12 \\ \hline 80 \\ 72 \\ \hline \end{array}$$

Step 2. $\dfrac{\# \text{ ml/hr} \times \text{TF}}{60} = \text{gtt/min}$

Macrodrip   *Microdrip*

$$\frac{\overset{7}{42} \times 10}{\underset{1}{60}} = 7 \text{ gtt/min}$$ Remember ml/hr = gtt/min, so microdrip is 42 gtt/min.

Proof: $\dfrac{42 \times 60}{60} = 42$ gtt/min

Use microdrip at 42 gtt/min.

17. $\dfrac{D}{H} \times S = A$ $\dfrac{\overset{3}{12 \text{ mg}}}{\underset{1}{4 \text{ mg}}} \times 5 \text{ ml} = 15 \text{ ml}$

18. $\dfrac{D}{H} \times S = A$ 0.5 g = 500 mg

$$\frac{\overset{2}{500 \text{ mg}}}{\underset{1}{250 \text{ mg}}} \times 1 \text{ cap} = 2 \text{ capsules}$$

19. Diluting fluid and # ml; 6.8 ml sterile water for injection
Solution made and new stock: 250 mg/ml
Rule and arithmetic: 0.6 g = 600 mg

$\dfrac{D}{H} \times S = A$ $\dfrac{\overset{12}{600 \text{ mg}}}{\underset{5}{250 \text{ mg}}} \times 1 \text{ ml} = \dfrac{12}{5}$ $5\overline{)12.0}\;\dfrac{2.4}{}$

$$\begin{array}{r} 10 \\ \hline 2\,0 \\ 20 \\ \hline \end{array}$$

Give: 2.4 ml IM
Write on label: Nothing. Cannot use. Label states entire contents must be withdrawn.
Storage: No. Discard vial in the proper receptacle.

20. No calculation necessary.
Use the U 100 insulin syringe.
Draw up 20 units of NPH insulin and give SC.

TEST 9. ASSORTED DOSAGE PROBLEMS: II

1. $\dfrac{D}{H} \times S = A$ $\dfrac{30 \text{ mcg}}{40 \text{ mcg}} \times 30 \text{ ml} = \dfrac{90}{4}$ $\begin{array}{r} 22.5 \\ 4\overline{)90.0} \\ \underline{8} \\ 10 \\ \underline{8} \\ 20 \\ \underline{20} \end{array}$

Give 22.5 ml PO.
You can use a syringe to obtain the exact amount.

2. Equivalent 0.06 Gm = 60 mg
Use the 30-mg tablets, which are closer in strength to the order.

$\dfrac{D}{H} \times S = A$ $\dfrac{\overset{2}{\cancel{60 \text{ mg}}}}{\underset{1}{\cancel{30 \text{ mg}}}} \times 1 \text{ tab} = 2 \text{ tablets}$

3. $\dfrac{D}{H} \times S = A$ $\dfrac{\overset{2}{\cancel{0.250 \text{ mg}}}}{\underset{1}{\cancel{0.125 \text{ mg}}}} = 2 \text{ tablets}$

4. Step 1. $\dfrac{\# \text{ ml}}{\text{hr}} = \text{ml/hr}$ $\dfrac{500 \text{ ml}}{6 \text{ hr}} = $ $\begin{array}{r} 83.3 \\ 6\overline{)500.0} \\ \underline{48} \\ 20 \\ \underline{18} \\ 20 \\ \underline{18} \\ 2 \end{array}$ Will administer 83 ml/hr

Step 2. $\dfrac{\# \text{ ml/hr} \times \text{TF}}{60 \text{ min}} = \text{gtt/min}$

Macrodrip

$\dfrac{83 \times 10}{60} = $ $\begin{array}{r} 13.8 \\ 6\overline{)83.0} \\ \underline{6} \\ 23 \\ \underline{18} \\ 50 \\ 48 \end{array}$

Microdrip

$\dfrac{83 \times \cancel{60}}{\cancel{60}} = 83 \text{ gtt/min}$

a. Choose microdrip tubing.
b. Drip rate at 83 gtt/min provides a better flow rate than 14 gtt/min.

5. Diluting fluid and # ml: 2 ml of sterile water for injection
Solution made and new stock: 400 mg/ml
Rule and arithmetic:

$\dfrac{D}{H} \times S = A$ Equivalent 0.4 g = 400 mg

No arithmetic needed
Give: 1 ml IM
Write on label: 400 mg/ml; date; initials
Storage: refrigerator

6. $\dfrac{D}{H} \times S = A$ $\dfrac{0.\overset{1}{\cancel{125}}\ \cancel{mg}}{0.\underset{4}{\underset{1}{\cancel{500}}}\ \cancel{mg}} \times \overset{5}{\cancel{20}}\ ml = 5\ ml$

7. a. $\dfrac{\#\ ml\ ordered}{\#\ ml/hr} = $ number of hours to run $\dfrac{\overset{5}{\cancel{250}}\ \cancel{ml}}{\underset{1}{\cancel{50}}\ \cancel{ml}/hr} = 5\ hr$

   b.   No calculation is required. The doctor ordered 50 ml/hr. Set the pump at 50 ml/hr.

8. a. $\dfrac{D}{H} \times S = A$ $\dfrac{\overset{5}{\cancel{50,000}\ \cancel{units}}}{\underset{1}{\cancel{10,000}\ \cancel{units}}} \times 1\ ml = 5\ ml$

   Add 5 ml to the IV fluid and label

   b. $\dfrac{\#\ units\ in\ IV}{\#\ units/hr} = $ number of hours to run

   $\dfrac{\overset{100}{\cancel{50,000}\ \cancel{units}}}{\underset{3}{\cancel{1,500}\ \cancel{units}/hr}} = \overset{33.3}{3\overline{)100.}} = $ approximately $33\dfrac{1}{3}$ hours

   c.   Step 1. $\dfrac{\#\ units}{\#\ ml} = units/ml$

   $\dfrac{\overset{100}{\cancel{50,000}\ units}}{\underset{1}{\cancel{500}\ ml}} = 100\ units/ml$

   Step 2. $\dfrac{\#\ units/hr}{\#\ units/ml} = ml/hr$

   $\dfrac{1500\ \cancel{units}/hr}{100\ \cancel{units}/ml} = 15\ ml/hr$

   Set infusion pump at 15 ml/hr.

9. $\dfrac{D}{H} \times S = A$ $\dfrac{0.02\ \cancel{Gm}}{0.01\ \cancel{Gm}} = 2\ tablets$

10. $\dfrac{D}{H} \times S = A$ $\dfrac{\overset{3}{\cancel{15}}\ \cancel{mg}}{\underset{4}{\cancel{20}}\ \cancel{mg}} \times 1\ ml = \overset{3}{\cancel{}} \overset{.75}{4\overline{)3.00}}$
                                                                          $\underline{2\ 8}$
                                                                          20
                                                                          $\underline{20}$

Give 0.8 ml IM.

11. a.   Choose the 250 mg/ml. If you chose 125 mg/ml you would have to give 4 ml to the patient.

    b.   Diluting fluid and # ml: 3.4 ml sterile water for injection

          Solution made and new stock: 250 mg/ml

          Rule and arithmetic: 0.5 g = 500 mg

$$\frac{D}{H} \times S = A \qquad \frac{\overset{2}{\cancel{500 \text{ mg}}}}{\underset{1}{\cancel{250 \text{ mg}}}} \times 1 \text{ ml} = 2 \text{ ml}$$

          Give: 2 ml IM

          Write on label: Nothing. Discard the vial. The reconstituted material loses its potency after 1 hour.

          Storage: No. Discard in an appropriate receptacle.

12.   a.   The low-dose insulin syringe because the number of units is an odd number and the dose is small.

       b.   No calculation is necessary. Use the U 100 Humulin insulin and the U 100 low-dose insulin syringe and draw up 7 units.

13.   Logic: Solution is 200 mg in 250 ml. You want 200 μg/min. As 1 mg = 1000 μg, first change 200 mg to micrograms by multiplying by 1000.

$$\begin{array}{r} 1000 \ \mu g \\ \times \ 200 \ mg \\ \hline 200{,}000 \ \mu g \end{array}$$

          The solution is 200,000 μg in 250 ml. This number can be reduced.

$$\frac{\overset{800}{\cancel{200{,}000 \ \mu g}}}{\underset{1}{\cancel{250 \ ml}}} = 800 \ \mu g/ml$$

          The solution is now expressed as 800 μg/ml.

          When micrograms are given IV without a pump, use microdrip tubing (60 gtt = 1 ml). Therefore, we can express 800 μg/ml in another way—800 μg/60 gtt/min.

          The order calls for 200 μg/min. Solve this using $\frac{D}{H} \times S = A$

          D = 200 μg; H = 800 μg; S = 60 gtt

$$\frac{\overset{1}{\cancel{200 \ \mu g}}}{\underset{\underset{1}{\cancel{4}}}{\cancel{800 \ \mu g}}} = \overset{15}{\cancel{60}} \text{ gtt} = 15 \text{ gtt}$$

          200 μg/15 gtt/min

          Set the initial rate at 15 gtt/min.

14. $\dfrac{D}{H} \times S = A$ $\dfrac{\cancel{300{,}000 \text{ units}}}{\cancel{100{,}000 \text{ units}}} \times 5 \text{ ml} = 15 \text{ ml}$

15.   a.   Aseptically withdraw 50 ml from the 250 ml bag.

       b.   Use the reconstitution device to add the 1 g of drug to the 200 ml. Label the bag.

       c. $\dfrac{\text{\# ml} \times TF}{\text{\# min}} = \text{gtt/min}$ $\dfrac{\overset{100}{\cancel{200}} \times 10}{\cancel{60}} = \dfrac{\cancel{100}}{3} \ \dfrac{33.3}{\overline{)100.0}} = 33 \text{ gtt/min}$

                                  3

16. $\dfrac{D}{H} \times S = A$ $\dfrac{\overset{2}{\cancel{25\!\!\!0} \text{ mg}}}{\underset{1}{\cancel{12\!\!5} \text{ mg}}} \times 5 \text{ ml} = 10 \text{ ml}$

17. $\dfrac{D}{H} \times S = A$ $\dfrac{\overset{3}{\cancel{15 \text{ mg}}}}{\underset{4}{\cancel{20 \text{ mg}}}} \times 1 \text{ ml} = \dfrac{3}{4} \overset{.75}{\overline{)3.00}} = 0.8 \text{ ml}$

18. Solve for macrodrip and microdrip and then decide

Step 1. $\dfrac{\text{Total \# ml}}{\text{\# hr}} = \text{ml/hr}$ $\dfrac{500}{24}\overset{20.8}{\overline{)500}} = 21 \text{ ml/hr}$

Step 2. $\dfrac{\text{\# ml/hr} \times TF}{\text{\# min}} = \text{gtt/min}$

Macrodrip   *Microdrip*

$\dfrac{21 \times \cancel{10}}{\cancel{60}} =$ $\dfrac{21 \times \cancel{60}}{\cancel{60}} = 21 \text{ gtt/min}$

$\dfrac{\cancel{21}}{6}\overset{3.5}{\overline{)21.0}} = 4 \text{ gtt/min}$
$\phantom{\dfrac{21}{6)}}\underline{18}$
$\phantom{\dfrac{21}{6)21.}}3\,0$

Use microdrip at 21 gtt/min.

19.   a.   Aseptically remove 50 ml from the IV bag of 250 ml.
    b.   Use the reconstitution device to add the medication to the 200 ml. Label the bag.

    c. $\dfrac{\text{\# ml} \times TF}{\text{\# min}} = \text{gtt/min}$ $\dfrac{\overset{4}{\cancel{200}} \times 10}{\underset{1}{\cancel{50}}} = 40 \text{ gtt/min}$

20. 1:1000 means 1 g in 1000 ml, but 1 g = 1000 mg; hence, we can say the solution is 1000 mg in 1000 ml. This reduces to 1 mg in 1 ml.

$\dfrac{D}{H} \times S = A$ $\dfrac{0.5 \text{ mg}}{1 \text{ mg}} \times 1 \text{ ml} = 0.5 \text{ ml}$

TEST 10. MENTAL DRILL FOR ASSORTED DOSAGE PROBLEMS

1. Give 1.5 cc IM.

2.   a.   Add 25,000 units of heparin sodium to an IV bag of 250 ml. This makes a solution of 100 U/ml.
    b.   You want 1200 units/hr; set the rate at 12 ml/hr.

3. Give 10 ml PO.

4. Give 2 tablets.

5. Give 0.67 ml.

6. Give 1.5 ml. Label vial 400 mg/ml; date; initials.

7. $\dfrac{150 \times 10}{60} = 25 \text{ gtt/min}$

8. Give 1 ml IM.

9. Give 2 tablets PO.

10. $\dfrac{4}{3} \times 5 = \dfrac{20}{3} = 6.7$ ml PO

11. Give 1.5 ml IM. Label the vial 250 mg/1.5 ml; date; initials.

12. Give 10 ml PO.

13. $\dfrac{\cancel{500}}{12} \overset{41.6}{\overline{)500.0}} = 42$ ml/hr; use microdrip tubing at 42 gtt/min.

14. Give $1\dfrac{1}{2}$ tablets.

15. $\dfrac{\overset{8}{\cancel{40}}}{\underset{5}{\cancel{25}}}$ Give 1.6 cc; Label 250,000 U/ml; date; initials.

16. Give 0.4 ml IM.

17. a. Aseptically remove 25 ml from the bag of D5W 150 ml.
  b. Add the 80 mg of Bactrim to the 125 ml D5W using sterile technique and label.

  c. $\dfrac{125}{\cancel{60}} \times \cancel{10} = 20.8 = 21$ gtt/min

18. 8 PM

19. a. Aseptically remove 50 ml of solution from the bag of 250 ml D5W.
  b. Use the reconstitution device to place the 1 g dose of kanamycin in the 200 ml D5W and label.

  c. $\dfrac{200 \times \overset{1}{\cancel{20}}}{\underset{6}{\cancel{120}}} = 33.3 = 33$ gtt/min.

20. Give 2 ml deep IM. Label 250 mg/ml; date; initials.

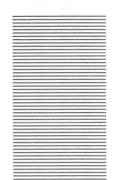

12

Information Basic to Administering Drugs

In previous chapters we have learned drug forms and preparations, how to read prescriptions, and how to calculate dosages. This chapter provides the opportunity to focus on some of the nurse's responsibilities for drug therapy—drug knowledge, legal and ethical considerations, and, finally, specific points that may prove helpful in giving medications.

DRUG KNOWLEDGE

Although a current *Physician's Desk Reference* (*PDR*) and the package insert are the best references for dosage, nursing drug handbooks are the best references for the nurse practitioner who needs a variety of information specifically designed to help assess, manage, evaluate, and teach the patient. The following headings represent the type of information found in a nursing handbook.

Generic and Trade Names

The generic name is the official name given the drug. It is usually followed by the letters USP or NF. The abbreviations stand for *United States Pharmacopeia* and *National Formulary*. A drug has only one generic name in the United States. It may have different generic names in other countries.

A trade name is the brand name under which a company manufactures a generic drug. A drug may have several trade names, but still only one generic name.

Consumer groups have advocated that drugs be prescribed by generic name only so that the pharmacist may dispense the least expensive drug available on the market. The nurse should understand that generic drugs, manufactured by different companies, are not exactly the same. The active ingredient in the drug meets standards of uniformity and purity, but manufacturers use different fillers and dyes. These substances can cause adverse effects (e.g., severe nausea caused by the dye used in coloring). Additionally, when a different trade name is prescribed a patient may become confused and distressed about receiving medication that looks different from previous doses. The active ingredient is the same, but size, shape, or color may vary.

Drug Class

The class of drug is a quick reference to the therapeutic action, use, and adverse effects of a drug. As the nurse develops a knowledge base, the drug class will identify general nursing implications and precautions in administering a drug.

Pregnancy Category

The Federal Drug Administration (FDA) has established the following categories:

   A.   No risk to the fetus in any trimester.
   B.   No adverse effect demonstrated in animals; no human studies available.
   C.   Animal studies have shown adverse reactions. No human studies are available. Given only after risks to the fetus have been considered.
   D.   Definite fetal risk exists; may be given in spite of risk to the fetus if needed for a life-threatening condition.
   E.   Absolute fetal abnormality; not to be used anytime in pregnancy.

A nurse administering a drug to a woman of childbearing age should be aware of the pregnancy category of a drug, to teach the patient and protect the fetus. In addition, this knowledge will aid in discussing the use of over-the-counter (OTC) drugs in pregnancy.

Dosage and Route

Information about the dosage and route of administration is crucial to protect against medication error. Most handbooks will give a dosage range for the adult, the elderly, and the child.

Action (Pharmacokinetics)

The nurse should understand how the drug is absorbed into the bloodstream, distributed to the cells, metabolized, and excreted. Some drugs should be taken between meals; some with food; some may not be combined because of incompatibility or interaction; some may not be taken orally.

Patients with liver or kidney disease may not be able to metabolize or excrete certain drugs. The drug accumulates in the body, leading to adverse effects. The nurse who knows the pharmacokinetics of a drug can better assess, manage, and evaluate drug therapy.

Uses

One of the most common questions asked of nurses is, "Why am I getting this drug?" The nurse relates the use of the drug to the expected therapeutic outcome. This information aids in observing for expected effects and in patient teaching.

Side Effects or Adverse Effects

Side effects are transient, nontherapeutic reactions to a drug. *Adverse effects* are untoward, nontherapeutic effects that may be harmful to the patient and that require lowering the dosage or discontinuing the drug. An example of a side effect is drowsiness, which occurs with some antihistamines. An example of an adverse effect is a serious decrease in white blood cells that results in decreased resistance to infection. The nurse must observe for these effects, know how to manage them, and teach the patient necessary information.

Contraindications and Precautions

These refer to conditions in which a drug should be given with caution or not given at all. For example, patients who have exhibited a previous reaction to penicillin should be cautioned against taking it again. Certain antibiotics must be administered with caution to patients who have poor kidney function. The nurse has a responsibility to know this information in order to safeguard the patient and carry out effective nursing care.

Interactions and Incompatibilities

When more than one drug is administered at a time, unexpected or nontherapeutic responses may occur. Some interactions are desirable. For example, naloxone (Narcan) is a narcotic antagonist that reverses the effects of a morphine overdose. Other interactions, however, are undesirable. For example, aspirin should not be taken with an oral anticoagulant because the possibility of an adverse effect is increased.

Some drugs may be incompatible and should not be mixed. This information is especially important when medications are combined for injection in IV administration. Chemical incompatibility is usually indicated by a visible sign, such as precipitation or color change. Physical incompatibility can occur without any visible sign; therefore, the nurse should check a suitable reference before combining drugs. A good rule of thumb is: when in doubt, do not mix.

Nursing Implications

This is information the nurse needs to administer the drug safely and to assess, manage, and teach the patient. This is not found in the *PDR*.

Evaluation of Effectiveness

Few drug references actually list this heading, yet the nurse is expected to evaluate the drug regimen and to record and report observations. Knowledge of the drug's class, its action, and its use leads to an understanding of expected therapeutic outcomes.

For example, ampicillin sodium is a broad-spectrum antibiotic that is used for urinary, respiratory, and other infections. Signs of effectiveness might include: normal temperature; the laboratory report of the white blood cell (WBC) count indicates a normal result; urine is clear; no pain on urination; no WBC in urine; an infected wound has decreased pus; wound is healing; the patient is more alert and interested in surroundings; appetite is improved.

Patient Teaching

The patient has a right to know the name and dose of the drug, why the drug is ordered, and what effects to expect or watch for. In addition, the patient who is to take a drug at home needs specific information. This is a professional responsibility shared by the physician and the nurse.

DRUG ACTION

When a drug is taken orally, it is absorbed through the villi of the small intestine, distributed to the cells by the blood stream, eventually metabolized, and then excreted from the body.

Absorption

Absorption of an oral drug depends upon the degree of stomach acidity, the time it takes for the stomach to empty, whether or not food is present, the amount of contact with villi in the small intestine, and blood flow to the villi.

Absorption of a drug may be affected in many ways. Enteric-coated (EC) tablets are not meant to dissolve in the acidic stomach. They ordinarily pass through the stomach to the duodenum. When an antacid is administered with an EC tablet, the pH of the stomach is raised, and the tablet may dissolve prematurely. The drug may become less potent, or it may irritate the gastric lining. Timed-release EC capsules that dissolve prematurely can deliver a huge dose of drug, causing adverse effects.

Laxatives increase gastrointestinal movement and decrease the time a drug is in contact with the villi of the small intestine where most absorption occurs. The presence of food in the stomach can impair absorption. Penicillin is a good example of a drug that should be taken on an empty stomach. Foods that contain calcium, such as milk and cheese, form a complex with some drugs and inhibit absorption.

Distribution

Distribution is the movement of a drug through body fluids, chiefly the bloodstream, to cells. Drugs do not travel freely in the blood. Most travel attached to plasma proteins, especially albumen. Drugs that are free can attach to cells, on which they produce an effect.

When more than one drug is present in the blood stream, they may compete for protein-binding sites. One drug may displace another. The displaced drug is now free to act with the cells, and its effect will be more pronounced. Aspirin is a common drug for displacement; it should not be given with oral anticoagulants, which are 99% bound to albumin. Aspirin displaces the anticoagulant; more is free to act at the cellular level, and a toxic effect may occur—bleeding.

Metabolism

Metabolism refers to the chemical biotransformation of a drug to a form that can be excreted. Most biotransformation occurs in the liver. Because oral drugs are carried first to the liver, this process begins once the drug is absorbed. Here, too, one drug can interfere with the effects of another. Barbiturates increase the activity of the liver enzymes. Because drugs are metabolized more quickly, their effect is reduced. Conversely, acetaminophen (Tylenol) will block the breakdown of penicillin in the liver, thereby increasing its activity.

Excretion

Excretion refers to the removal of a drug from the body. The major organ of excretion is the kidney. Drug interactions may also occur at this level; for example, probenecid inhibits the excretion of penicillin and increases its length of action, and furosemide (Lasix), a diuretic, blocks the excretion of aspirin and can lead to adverse effects by aspirin.

Drug interactions are not necessarily harmful. For example, narcotic antagonists are used to reverse the adverse effects of general anesthetics. This action is termed *antagonism. Synergism* is a term used when a second drug increases the intensity or prolongs the effect of a first drug. For example, a narcotic and a minor tranquilizer produce more pain relief than the narcotic alone. The nurse administering medications needs to be aware of possible interactions and evaluate the patient's response.

To minimize adverse interactions, the nurse should know the patient's drug profile, give as low a dose as possible, know the actions and adverse effects of the drugs administered, and monitor the patient. Some drug interactions may take several weeks to develop.

Tolerance

When a pain or sleeping medication is given frequently, the liver enzymes become skilled in biotransforming more quickly. Less drug is available, and thus the drug is less effective in relieving pain or in aiding sleep. Some nurses call this reaction "addiction," because the patient complains that the drug is not working and asks for more drug. In fact, it is a physiologic response. The patient requires more of the drug or a drug with a different molecular structure.

Cumulation

When biotransformation or excretion are inhibited, as can occur in liver or kidney disease, the drug accumulates in the body and an adverse effect can occur. Cumulation can also result from taking too much drug or from taking a drug too frequently.

Other factors that affect drug action include:

- Weight: larger individuals need a higher dose.
- Age: extremes of life respond more strongly. The livers and kidneys of infants are not well developed; in the aged, systems are less efficient.
- Pathologic conditions: especially of liver and kidney.
- Hypersensitivity to a drug: allergic reaction.
- Psychological and emotional state: depression or anxiety can decrease or increase body metabolism and affect drug action.

Adverse reactions may occur in any system or organ. Drug knowledge will enhance the nurse's observational skills and lead to responsible and appropriate intervention.

LEGAL CONSIDERATIONS

There are two types of law that affect nursing practice—criminal and civil.

Criminal Law

Criminal law relates to offenses against the general public that are detrimental to society as a whole. Criminal actions are prosecuted by governmental authorities. If the defendant is judged guilty, the penalty may be a fine, imprisonment, or both.

Nurses must know the scope of nursing practice in the state in which they function. They should be familiar with government regulations—federal, state, and local—that affect nursing. The policies and procedures of the agency in which they practice also have legal status. Failure to follow guidelines or lack of knowledge can lead to liability.

Criminal charges include unlawful use, possession, or administration of a controlled substance. The Comprehensive Drug Abuse, Prevention and Control Act of 1970 classified drugs that are subject to abuse into one of five schedules according to their medical usefulness and abuse potential.

Schedule I drugs have no valid use and are not available for prescription use (e.g., LSD).

Schedule II drugs have a valid medical use and are available for prescriptions, but exhibit a high abuse potential. Misuse can lead to physical and psychological dependence. Labels for these drugs are marked with the symbol Ⓒ (Fig. 12-1). Controlled drugs are counted each shift, and discrepancies are reported. Government and institutional regulations specify how these drugs are stored and protected. For example, an order for a narcotic in a hospital setting might be valid for 2 days. When the 2 days have elapsed, the order must be rewritten. A nurse who administers a controlled drug after the order has expired commits a medication error. Figure 12-2 is an example of a hospital policy on controlled drugs.

Schedule III, IV, and V drugs are classed as having less abuse potential than Schedule II drugs, but they can cause some physical and psychological dependence. Figure 12-3 lists

St. Vincent's Hospital & Medical Center
of New York
Department of Pharmacy

CONTROLLED DRUG REQUISITION FORM

NURSING UNIT

QUANTITY	UNIT OF ISSUE	CONTROLLED DRUG	DOSAGE FORM	STRENGTH
	25	Codeine	Tablet	15 mg/30 mg
	10	Codeine	Syringe	30 mg/60 mg
	10	Fentanyl (Sublimaze)	Ampules	5 ml
	10	Hydromorphone (Dilaudid)	Tablet	2 mg/4 mg
	10	Hydromorphone (Dilaudid)	Syringe	2 mg
	10	Levorphanol (Levo-Dromoran)	Tablet	2 mg
	10	Levorphanol (Levo-Dromoran)	Ampule	2 mg
	25	Meperidine (Demerol)	Tablet	50 mg
	10	Meperidine (Demerol)	Syringe	25 mg/50 mg/ 75 mg/100 mg
	10	Methadone	Tablet	5 mg/10 mg
	20 ml	Methadone	Vials	10 mg/ml
	10	Morphine	Syringe	4 mg/10 mg/ 15 mg
	10	Methylphenidate (Ritalin)	Tablet	5 mg/10 mg
	10	Pentobarbital (Nembutal)	Syringe	100 mg
	25	Pentobarbital (Nembutal)	Capsules	50 mg/100 mg
	25	Percodan	Tablets	
	25	Secobarbital (Seconal)	Capsules	50 mg/100 mg
	10	Secobarbital (Seconal)	Syringe	50 mg/100 mg
	10	Tuinal	Capsules	

Ordered By _____   Date _____
                          Nurse
Received By _____   Date _____
                          Nurse
Dispensed By _____   Date _____
                        Pharmacist

Figure 12-1. *Nursing Controlled Drug Requisition Form for Schedule II drugs. (Courtesy of Pharmacy Department, St. Vincent's Hospital and Medical Center, New York City.)*

Nursing Responsibilities

1. Count will be done each shift by two (2) registered nurses.
   a. The oncoming nurse should handle and physically count the controlled drugs.
   b. The off-going nurse should verify the count and record the number on hand on the controlled drug sheets.
   c. Both nurses should sign the controlled drug sheets.
2. All controlled drugs will be stored in a double-locked cabinet specifically designated for this purpose.
3. At all times, the narcotic keys must be in the possession of a staff nurse who is physically present on the unit.
4. A written physician's order must precede administration of any controlled substance, except in a dire emergency (emergency intubation, acute control of seizures, etc.), in which case the order will be written as soon as the emergency is over.
5. All controlled substances must be signed for by the nurse administering the medication at the time it is removed from the cabinet. The name of the prescribing physician should be inserted in the appropriate space.
6. If a controlled substance is removed from the cabinet in preparation for administration and is not used, or if part is wasted, the waste should be witnessed by another nurse and recorded as such on the controlled substance sheet. The signatures of both nurses are required.
7. In the event of a discrepancy at the time of count, the Nursing Care Coordinator or Divisional Nursing Coordinator is notified, and the loss section of the controlled drug order form is completed.
8. Controlled substances delivered by Pharmacy will not be accepted if the bag is opened or tampered with in any manner.
9. Upon receipt of the drugs, the nurse will verify the count/delivery and complete the addition to the controlled drug sheet.
10. Narcotics must be reordered every seventy-two (72) hours. Barbiturates must be ordered every seven (7) days.

Figure 12-2. *A hospital policy for signing and counting controlled drugs. (Courtesy of Nursing Department, St. Vincent's Hospital and Medical Center, New York City.)*

some generic and trade names of controlled drugs in Schedules III, IV, and V. Note that C III, C IV, and C V symbols identify these drugs.

Nurses who become impaired (unable to function) owing to alcohol or drug abuse leave themselves open to criminal action, as well as to disciplinary action by the state board of nursing. Many states have laws requiring mandatory reporting of impaired nurses.

Civil Law

Civil law is concerned with the legal rights and duties of private persons. When an individual believes that wrong was committed against him or her personally, that individual can sue for damages in the form of money.

The legal wrong is called a *tort. Malpractice* refers to negligence on the part of the nurse. There are four elements of negligence:

1. A claim that the nurse owed the patient a special duty of care, that is, a nurse–patient relationship existed.
2. A claim that the nurse was required to meet a specific standard of care in carrying out the action or function. To prove or disprove this element, both sides bring in expert witnesses to testify.
3. A claim that the nurse failed to meet the required standard.
4. A claim that harm or injury resulted for which compensation is sought.

The nurse–patient relationship is a legal status that is created the moment a nurse actually provides nursing care to another person.

For administration of medications, *a nurse is required by law to exercise the degree of skill and care that a reasonably prudent nurse with similar training and experience, practicing in the same community, would exercise under the same or similar circumstances.* When a nursing

St. Vincent's Hospital & Medical Center
of New York
Department of Pharmacy

CONTROLLED DRUG REQUISITION FORM

NURSING UNIT

QUANTITY	UNIT OF ISSUE	CONTROLLED DRUG	DOSAGE FORM	STRENGTH
	10	Chloral Hydrate	Capsule	500 mg
	60 ml	Chloral Hydrate	Solution	500 mg/5 ml
	25	Chlordiazepoxide (Librium)	Capsule	5 mg/10 mg/ 25 mg
	10	Chlordiazepoxide (Librium)	Ampule	100 mg
	25	Clorazepate (Tranxene)	Capsule	3.75 mg/7.5 mg
	25	Diazepam (Valium)	Tablets	2 mg/5 mg/ 10 mg
	10	Diazepam (Valium)	Ampules	10 mg
	25	Flurazepam (Dalmane)	Capsules	15 mg/30 mg
	10	Hycodan	Tablets	
	60 ml	Hycodan	Syrup	
	10	Lomotil	Tablets	
	60 ml	Lomotil	Liquid	
	25	Oxazepam (Serax)	Capsules	10 mg/15 mg
	25	Phenobarbital	Tablets	15 mg/30 mg
	120 ml	Phenobarbital	Elixir	20 mg/5 ml
	10	Phenobarbital	Ampules	120 mg
	10	Pentazocine (Talwin)	Tablets	50 mg
	10	Pentazocine (Talwin)	Syringe	30 mg
	25	Propoxyphene (Darvon)	Capsules	65 mg
	25	Temazepam (Restoril)	Capsules	15 mg/30 mg

Ordered By _____ Date _____
                    Nurse
Received By _____ Date _____
                    Nurse
Dispensed By _____ Date _____
                  Pharmacist

Figure 12-3. *Controlled Drug Requisition Form for Schedule III, IV, and V drugs. (Courtesy of Pharmacy Department, St. Vincent's Hospital and Medical Center, New York City.)*

student performs duties that are customarily performed by a registered nurse, the courts have held the nursing student to the higher standard of care of the registered nurse.

Mistakes in administering medications are among the most common causes of malpractice. Liability may result from administering the wrong dose, giving a medication to a wrong patient, giving a drug at the wrong time, or failing to administer a drug at the right time or in the proper manner.

A frequent cause of medication errors is misreading the physician's order or failing to check with the physician when the order is questionable. Faulty technique in administering medications, especially injections that result in injury to the patient, is another common medication error.

Not all malpractice is a result of negligence. Malpractice claims are also founded upon the daily interaction between the nurse and the patient; consequently, the nurse's personality plays a major role in the fostering or prevention of malpractice claims. All nurses should be familiar with the principles of psychology. The surest way to prevent claims is to recognize the patient as a human being who has emotional, as well as physical, needs and to respond to these needs in a humane and competent manner.

Should an error occur, primary consideration must be given to the patient. The nurse notifies the physician and the immediate nursing supervisor; students notify the instructor. Error-in-medication forms are filled out and appropriate action is taken under the direction of the physician.

To prevent malpractice claims, the nurse must render, as consistently as possible, the best possible care to patients. Every nurse involved in direct care should regard prevention of malpractice claims as an integral part of daily nursing responsibilities for two fundamental reasons:

1. Such measures result in higher quality care.
2. All affirmative measures taken to minimize malpractice will minimize the nurse's exposure to personal liability.

How can liability claims be avoided?

- Know and follow institutional policies and procedures.
- Look up what you do not know.
- Do not leave medicines at the bedside.
- Chart carefully.
- Listen to the patient: "I never took that before," and the like.
- Check.
- *Double check* when a dose seems high. Most oral tablet doses range from $\frac{1}{2}$ to 2 tablets. Most injections are less than 2 ml.
- Label any powder you dilute. Label any IV bag you use.
- When necessary, seek advice from competent professionals.
- Do not administer drugs poured by another nurse.
- Keep drug knowledge up to date—attend continuing education programs; update nursing skills.

It is possible to render high-quality nursing care and never commit a medication error. Safe, effective drug therapy is a combination of knowledge, skill, carefulness, and caring.

ETHICAL PRINCIPLES IN DRUG ADMINISTRATION

A moral as well as legal dimension is involved in the administration of medications. There is a difference between actions that are right and actions that are wrong. Nurses are responsible for their actions.

The American Nurses Association Code of Ethics contains several statements that apply to drug therapy. Briefly stated, they are

1. The nurse provides services with respect for the human dignity and the uniqueness of the patient.

2. The nurse safeguards the patient's right to privacy.
3. The nurse acts to safeguard the patient from incompetent, unethical, or illegal practice.
4. The nurse assumes responsibility and accountability for nursing judgments and actions.
5. The nurse maintains competence in nursing.

Several principles can be used as guides when an ethical decision must be made. These principles are autonomy, truthfulness, beneficence, nonmaleficence, confidentiality, and justice.

Autonomy

Autonomy is a form of personal liberty in which an individual has the freedom to decide, knows the facts and understands them, and acts without outside force, deceit, or constraint. For the patient, this implies a right to be informed about drug therapy and a right to refuse medication. For the nurse, autonomy brings a responsibility to discuss drug information with the patient and to accept the patient's right to refuse. Autonomy also gives the nurse the right to refuse to participate in any drug therapy deemed to be unethical or unsafe.

Truthfulness

The nurse has an obligation to tell the truth. Some ethicists hold that this is not an absolute obligation and argue that it may be more beneficial not to give all the facts or, sometimes, even to deliberately deceive. In drug therapy, this principle can lead to a dilemma when a *placebo* is ordered.

A placebo is a nondrug or a dummy drug that produces a therapeutic effect, not because of any chemical property, but because of the positive relationship that exists between the patient who receives it and the nurse who administers it. Placebos are sometimes ordered in place of pain medication. The nurse administers the placebo, stating that it will relieve pain. "Cooperative" patients are said to produce *endorphins,* chemical mediators that block pain impulses. Patients who do not have a positive relationship with the nurse experience no relief. The dilemma is that some nurses see the use of a placebo as lying to the patient, whereas others see it as a benevolent way of providing relief without pharmacologic intervention. To act in an ethical manner, the nurse who administers a placebo should respect the patient and believe that this therapy can be effective. The nurse should not use the placebo with the intent of tricking or punishing the patient.

The principle of truthfulness also applies when giving drug information to a patient. It is generally held that patients should be informed, to some extent, about drug therapy. There is disagreement about the extent of disclosure.

Beneficence

This concept holds that the nurse must contribute to the good health and welfare of the patient. Every action has both benefits and costs. Do the benefits outweigh the cost? Relative to disclosure of drug information, do the principles of autonomy and veracity outweigh the possible negative effects of revealing all the consequences of taking a drug? Might the patient refuse a drug that, in the end, would be beneficial? In the use of chemotherapy (for cancer), informed consent is required, and the patient is given detailed information. Disclosure is not so complete in other areas of medical care.

Nonmaleficence

Nonmaleficence holds that the nurse must not inflict harm on the patient and must prevent harm whenever possible. Doing something good may lead to a secondary effect that is harmful. For example, giving morphine may relieve pain—a good effect—but may hasten death. It is moral to act for the benefit and to permit the harm, provided the intent is the benefit.

Confidentiality

Confidentiality is respect for information learned from professional involvement with patients. A patient's drug therapy and responses should be discussed only with those individuals who have a right to know, that is, other professionals caring for the patient. To what extent the family or significant others have a right to know depends on the specific situation and wishes of the patient and sometimes may cause conflict.

Justice

Justice refers to the patient's right to receive the right drug, the right dose, by the right route, at the right time. In addition, the patient has a right to the nurse's careful assessment, management, and evaluation of drug therapy and to those nursing actions that promote the patient's safety and well-being. The nurse's obligation is to maintain a high standard of care.

SPECIFIC POINTS THAT MAY BE HELPFUL IN GIVING MEDICATIONS

Medication Orders

A correct medication order has the patient's name and room number, the date, the name of the drug (generic or trade), the dose of the drug, the route of administration, and the times to administer the drug. It ends with the physician's signature.

There are several types of orders:

1. Standing order with termination

   | | *EXAMPLE:* thyroxin 4 mg qd × 5 days

2. Standing order without termination

   | | *EXAMPLE:* digoxin 0.5 mg po qd

3. A prn order

   | | *EXAMPLE:* demerol 50 mg IM q4h prn

4. Single-dose order

   | | *EXAMPLE:* atropine SO$_4$ 0.3 mg SC 7:30 AM on call to OR

5. Stat order

   | | *EXAMPLE:* morphine sulfate, 10 mg SC stat

Hospital guidelines provide for an automatic stop time on some classes of drugs; for example, narcotic orders may be valid for only 3 days, antibiotics for 10 days. When the nurse first picks up and transfers the order, care must be taken to note the expiration time so that all staff who pour medications are alerted. State laws and hospital policies vary.

- Medical students may write orders on charts, but they must be countersigned by a house physician before they are legal. Medical students are not licensed.
- In states that allow nurses or paramedical personnel to prescribe drugs, hospital guidelines must be followed in carrying out orders.
- Do not carry out an order that is not clear or that is illegible. Check with the physician who wrote the order. Do not assume anything.
- Do not carry out an order if a conflict exists with nursing knowledge; for example, Demerol 500 mg IM is above the average dose.
- Nursing students should not accept oral or telephone orders. They should refer the physician to the charge nurse.
- Professional nurses may take oral or telephone orders in accord with institutional policy. These orders must be written and signed by the physician within 24 hours. Two nurses should listen to and verify the order.

Knowledge Base

- Nurses should know generic and trade names of drugs to be administered, class, average dose, routes of administration, use, side and adverse effects, contraindications, and nursing implications in administration. Nurses should also know what signs of effectiveness to look for and what drug interactions are possible. New or unfamiliar drugs should be researched.
- The nurse should be aware of the patient's diagnosis and medical history, especially relative to drugs taken. Be especially alert to over-the-counter (OTC) drugs, which the patient often does not consider important. Check for allergies.
- Assess the patient's need for drug information. Be prepared to implement and evaluate a nursing care plan in drug therapy.

Pouring Medications

- The patient has a right to considerate and respectful care and the right to refuse a medication. The patient also has a right to know the name of the medication, what it is supposed to do, any side effects that may occur, and what to do should these occur.
- In the ticket system, the Kardex is the main check against the medication ticket. If the ticket does not agree with the Kardex, go to the chart and find the original order. Check through every order to the current date to identify changes in orders.
- In the unit-dose, mobile cart system, the nurse has the medication sheets of each patient together in a folder or on a computer printout. If you are unsure of an order, take the sheet to the patient's chart and check from the date ordered to the current date.
- Do not pour and administer a drug for which any doubt exists. Check further with the physician, the pharmacist, or a supervising nurse.
- Quiet and concentration are needed to pour drugs. Follow a routine in pouring. Methodology is the best safeguard in preventing error.
- Keys are needed to obtain controlled drugs (e.g., narcotics) and to prevent others' access to medications.
- Pour oral medications first, then injections. Medical asepsis (clean technique) is used for oral administration. Injections require sterile technique.
- Read labels three times: (1) when removing the drug from storage, (2) when calculating the dose, and (3) after pouring the drug and before returning the stock to storage.

- Orders issued as "stat" take precedence and must be carried out immediately.
- Perform indicated nursing actions before administering certain medications; for example, digitalis preparations require an apical heart rate, whereas antihypertensives require a blood pressure reading.
- Medications should be administered within 30 minutes of the time given. They may be prepared before then in the ticket system. When the mobile cart is used, medications are prepared at the patient's bed and administered.
- Keep medications within sight at all times. Never leave medications unattended. The mobile cart or the medication tray must be kept in view.
- Administer irritating oral drugs with meals or a snack to decrease gastric irritation.
- Break a tablet only if it is scored.
- Never open capsules or break enteric-coated tablets. If the patient cannot swallow them, ask the physician to order a liquid, or check with the pharmacist.
- Check tablets in a stock container. Are they the same size? Same color? If not, return them to the pharmacy.
- It is a fallacy that the nurse is no longer required to calculate or prepare drugs dispensed as unit-dose. Fractional doses may still be necessary. The pharmacy may not have the exact dose. Antibiotics must be prepared. The label must still be read three times.
- Labels must be clear. If not, return them to the pharmacy.
- Never return any poured drug to a stock bottle once you have left the medication room.
- Never combine medications from two stock bottles. Return both bottles to the pharmacy. It is the responsibility of the pharmacist to combine drugs.
- Hydrophilic capsules are not medications. They are labeled DO NOT EAT and are placed in stock containers of tablets and capsules to absorb dampness and maintain the drug in a solid state.
- If the patient is nauseous or vomiting, hold oral medications and notify the physician or your immediate superior. Be sure to chart this action. Also hold medications if you suspect that an adverse effect has occurred or if the drug is contraindicated.
- Some liquid medications require dilution. Check references for directions.
- Some liquids may have to be administered through a straw; for example, liquid iron preparations discolor teeth and should not contact them.
- Liquids are poured at eye level using a medicine cup. Measure at the *center* of the meniscus—pour with the label up to prevent soiling.
- After the patient has taken a liquid antacid, add 5–10 ml of water to the cup, mix, and have patient drink it as well. Antacids are thick and medication often remains in the cup.
- The nurse who pours medications is responsible for administering and charting.
- Do not give drugs that another nurse has poured.

Giving Medications

- Follow the universal safeguards in administration of medications.
- *Always* check the patient's ID band before administering medications. If the patient does not have an ID band, have a responsible person identify the patient for you and be sure to notify the ward clerk to obtain an ID band for the patient.
- Listen to the patient's comments and act on them, for example, "Not mine" or "Never took this before." Check carefully, then return to the patient with the result of your investigation. Failure to do this will result in loss of the patient's trust and confidence and may also result in a medication error.
- If a patient refuses a drug, find out why. Then implement nursing action to correct the situation. Chart the reason for refusal.
- Watch to make sure the patient takes the drugs. Stay until oral drugs are swallowed.
- Keep drugs within your view at all times.
- Do not administer drugs prepared by other nurses.

■ Never leave any drug at the bedside stand unless hospital policy permits you to do so. If you do leave a medication, inform the patient why the drug is ordered, how to take it, and what to expect. Check to determine if the drug was taken and record your findings.

Charting

■ Chart single doses, stat doses, and prn medications immediately and use the *exact time* when administered.
■ Chart standing orders using *standard time* (e.g., tid).
■ If you hold a drug or the drug was refused, write the reason on the nurse's notes.
■ Chart any nursing actions preliminary to administering drugs, for example, apical heart rate or blood pressure.

Evaluation

■ Check for the expected effect of the drug. Did side effects or adverse effects occur? Perform indicated nursing actions. Record your observations.

Error in Medication

■ Report an error immediately to the charge nurse and the physician.
■ Primary concern must be given to the patient.
■ Error-in-medication forms should be filled out. Follow the physician's directions in caring for the patient.

SELF-TEST 1

Give the information requested. Answers may be found at the end of the chapter.

1. List ten kinds of information the nurse needs to know to give drugs safely.

_____   _____
_____   _____
_____   _____
_____   _____
_____   _____

2. List the five pregnancy categories used to identify the safety of drugs for the fetus and briefly define each.

_____
_____
_____
_____
_____
_____

3. Name the major organ for these drug activities.
    a. Absorption _____   **c.** Biotransformation _____

    b. Distribution _____   **d.** Excretion _____

(continued)

SELF-TEST 1 *(Continued)*

4. Define:

a.   Tolerance _____

_____

_____

b.   Cumulation _____

_____

_____

5. List the 4 elements of negligence.

_____ ,

_____ ,

_____ , and

_____

6. What is the standard by which a tort is judged?

_____

_____

_____

7. List five positive actions to avoid liability.

_____

_____

_____

_____

_____

8. List and briefly describe five ethical principles in drug therapy.

_____

_____

_____

_____

_____

9. What are the seven elements of a correct medication order?

_____   _____

_____   _____

_____   _____

_____

10. What action should a nurse take when an order is not clear?

_____

SELF-TEST 2

Choose the correct answer. Answers will be found at the end of the chapter.

1. Two drugs are given for different reasons, but drug Y interferes with the excretion of drug X. The effect of drug X would be
   a. increased
   b. decreased
   c. unchanged
   d. stopped

2. Major biotransformation of drugs occurs in the
   a. lungs
   b. kidney
   c. liver
   d. urine

3. Toxicity to a drug is more likely to occur when
   a. elimination of the drug is rapid
   b. the drug is bound to the plasma protein, albumen
   c. the drug will not dissolve in the lipid layer of the cell
   d. the drug is free in the blood circulation

4. The term USP after a drug name indicates that the drug
   a. is made only in the United States
   b. meets official standards in the United States
   c. cannot be made by any other pharmaceutical company
   d. is registered by the U.S. Public Health Service

5. When an order is written to be administered "as needed" it is called a
   a. standing order
   b. prn order
   c. single order
   d. stat order

6. Signs of effectiveness of a drug are based on what information?
   a. Action and use
   b. Untoward effects
   c. Generic and trade names
   d. Drug interaction

7. Drug classification is an aid in understanding
   a. use of the drug
   b. drug idiosyncrasy
   c. the trade name
   d. the generic name

8. Names of many drugs include
   a. several generic, several trade names
   b. several generic, one trade name
   c. one generic, one trade name
   d. one generic, several trade names

(continued)

SELF-TEST 2 (*Continued*)

9. Which pregnancy category is considered safe for the fetus?
    a. A
    b. B
    c. C
    d. D

10. What is the primary purpose of enteric-coating medications?
    a. Improve taste
    b. Delay absorption
    c. Code the drug for identification
    d. Make the drug easier to swallow

11. Which of the following drug preparations does *not* have to be shaken before pouring?
    a. Emulsion
    b. Gel
    c. Suspension
    d. Aqueous solution

12. Most oral drugs are absorbed in the
    a. mouth
    b. stomach
    c. small intestine
    d. large intestine

13. Nursing legal responsibilities associated with controlled substances include
    a. storage in a locked place
    b. assessing vital signs
    c. evaluating psychological response
    d. establishing automatic 24-hour stop orders

14. Characteristics of a Schedule II drug include
    a. accepted medical use with a high abuse potential
    b. medically accepted drug with low-dependence possibility
    c. no accepted use in patient care
    d. unlimited renewals

15. The responsibilities of the medication nurse in the hospital include
    a. prescribing drugs
    b. teaching patients
    c. regulating automatic expiration times of drugs
    d. preparing solutions

16. Under what condition does a nurse have a right to refuse to administer a drug?
    a. The pharmacist ordered the drug.
    b. The drug is manufactured by two different companies.
    c. The drug is prescribed by a licensed physician.
    d. The dose is within the range given in the *PDR.*

17. When administering medication in the hospital, the nurse should
    a. chart medications before administering them
    b. chart only those drugs that she or he personally gave the patient
    c. chart all medications given for the day at one time
    d. determine the best method for giving the drugs

18. Which of the following illustrates a medication error?
    a. Administering a 10 AM dose at 10:20 AM
    b. Giving 2 tablets of Gantrisin 500 mg when 1 g is ordered
    c. Pouring 5 ml of cough syrup when 1 tsp is ordered
    d. Giving digoxin IM when digoxin 0.25 mg is ordered

19. A nurse reads a medication order that is not clear. What action is indicated?
    a. Ask the charge nurse to explain the order.
    b. Ask a doctor at the nurses' station for help.
    c. Check the *PDR* on the unit.
    d. Check with the doctor who wrote the order.

20. Which nursing action is illegal?
    a. Pouring medication from one stock bottle into another
    b. Counting control drugs in the narcotic closet each shift
    c. Labeling a vial of powder after dissolving it
    d. Refusing to carry out an order that is confusing

ANSWERS

Self-Test 1

1. Generic/trade name; class; pregnancy category; dose and route; action; use; side/adverse effects; contraindications/precautions; interactions/incompatibilities; nursing implications; evaluation of effectiveness; patient teaching

2. **A.** No risk to fetus
   B. No adverse effects in animals, but no human studies
   C. Animals show adverse effects; calculated risk to fetus
   D. Fetal risk exists
   E. Absolute fetal abnormality

3. **a.** Small intestines   **c.** liver
   b. blood   **d.** kidney

4. **a.** Repeated administration of a drug increases microsomal enzyme activity in the liver. The drug is broken down more quickly and its effectiveness is decreased.
   b. Biotransformation is inhibited and the drug level remains high. Adverse effects are more likely to occur.

5. A claim that a nurse–patient relationship existed
   The nurse was required to meet a standard of care
   A claim that the nurse failed to meet that standard
   A claim that this resulted in injury

6. Did the nurse exercise the degree of skill and care that a reasonably prudent nurse with similar training and experience, practicing in the same community, would exercise under the same or similar circumstances?

7. Know policies and practices of the institution.
   Research unfamiliar drugs.
   Do not leave medicines at the bedside.
   Chart carefully.
   Listen to the patient's complaints.
   Check yourself (e.g., read labels three times).
   Label anything you dilute.
   Keep up to date.

8. Autonomy: freedom to decide based on knowledge with no constraint
   Truthfulness: truth telling that can create a dilemma. Is it absolute or is there a beneficent deceit?
   Beneficence: obligation to help others
   Nonmaleficence: do no harm
   Confidentiality: keep secrets
   Justice: rights of an individual

9. Patient's name and room; date; name of drug; dose; route; times of administration; doctor's signature

10. The nurse does not administer the drug and checks with the physician who wrote the order.

Self-Test 2

1.	a	11.	d
2.	c	12.	c
3.	d	13.	a
4.	b	14.	a
5.	b	15.	b
6.	a	16.	a
7.	a	17.	b
8.	d	18.	d
9.	a	19.	d
10.	b	20.	a

13

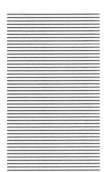

Administration Procedures

Throughout this text we have calculated dosages and studied information related to drug therapy. Finally, we arrive at the "how to" chapter—methods of administering drugs orally, parenterally, and topically. The adages "practice makes perfect" and "one picture is worth a thousand words" apply. Learning to administer medications is a skilled activity that requires practice, with supervision, to ensure correct technique.

Every institution has a standard procedure for administering medications, which depends on the way the drugs are dispensed—unit-dose, multidose containers, or a combination of the two. Institutional procedure may call for the use of a tray and medication tickets or for a mobile cart with medication sheets.

Whatever the procedure is, follow it carefully. Do not look for shortcuts. *Methodology*—a step-by-step attention to detail—is the best safeguard to assure the patient's five rights. Research has proved time after time that most medication errors occur because the nurse violated procedural guidelines.

UNIVERSAL SAFEGUARDS APPLIED TO ADMINISTRATION OF MEDICATIONS

In administering drugs, there is a risk of potential exposure to hepatitis B virus (HBV) and the human immunodeficiency virus (HIV) through contact of the nurse's skin or mucous membranes with patient blood, body fluids, or tissues. The Centers for Disease Control (CDC) in Atlanta advocate that *Universal Safeguards be employed in caring for all patients when handling equipment contaminated with blood or blood-streaked body fluids.*

The following points that are based on CDC guidelines are offered to aid in determining appropriate safeguards in giving medications. These points are *dependent upon the type of contact you have with patients.*

General Safeguards in Administering Medications

1. Oral medications: Handwashing is adequate unless there is a possibility of exposure to blood or body secretions.
2. Injections: Handwashing is adequate. If there is a possibility of exposure to blood or body secretions, gloves may be worn. Use nursing judgment. Place used equipment in a puncture-proof container.

3. Heparin locks, intravenous catheters, and intravenous needles: Wear gloves when inserting or removing intravenous needles and catheters. The use of a clamp is recommended to hold contaminated IV needles and catheters being carried to a puncture-proof container.
4. Secondary administration sets or intravenous piggyback sets: Handwashing is adequate after removing this equipment from the main IV tubing because there is no direct exposure to blood or body secretions. Used needles should be placed in a puncture-proof container.
5. Application of medication to mucous membranes: Gloves should be worn (see the following guidelines in using gowns, masks, goggles).
6. Applications to skin: Exercise nursing judgment. Handwashing may be sufficient protection when applying such drug forms as transdermal patches. Use gloves when the patient's skin is not intact. Use gloves when applying lotions, ointments, or creams to areas of rash or to skin lesions.

HANDS

1. Hands must be washed before preparing medications and after administering medications to each patient.
2. Hands must be washed *after* removing gloves, gowns, masks, goggles, and *before* leaving the room of any patient for whom they are used.
3. Hands must be washed immediately when soiled with patient blood or body fluids.
4. Hands must be washed *after* handling equipment soiled with blood or body fluids.

GLOVES

1. Gloves must be worn for any direct ("hands-on") contact with patients' blood, bodily fluids, or secretions while administering medications.
2. Gloves must be worn when handling materials or equipment contaminated with blood or body fluids.
3. When gloves are used, they must be changed upon completion of procedures for each patient *and* between patients.

GOWNS

When administering medications, gowns are required *only* if the nurse's clothing may become contaminated with a patient's blood or body fluids.

MASKS

Masks *are not required* except in the following instances:

1. The patient is placed on *strict* or *respiratory* isolation precautions.
2. Carrying out a medication procedure may cause blood or body fluids to splash directly onto the nurse's face.

GOGGLES (PROTECTIVE EYEWEAR)

Goggles should be worn during the performance of any medication procedure in which the nurse would be in *extremely close contact* with the patient and there is possibility of splashing or aerolization of blood or blood-tinged fluids into the nurse's eyes or mucous membranes (e.g., use of power spray apparatus).

MANAGEMENT OF USED NEEDLES AND SHARPS

1. All used needles, syringes, sharps, and IV catheters must be placed in appropriate, labeled, puncture-proof containers.
2. Do not break, bend, or recap needles after use. Place needles immediately into a puncture-proof container.
3. Exercise caution in removing heparin locks, intravenous catheters, and intravenous needles. Gloves should be worn. The use of a clamp is advisable to hold the used IV needle being transported to a puncture-proof container. *Do not remove the IV needle from the IV tubing by hand; use a clamp.*
4. If *reusable* needles and syringes are employed, the needle should be separated from the syringe with a clamp. *Never manipulate a used needle by hand.* Place the needle and syringe in appropriate puncture-proof containers for sterilization. *It is strongly recommended that disposable needles and syringes be used.*

MANAGEMENT OF MATERIALS OTHER THAN NEEDLES AND SHARPS

Paper cups, plastic cups, and other equipment not contaminated with blood or body fluids may be discarded according to routine hospital procedure. In cases of *strict* or *respiratory* isolation precautions, follow the protocol established by the institution.

MANAGEMENT OF NURSE CONTAMINATED WITH BLOOD OR BODY FLUIDS

The nurse who is exposed to blood or blood-streaked body fluids of any patient through a personal needlestick or injury or through laceration of the skin should immediately squeeze the area if this is indicated, wash the area with soap and water, and scrub the area with povidone–iodine (Betadine) or another acceptable antiseptic. The protocol established by the health care institution for management of needlestick injury or accidental exposure to blood or body fluids should be followed.

SYSTEMS OF ADMINISTRATION

The ticket system is used when drugs are dispensed in multidose containers. Drugs are prepared in a medication room and carried to the patient on a tray. When unit-dose packaging is available, drugs are placed in individual patient drawers on a mobile cart. The cart is wheeled into the patient's room and medications are prepared at the bedside for administration.

Ticket System (Universal Safeguard: Handwashing)

In this system, a medication order is transferred to three places: a medication ticket, the patient's medication sheet, and the patient's Kardex file, which contains the nursing care plan.

Tickets for all patients are kept in a central location. The nurse sorts them according to time of administration. Each ticket is compared with the Kardex entry. If there is a discrepancy, the nurse checks the original order on the patient's chart. When all tickets have been verified, the nurse obtains the keys to the medication room, washes his or her hands, and enters the room. Quiet and concentration are essential.

The first patient's tickets are separated and placed together in a pile one on top of another, so that only one ticket is visible at a time. The ticket is read, the multidose container is located, and the stock label is verified with the ticket (first check).

The dose on the ticket is compared with the stock measure, and the amount of drug is calculated and poured (second check).

Before returning the multidose container to the shelf, the order and the label are read again and the poured dose is verified (third check).

Example:

> I want digoxin 0.125 mg. I have a stock of scored tablets of digoxin 0.25 mg. I pour ½ tablet.

The medication is placed on a tray with the ticket in front to identify it (Fig. 13-1). When all medications have been prepared, the nurse locks the door to the medication room and proceeds to each patient.

The patient is greeted and the tray is placed on a flat surface within the nurse's view. The tray must never be out of sight.

The nurse picks up the patient's tickets and medicines. The name on the ticket is compared with the patient's ID band. Any required nursing assessment is carried out. For example, an apical heart rate is required before digoxin can be administered. The nurse will make a decision to withhold or to give the drug on the basis of this assessment. The nurse administers the drugs, watches to be sure the patient has taken them, carries out comfort measures as necessary, washes his or her hands, picks up the tray, and moves to the next patient.

When all medications have been given, the tray is cleaned and put away and the medication tickets are brought to the nurse's station and used to record doses on each patient's chart.

There are several disadvantages to this system. Every order must be transcribed to three different places. Each time the order is rewritten an error is possible. Tickets may be lost or misplaced. An error may occur in choosing the stock. The tickets may become mixed, so that the wrong patient receives a medication. Medications that require assessment must be tagged in some way to identify them. It is time-consuming to locate the chart of each patient.

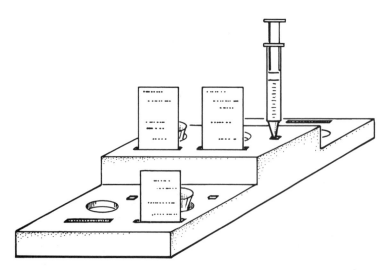

Figure 13-1. A medication tray with tickets and drugs in place.

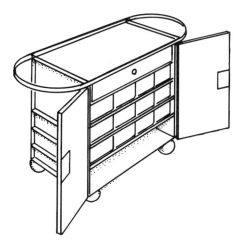

Figure 13-2. *A mobile cart: Each drawer is labeled with a patient's name. Unit-dose drugs are placed in the drawers by the pharmacist. The nurse administers the drugs.*

Mobile-Cart System (Universal Safeguard: Handwashing)

Compared with the ticket system, the mobile-cart system has many advantages. The pharmacist dispenses unit-dose medications directly to the patient's drawer (Fig. 13-2). Each drawer is labeled with the patient's name. The cart contains all the equipment the nurse might require to administer medications.

When a drug is ordered, the nurse transcribes the order to one place—the patient's medication sheet, found in a medication book on the cart. This book contains the medication sheets for every patient on the unit.

When it is time to administer medications, the nurse washes his or her hands and rolls the cart to the bedside of the first patient, unlocks the cart, and opens the medication book to the first patient's medication sheet.

The sheet is checked for special nursing actions required before giving medication. These are carried out, the results are recorded, and the decision is made to withhold or to administer the medication.

The patient's drawer is placed on the top of the cart. The nurse reads each medication order, starting with the first medication listed. When a dose is to be given, the nurse chooses the unit dose from the drawer and compares the label with the order (first check).

The dose is computed after comparing the order with the unit measure, the unit dose is opened, and the amount is poured (second check).

The unit-dose label and the order are again read and the dose is verified (third check). The unit-dose package is then discarded in a waste receptacle on the cart. When all the patient's medications have been prepared, the nurse reads the name on the medicine sheet, checks the patient's ID band, and administers the drugs. The nurse remains with the patient until the medications are taken, provides any comfort measures, washes his or her hands, and returns to the cart to chart the drugs administered. The patient's drawer is replaced and the cart is rolled to the next patient. When all medications have been administered, the mobile cart is returned to its designated area.

This system has several advantages. There are two professionals involved in checking the medication in the drawer—the pharmacist and the nurse. All the medication sheets are together on the cart. This is time-saving. Nursing assessment can be carried out and results charted before any medication is poured. The drugs can be signed for immediately after administration.

Note, however, that in both systems, the nurse checks the label three times—when choosing the drug, when calculating and pouring the dose, and before replacing the stock.

Some hospitals have computerized medication procedures. Doctors input orders directly on the computer. The nurse receives the printout of drugs to be administered to patients at specific times. When the task is completed, the nurse signs for medications using the computer. Paperwork is eliminated. The hard disk contains the patient's chart.

ROUTES OF ADMINISTRATION

Oral Route (Universal Safeguard: Handwashing)

Regardless of the system used to pour the medications, the procedure for administering drugs contains specific steps. The nurse greets the patient orally and checks the ID band. The patient is assisted to a sitting position. The patient should be alert and able to swallow. Oral solids are given first, together with a full glass of water whenever possible, followed by oral liquid medications. The nurse watches to be sure the patient has swallowed all of the drugs before leaving. The paper and plastic cups may be discarded according to routine hospital procedure, unless the patient is on strict or respiratory isolation. For this, special isolation bags are utilized. The nurse makes the patient comfortable, washes his or her hands, and charts the doses given.

Special considerations for oral administration include the following:

- If the patient is NPO (nothing by mouth), check with the doctor to determine if oral medication can be administered with a small amount of water. The doctor may not wish to withhold certain drugs (for example, an anticonvulsant for a patient with epilepsy).
- When a patient refuses a drug, find out why, chart the reason, and initiate action to correct the situation.
- Solid stock medications are poured first into the container lid and then into a paper cup, using medical asepsis. The medication is not touched. Several solids may be combined in the cup, but each medication should first be poured into a separate cup until the third check is completed.
- Medical asepsis is followed to break a scored tablet. This means that clean, not sterile, technique is required. One method is to place the tablet in a paper towel, fold the towel over and, with thumbs and index fingers in apposition, break the tablet along the score line. Tablets that are not scored should not be broken.
- Check expiration dates on all labels.
- If the patient has difficulty swallowing solids, first determine if the medication is available in a liquid form. Enteric- and film-coated tablets should not be crushed. Ordinarily, capsules should not be opened. Check with the pharmacist for alternative forms.
- If a medication can be crushed, it is best to use a "pill" crusher, with the medication placed between two paper cups. If a mortar and pestle is used, be sure it is cleaned before and after crushing so there is no residue. If no equipment is available, place the tablet between two paper cups and use the edge of a bottle or other hard surface to crush the drug. A crushed drug may be mixed with water or semisolids, such as apple sauce or custard, for ease in swallowing.
- Some drugs are best taken on an empty stomach; others may be taken with food. The nurse should be aware of foods or fluids that may be ingested with the drug and of those that are contraindicated.
- Check patients for allergies to drugs. This should be a routine procedure.
- The nurse should be knowledgeable about food–drug and drug–drug interactions and act to safeguard the patient.
- Failure to shake some liquid medications can result in a wrong dose. The drug settles to the bottom, and only the weak diluent is poured.
- Pour liquids at eye level, with the thumb indicating the meniscus. In pouring liquids, the label should be up so it will not be stained. Wipe the lip of the bottle with a paper towel before recapping.
- Note any presence of an unusual color change or precipitate in a liquid. If such a change

is present, do not use. Send the container to the pharmacy with a note indicating your observation.

- Check references to determine how to disguise liquids that are distasteful or irritating. Two possibilities are to mix with juice or give through a straw after diluting well. Liquid iron preparations stain the teeth and are taken through a straw placed in the back of the mouth. Tinctures are always diluted.
- Liquid cough mixtures are not diluted. They have a secondary soothing (demulcent) effect on the mucous membranes in addition to the antitussive action.
- The oral route is the least expensive, the safest, and the easiest to take.

Parenteral Route

Medications may be given by the IM, SC, IVPB, or IV route or intradermally. The parenteral route is used when a drug cannot be given orally, when it is necessary to obtain a rapid systemic effect, or when a drug would be rendered ineffective or destroyed by the oral route.

CHOOSING THE SITE

The following areas should be avoided: bony prominences, large blood vessels, nerves, sensitive areas, bruises, hardened areas, abrasions, and inflamed areas. The site for IM injections should be able to accept 3 ml; rotate sites when repeated injections are given.

PREPARATION OF THE SKIN

Cleanse the site with an alcohol pad while using a circular motion from the center out. Grasp the area firmly between the thumb and forefinger and insert the needle with a dartlike motion (Fig. 13-3). If the area is obese, the skin may be spread rather than pinched together.

SYRINGES FOR INJECTION

The most common syringe used for injections is a standard 3-ml size, marked in minims and in milliliters (ml or cc) to the nearest tenth. The precision (tuberculin) syringe is marked in half-

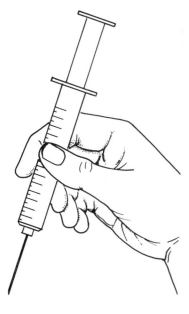

Figure 13-3. *An injection is administered with a quick dartlike motion into taut skin that has been spread or pinched.*

minims and milliliters to the nearest hundredth. There are two insulin syringes: a regular 1-ml size, marked to the U 100 and a 0.5-ml size (low-dose) insulin syringe marked to U 50.

NEEDLES FOR INJECTIONS

Needles are chosen for their gauge and their length. *Gauge* is the diameter of the needle opening. The principle is: the higher the gauge number, the finer the needle.

The 28-gauge needle on the insulin syringe is the finest needle currently available for injections. Numbers 25, 26, 28 are used for SC injections for adults and for IM injections for children and emaciated patients. Numbers 23 and 22 are used for IM injections; 20 and 21 for IV therapy; and 15 and 18 for blood transfusions.

ANGLE OF INSERTION

Intramuscular.   For IM injection use a 22-gauge, $1\frac{1}{2}$-inch-long needle for adults and a 23-gauge, 1-inch-long needle for children or emaciated adults, inserted at a 90° angle.

Subcutaneous.   For SC injection use a 25-gauge, $\frac{1}{2}$-inch needle, a 26-gauge, $\frac{3}{4}$-inch or $\frac{5}{8}$-inch needle, or a 28-gauge, $\frac{1}{2}$-inch insulin syringe inserted at a 45° angle. Some injections may be given at a 90° angle if the subcutaneous layer of fat is thick and the needle is short.

Care must be exercised to reach the correct site. Intramuscular sites have a good blood supply and absorption is rapid; subcutaneous sites have a poor blood supply, and absorption is prolonged.

Intradermal.   For intradermal injection the angle is parallel to the skin. A 26-gauge, $\frac{5}{8}$-inch or $\frac{3}{4}$-inch needle is used for skin testing for allergy and tuberculosis.

PREPARING THE DOSE

Ordinarily, to prevent incompatibility of drugs only one medication should be drawn up in a syringe. When two drugs are given in one syringe, follow the procedure for mixing after determining that the drugs are compatible.

Drugs That Are Liquids in Vials

1. Cleanse the top of the vial with an alcohol sponge.
2. Draw the amount of air equivalent to the amount of solution desired into the syringe.
3. Inject the needle through the rubber diaphragm into the vial.
4. Expel air from the syringe into the vial. This increases the pressure in the vial and makes it easier to withdraw medication.
5. The medication can be drawn up in one of two ways (Fig. 13-4): Invert the vial and draw up the desired amount into the syringe, or leave the vial on the table and pull up the medication.
6. Withdraw the needle quickly from the vial.
7. The rubber diaphragm will seal.

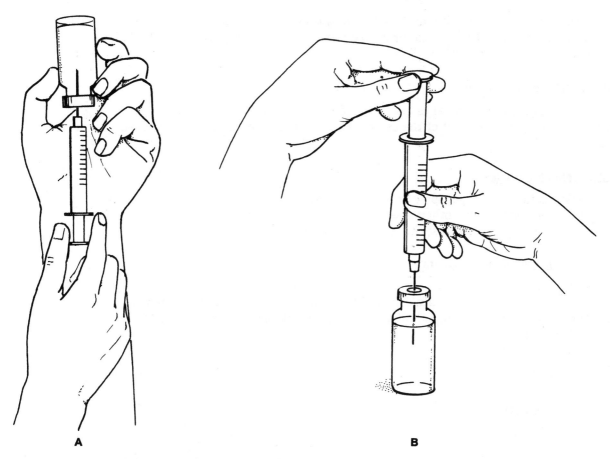

Figure 13-4. *Two methods of withdrawing medication from a vial: (A) Invert the vial and draw up the desired amount into the syringe. (B) Leave the vial on the table and pull up the medication.*

Drugs That Are Powders in Vials

1. Cleanse the top of the vial with an alcohol sponge.
2. Draw up the amount of calculated diluent from a 10-ml vial of distilled water or normal saline for injection. (Saline is less painful.) Follow pharmaceutical directions if another solvent is indicated.
3. Add diluent to the powder and roll the vial between your hands to dissolve the powder.
4. Label the vial with the solution made, your initials, and the date.
5. Cleanse the top of the vial again.
6. Draw up the amount of air equivalent to the amount of solution you desire into the syringe.
7. Inject the needle through the rubber diaphragm into the vial.
8. Expel the air into the vial. Invert the vial and draw up the desired amount of medication into the syringe.

Drugs in Glass Ampules

1. Tap the top of the ampule with your finger to clear out any drug.
2. Place an opened alcohol pad around the neck of the ampule.
3. Hold the ampule sideways.
4. Place thumbs in apposition above and index fingers in apposition below the ampule neck.
5. Press down with thumbs to break the ampule.

6. Insert the syringe needle into the solution, tilt the ampule, and withdraw the dose (Fig. 13-5). *Important: Do not add air before removing dose.* This will cause medication to spray from the ampule.

Unit-dose Cartridge and Holder

Insert the cartridge into the metal or plastic holder and screw into place. Move the plunger forward until it engages the shaft of the cartridge. Twist the plunger until it is locked into the cartridge.

Unit-dose Prefilled Syringes

The medication is in the syringe. Some prefilled syringes are simple and require no action other than removing the needle cover; others are packaged for compactness and directions are given to prepare the syringe for use. These syringes are disposable.

Mixing Two Medications in One Syringe

General Principles
1. Determine that the drugs are compatible by consulting a standard reference.
2. When in doubt about compatibility, prepare medications separately and administer into different injection sites.

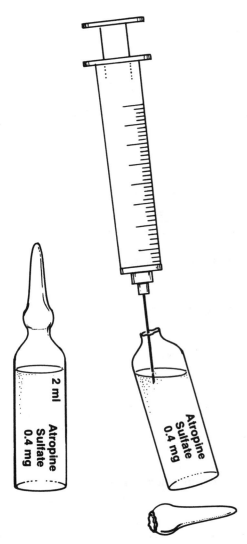

Figure 13-5. *Withdrawing medication from an ampule.*

3. When medications are in a vial and an ampule, draw up the medication from the vial first, then add the medication from the ampule. Discard any medication left in the ampule.

4. In preparing two types of insulin in one syringe, the vial containing *regular insulin must be drawn first* into the syringe. Regular insulin has not been adulterated with protein as have other insulins such as protamine zinc insulin.

Method 1

1. Once compatibility has been determined, the *easiest way* to mix medications for injection is to use an empty, sterile cartridge.

2. Carefully remove the covered needle from the cartridge. A rubber diaphragm is now visible.

3. Prepare the two compatible medications in separate syringes.

4. Clean the empty cartridge rubber with an alcohol pad and inject both medications into the cartridge. Rotate the cartridge in your hands to mix the medication. Replace the needle on the cartridge with sterile technique.

4. Place the cartridge in the metal or plastic holder and screw into place.

Method 2

1. Clean both vials with an alcohol pad.

2. Choose one vial as *primary.* For example, with vials of a narcotic and a non-narcotic, the narcotic is primary. With two insulins, regular insulin is primary.

3. Draw up medication from the primary vial in the usual way. Be sure there are no air bubbles.

4. Insert a 25- to 26-gauge needle at an angle into the rubber diaphragm of the *second* vial. This needle will act as an air vent.

5. Remove the needle from the syringe containing the *primary* medication. Put that needle in a sharps container. Place a new, sterile needle on the syringe.

6. Insert the needle into the *second* vial and invert the vial. Slowly withdraw the needed amount of drug. As medication is withdrawn, air will enter through the vent to replace the medication.

7. *Do not push the plunger back into the barrel.* This may force the primary medication into the second vial and contaminate the vial.

8. If there are any air bubbles in the syringe, decide how many minims and withdraw that amount of medication over the amount desired.

9. Remove the two needles, check for air and the correct dose in the syringe, and cap the needle. Place the air vent needle in the sharps container.

RATIONALE

The 25- to 26-gauge needle acts as an air vent to equalize pressure both inside and outside the vial. As medication is drawn from the vial, air enters through the vent to keep the pressure equalized. Changing the needle on the syringe before withdrawing medication from the second vial will prevent contamination of the second vial.

Method 3

1. Prepare the injection from the primary vial.

2. Be sure the dose is accurate and there are no air bubbles.

3. Remove the needle from the syringe and place in a sharps container. Place a new, sterile needle on the syringe.

4. Clean the second vial and insert the needle and syringe with the primary medication. Slowly withdraw the needed amount of drug.

5. **Do not push the plunger back into the barrel.** This may force the primary medication into the second vial and contaminate the vial.
6. If there are any air bubbles in the syringe, decide how many minims and withdraw that amount of medication over the amount desired. Check to be sure the dose is accurate and there are no air bubbles. Cap the needle.

IDENTIFYING THE INJECTION SITE

Intramuscular

Common sites are dorsogluteal, ventrogluteal, vastus lateralis, and deltoid.

DORSOGLUTEAL SITE. The dorsogluteal site is composed of the thick gluteal muscles of the buttocks.

Position: The patient may be prone or in a side-lying position with both buttocks fully exposed.

Location of injection site: The area must be chosen very carefully to avoid striking the sciatic nerve, major blood vessels, or bone. The landmarks of the buttocks are the crest of the posterior ilium as the superior boundary and the inferior gluteal fold as the lower boundary. The exact site can be identified in either of two ways:

1. Diagonal landmark (Fig. 13-6): Find the posterosuperior iliac spine and the greater trochanter of the femur. Draw an imaginary diagonal line between these two points, and give the injection lateral and superior to that line at least 1 inch below the iliac crest to avoid hitting the iliac bone. Should you hit the bone, withdraw the needle slightly and continue the procedure.
2. Quadrant landmark (see Fig. 13-6): Divide the buttocks into imaginary quadrants. The vertical line extends from the crest of the ilium to the gluteal fold. The horizontal line extends from the medial fold of the buttock to the lateral aspect of the buttock. Locate the upper-outer aspect of the upper-outer quadrant. The injection should be given in this area, 1 to 2 inches below the crest of the ilium, to avoid hitting bone. *Note:* The crest of the ilium must be palpated for precise site selection.

VENTROGLUTEAL SITE. The ventral part of the gluteal muscle has no large nerves or blood vessels and less fat. It is identified by finding the greater trochanter, anterior superior iliac spine, and iliac crest (Fig. 13-7). Place the palm of the hand over the greater trochanter. Point the index finger toward the anterosuperior iliac spine. Point the middle finger toward the iliac crest. Give the injection in the center of the triangle between these fingers.

Position: The patient may be supine, lying on the side, sitting, or standing.

VASTUS LATERALIS SITE: LATERAL THIGH. Measure one hand's width below the greater trochanter and one hand's width above the knee (Fig. 13-8). Give the injection in the lateral thigh. Ask the patient to point the big toe to the center of his body. This relaxes the vastus muscle.

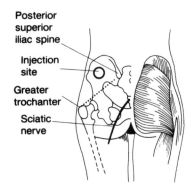

Posterior
superior
iliac spine

Injection
site

Greater
trochanter

Sciatic
nerve

Figure 13-6. *Identification of the dorsogluteal injection site. The injection is given in the upper outer area of the upper outer quadrant. (Smith, A. J., and Johnson, J. Y.: Nurses' Guide to Clinical Procedures. Philadelphia: J. B. Lippincott, 1990, p. 591.)*

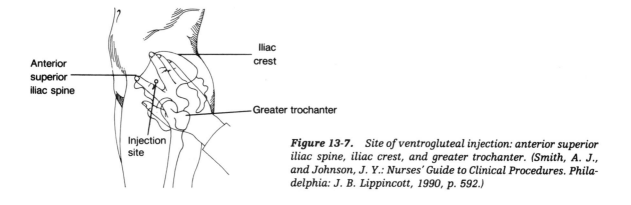

Figure 13-7. *Site of ventrogluteal injection: anterior superior iliac spine, iliac crest, and greater trochanter. (Smith, A. J., and Johnson, J. Y.: Nurses' Guide to Clinical Procedures. Philadelphia: J. B. Lippincott, 1990, p. 592.)*

Position: The patient may be supine, lying on the side, or standing.

DELTOID SITE.   The deltoid muscle on the lateral aspect of the upper arm is a small muscle close to the radial and brachial arteries. It should be used for IM injections only if specifically ordered, and no more than 2 ml should be injected. The boundaries are the lower edge of the acromion process (shoulder bone) and the axilla (armpit) (see Fig. 13-9C). Give the injection into the lateral arm between these two points and about 2 inches below the acromion process.

Position: The patient may be sitting or lying down.

Subcutaneous

Common injection sites include the upper arms, the thighs, or the abdomen (Fig. 13-9A, B). Only 1 ml or less should be injected. The injection is given at a 45° angle. If the needle is short or if the area is obese, a 90° angle may be used.

Intradermal (Intracutaneous)

The intradermal site is used for skin testing for allergies and diseases such as tuberculosis. Injecting an antigen causes an antigen–antibody sensitivity reaction if the individual is susceptible. If positive, the area will become raised, warm, and reddened.

The site is the inner aspect of the forearm. Prepare the skin with an alcohol pad and allow it to dry. Place your nondominant hand around the arm from below and pull the skin tightly to make the forearm tissue taut. Hold the syringe in your four fingers and thumb, with the bevel (opening) of the needle up, and insert the needle almost parallel to the skin (Fig. 13-10). It remains visible under the skin. Inject the solution such that it raises a small wheal (a raised bump). Remove the needle and allow the injection site to dry. *Do not massage the skin.* An alcohol pad or dry gauze pad may be used to gently wipe away any residue. Place the needle and syringe in a sharps container. Make the patient comfortable. Wash your hands. Chart the procedure.

ADMINISTERING INJECTIONS (UNIVERSAL SAFEGUARD: HANDWASHING)

1. Identify the patient orally.
2. Check ID band.
3. Perform any assessment before injection (e.g., vital signs, apical rate, site integrity).
4. Explain the procedure to the patient.
5. Ask the patient where the last injection was given. The sites should be rotated.
6. Prepare the area with an alcohol pad, using a circular motion from the center out.
7. Place the alcohol pad between your fingers or lay it on the patient's skin above the site.
8. Remove the needle cover.

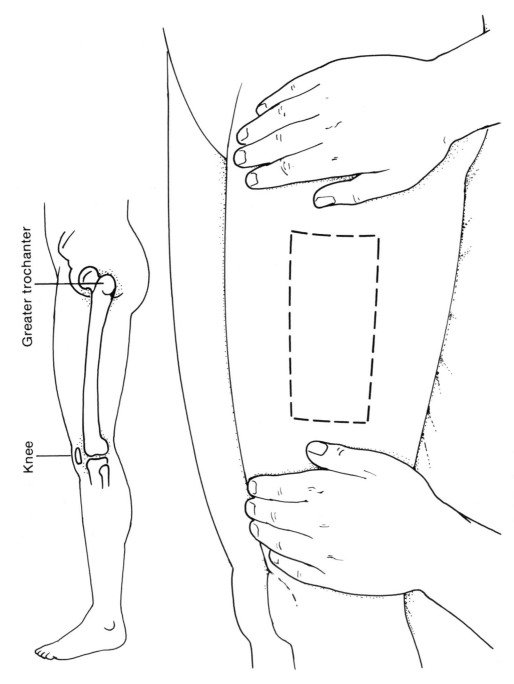

Figure 13-8. *Vastus lateralis injection site.*

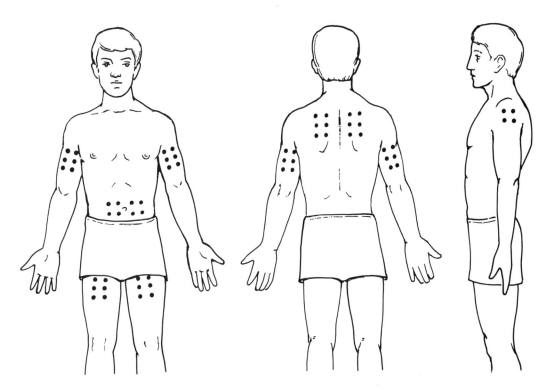

Figure 13-9. **(A, B)** *Sites for subcutaneous injection.* **(C)** *The deltoid muscle may be used for subcutaneous injections or, when ordered, small intramuscular injections.*

9. Make the skin taut by mounding the tissue between thumb and index finger or by spreading it firmly.
10. Dart the needle in quickly (Fig. 13-11).
11. Hold the barrel with your nondominant hand and with your dominant hand pull the plunger back. This is termed *aspiration* and is done to be sure the needle is not in a blood vessel.
12. If blood enters the syringe, withdraw the needle, discard the needle and syringe into a sharps container, and prepare another injection.
13. If no blood is aspirated, inject the medication slowly.
14. Remove the needle quickly.
15. Press down on the area with the alcohol pad or a dry gauze pad to inhibit bleeding.
16. Dispose of needle and syringe in a sharps container. *Do not recap the needle.* Make the patient comfortable. Wash hands. Chart the medication.

SPECIAL INJECTION TECHNIQUES

Subcutaneous Heparin

Prepare the medication in the usual way, using a syringe with a subcutaneous needle. This injection is given in the lower abdominal fold at least 2 inches from the umbilicus.

1. Make the tissue taut by pinching or spreading.
2. Inject the needle at a 90° angle.
3. *Do not aspirate.*
4. Inject slowly.
5. Remove needle quickly.
6. *Do not massage the area.*

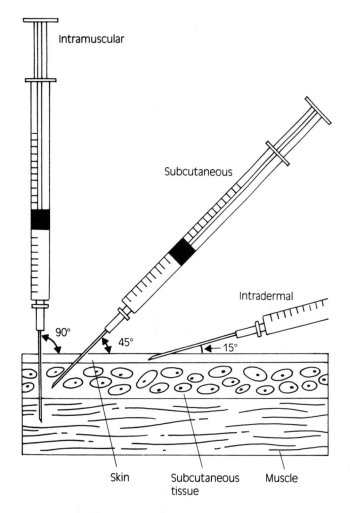

Figure 13-10. *An intradermal injection angle compared with IM and SC angles. (Taylor, C., Lillis, C., and LeMone, P.: Fundamentals of Nursing. Philadelphia: J. B. Lippincott, 1989, p. 1157.)*

Z-Track Technique for Intramuscular Injections

When medications, such as iron dextran (Imferon) and hydroxyzine (Vistazine), are irritating to the tissues and can stain the skin, this method may be used at the dorsogluteal site.

1. After preparing the medication, change the needle so that no medication is on the needle.
2. Add 0.2 cc of air to the syringe. As the medication is injected, the air will rise to the top of the syringe and will be administered last. This will seal off the medication and prevent its leakage to the skin.
3. Prepare the patient and the site in the usual manner.
4. Use the heel of your hand and retract the tissue to the side. *Hold this position during the injection* (Fig. 13-12).
5. Inject as usual at a 90° angle. Be sure to aspirate before injecting.
6. Count 10 seconds after giving the injection.
7. Remove the needle quickly.
8. Remove the hand that has been retracting the tissue.
9. *Do not massage the site.*
10. Use an alcohol pad or a dry gauze pad to press down on the area to inhibit bleeding.

Application to Skin and Mucous Membrane

Drug preparations are administered for their local effect or to act systemically. To achieve a systemic effect the drug must be absorbed into the circulation.

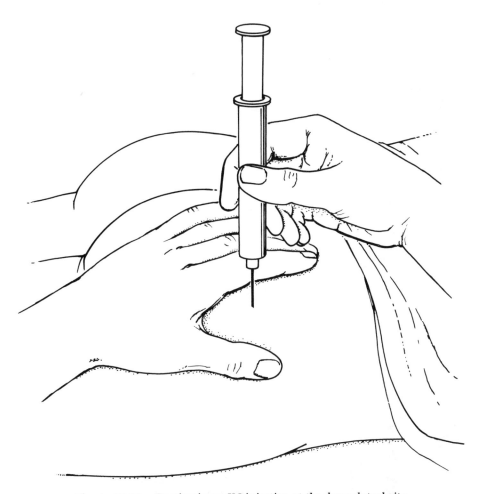

Figure 13-11. *Darting in an IM injection at the dorsogluteal site.*

BUCCAL TABLET (UNIVERSAL SAFEGUARD: HANDWASHING)

Identify the patient orally. Check the ID band. Explain the procedure and give the tablet to the patient. The patient should place the tablet between his gum and his cheek. The tablet should not be disturbed as it dissolves. Systemic absorption is rapid across mucous membranes. Doses should be alternated between cheeks to minimize irritation.

EAR DROPS (UNIVERSAL SAFEGUARD: HANDWASHING)

The ear drops will be labeled otic or auric. They should be warmed to body temperature. Greet the patient orally and check the ID band. Explain the procedure. Place the patient sitting in an upright position, with the head tilted toward his unaffected side, or lying on his side with the affected ear up. Be sure the patient is comfortable. With a dropper, draw the medication up. Straighten the ear canal by pulling the pinna up and back in the adult or down and back in a child 3 years or younger.

Place the tip of the dropper at the opening of the canal and instill the medication into the canal. The patient should rest on his unaffected side 10 to 15 minutes. A cotton ball may be placed in the canal if the patient wishes. Make sure the patient is comfortable. Wash hands. Chart the medication.

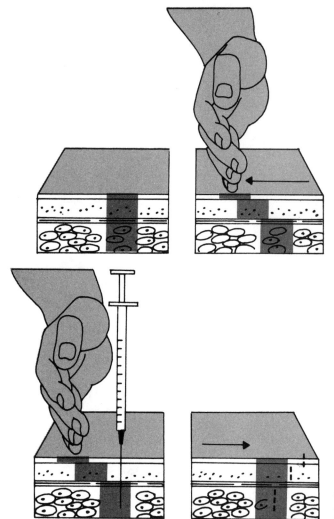

Figure 13-12. *"Z"-track technique—dorsogluteal site. The tissue is retracted to the side and held there while the injection is given. (Taylor, C., Lillis, C., and LeMone, P.: Fundamentals of Nursing. Philadelphia: J. B. Lippincott, 1989, p. 1161.)*

EYE DROPS OR OINTMENT (UNIVERSAL SAFEGUARD: GLOVES)

Greet the patient and check the ID band. Explain the procedure. Hand the patient a tissue. The patient may be sitting or lying down. If exudate is present, it may be necessary to cleanse the eyelid with cotton or gauze and either normal saline or distilled water for the eye.

Prepare the eye drops or uncap the ophthalmic ointment. Gently draw the lower eyelid down to create a sac (Fig. 13-13). Instruct the patient to look up. Instill the liquid medication into the lower conjunctival sac, taking care not to touch the membrane. The ophthalmic ointment should be placed from the inner to the outer canthus of the eye.

Instruct the patient to close his eyelids gently and rotate his eyes. The patient may use the tissue to wipe away excess medication. After instilling eye drops, have the patient apply gentle pressure with his index finger to the inner canthus for a minute. This action inhibits the medication from entering the tear duct.

When possible, each patient should have individual medication containers to prevent cross-contamination. Provide a safe environment if the medication impairs the patient's vision. Make the patient comfortable. Dispose of the gloves according to institutional procedure. Wash your hands and chart the medication.

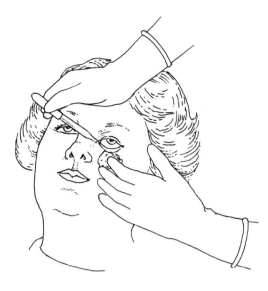

Figure 13-13. *Applying eye drops: Gently draw the lower eyelid down to create a pocket. Insert the medication into this pocket.*

NASOGASTRIC ROUTE (UNIVERSAL SAFEGUARD: GLOVES)

When possible, obtain the medication in liquid form. Before opening capsules or crushing tablets, check with the pharmacist for alternatives.

Dilute the medication with water. Greet the patient, check the ID band, and explain the procedure. Elevate the head of the bed when possible. Put on gloves. Insert the bulb syringe into the tube. Remove the clamp on the tube. Check the position of the tube in the stomach by (1) aspirating some stomach contents or (2) placing a stethoscope on the stomach and inserting about 15 ml of air. A swishing sound indicates proper placement.

Close off the tube by bending it on itself. Hold the bulb syringe and bent tube in your nondominant hand. Remove the bulb and leave the syringe in place.

Pour the medication into the bulb syringe. Release the tubing and allow the medication to flow in by gravity. *Do not force medication to flow by using pressure on the bulb.* If the patient shows discomfort, stop the procedure and wait until he or she appears relaxed.

Before all the medication flows in, flush the tube by adding 50 to 100 ml of water to the syringe. Shut the tube by bending it on itself before the bulb syringe completely empties. Clamp the tube and remove the bulb syringe. Make the patient comfortable. If possible, leave the head of the bed elevated. Dispose of gloves according to institutional procedures. Wash your hands. Chart the medication.

NOSE DROPS (UNIVERSAL SAFEGUARD: HANDWASHING)

Greet the patient, check the ID band, and explain the procedure. The patient may have to gently blow his nose to clear the nasal passageway. The patient may be sitting or lying down. Have the patient tilt his head back. In bed a pillow may be placed under the shoulders to hyperextend the neck. Draw up the medication. Insert the dropper about one-third into each nostril. Do not touch the nostril. Instill the nose drops. Instruct the patient to maintain the position 1 to 2 minutes. If the patient feels the medication flowing down his throat, he may sit up and bend his head down to allow the medication to flow into the sinuses.

The patient should have his own medication container to prevent cross-contamination. Make the patient comfortable. Wash your hands. Chart the medication.

RECTAL SUPPOSITORY (UNIVERSAL SAFEGUARD: GLOVES)

Greet the patient, check the ID band, and explain the procedure. Encourage the patient to defecate (unless the suppository is ordered for this purpose). Position the patient in the left lateral recumbent position (Fig. 13-14). Moisten the suppository with a water-soluble lubricant. Instruct the patient to breathe slowly and deeply through the mouth. Ask the patient to "bear down" as if having a bowel movement to open the anal sphincter. Insert the suppository past the sphincter, using a gloved finger. You will feel the suppository move into the canal. Wipe away excess lubricant. Encourage the patient to retain the suppository. Make the patient comfortable. Dispose of gloves according to institutional procedure. Wash your hands. Chart the medication.

The patient may insert his own suppository if he is able and wishes to do so. Provide a glove, lubricant, and suppository. Check to be sure the suppository was inserted and is not in the bed.

RESPIRATORY INHALER (UNIVERSAL SAFEGUARD: HANDWASHING)

An inhaler is a small, pressurized metal container that holds medication. It is accompanied by a mouthpiece. The following are general directions to teach the patient, who must carry out the procedure:

1. Shake the inhaler well immediately before use.
2. Remove the cap from the mouthpiece.
3. Breathe out fully; expel as much air as you can; hold your breath.
4. Place the mouthpiece in your mouth and close your lips around it. The metal inhaler should be upright.
5. While breathing in deeply and slowly, fully depress the metal inhaler with your index finger.
6. Remove the inhaler from your mouth and release your finger. Hold your breath for several seconds.
7. Wait 1 minute and shake the inhaler again. Repeat the steps for each inhalation prescribed. An order might read "Proventil Inhaler 2 puffs qid."
8. Cleanse the mouthpiece and cap by rinsing in warm running water at least once a day. When dry, replace the mouthpiece and cap.

The inhaler may be left at the bedside stand if the institution's policy permits. Make the patient comfortable. Wash your hands. Chart the medication.

SKIN APPLICATIONS (UNIVERSAL SAFEGUARD: GLOVES)

Greet the patient, check the ID band, and explain the procedure. Avoid personal contact with the medication to prevent absorption of drug. Apply the medication with a tongue blade, glove, gauze pad, or cotton-tipped applicator. Cleanse the area as appropriate before a new application.

Obtain the following information before proceeding, because many kinds of medicines are applied topically.

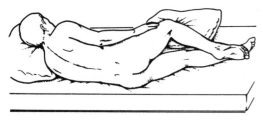

Figure 13-14. Left lateral recumbent position.

- The preparation of the skin
- The method of application
- Whether the skin should be covered or uncovered

Drug preparations include the following:

- Powders: sprinkle on your gloved hands and then apply. Use sparingly to avoid caking. Skin should be dry.
- Lotions: Pat on lightly. Use gloved hand or gauze pad.
- Creams: Rub into skin using gloves.
- Ointments: Use gloved hand or applicator. Apply an even coat and place a dressing on skin.

Make the patient comfortable. Dispose of gloves according to institutional policy. Wash your hands. Chart the medication.

Nitroglycerin Ointment (Universal Safeguard: Gloves)

Greet the patient, check the ID band, and explain the procedure. Take a baseline blood pressure and record. Don the gloves to protect yourself from contact with the drug, a potent vasodilator. Remove the previous dose and cleanse the skin.

Measure the prescribed dose in inches on the ruled paper that comes with the ointment. Select a nonhairy site on the trunk–chest, upper arm, abdomen, or upper back. If necessary, shave the area. (Seek advice before doing this.) Spread the measured ointment on the skin, using the ruled paper. Apply the ointment in a thin layer about 6 inches by 6 inches. **Do not rub.** Tape the ruled paper in place over the ointment. Cover the area with plastic wrap and tape the plastic in place. Check the patient's blood pressure within 30 minutes.

If a headache occurs or the blood pressure lowers, have the patient rest until the blood pressure returns to normal. Make the patient comfortable. Dispose of gloves according to institutional procedure. Wash your hands. Chart the medication.

Transdermal Disks, Patches, and Pads (Universal Safeguard: Handwashing)

These products are unit-dose adhesive bandages consisting of a semipermeable membrane that allows medication to be released continuously over time. Some patches are effective for 24 hours, some for 72 hours, and some last as long as 1 week.

The skin should be free of hair and not subject to excessive movement; therefore, avoid distal extremities. The site should be changed with each administration. If the patch loosens with bathing, apply a new pad.

Medications that can be administered by this route include hormones, antihypertensive drugs such as clonadine (Catapres), antimotion sickness drugs such as scopolamine, and nitroglycerin.

Greet the patient, check the ID band, and explain the procedure. Select the site. The skin should be clear and dry with no signs of irritation. Open the packet. Remove the cover from the adhesive transdermal drug. *Do not touch the inside of the pad.* Apply the pad to the skin. Press firmly to be certain all edges are adherent. Make the patient comfortable, wash your hands, and chart the medication.

SUBLINGUAL TABLETS (UNIVERSAL SAFEGUARD: HANDWASHING)

The most common sublingual medication is nitroglycerin, which is prescribed to abort an attack of angina pectoris. If relief is not felt in 5 minutes, a second and then a third tablet may be taken. Tolerance to nitroglycerin is common. If the pain is not relieved within 15 minutes, the physician should be notified.

To administer a sublingual tablet, greet the patient, check the ID band, and explain the procedure. Instruct the patient to sit down and place the tablet under the tongue. If the patient is unable to place the tablet under his tongue himself, wear a glove to place the tablet. The tablet should not be swallowed or chewed but allowed to dissolve. The patient should not eat or drink anything because this will interfere with the effectiveness of the medication. Stay with the patient until the pain is relieved. Consult an appropriate text for further information. Wash your hands and chart the medication.

URETHRAL SUPPOSITORY (UNIVERSAL SAFEGUARD: GLOVES)

Greet the patient, check the ID band, and explain the procedure. Encourage the patient to urinate. Leave the patient on the bedpan. Drape the patient, leaving the perineal area exposed. Put on sterile gloves. Cleanse the urinary meatus with an antiseptic solution. Place a sterile gauze pad over the meatus.

Remove the patient from the bedpan. Remove the first pair of gloves. Open a sterile gauze pad. Open the sterile suppository and aseptically place it on the gauze pad. Moisten the suppository with a sterile, water-soluble lubricant. Put on a second pair of sterile gloves.

Separate the labia and remove the gauze pad. Gently insert the urethral suppository. Cover the meatus with a gauze pad to collect secretions as the suppository melts. Make the patient comfortable. Dispose of gloves and equipment according to institutional policies. Chart the medication.

VAGINAL SUPPOSITORY OR TABLET (UNIVERSAL SAFEGUARD: GLOVES)

Greet the patient, check the ID band, and explain the procedure. Ask the patient to void in a bed pan. (If the perineal area has much secretion, it may be necessary to perform perineal care after the patient voids.) Insert the suppository or tablet into the applicator. Assist the patient into a lithotomy position (lying on the back with knees flexed and legs apart) and drape her, leaving the perineal area exposed. Put on sterile gloves.

Separate the labia majora and identify the vaginal opening. Insert the applicator up and back and eject the suppository or tablet into the vagina. (The patient may do this procedure herself if she wishes.) Place a 4 × 4 gauze pad at the opening to collect secretions. Make the patient comfortable before leaving.

Wash the applicator with soap and water, wrap it in a paper towel, and leave it at the bedside. Dispose of gloves and equipment according to institutional procedure. Chart the medication.

VAGINAL CREAM

The steps are the same as those for the vaginal suppository to the point at which the medication is inserted. The vaginal cream comes with its own applicator. Push the plunger of the applicator all the way into the barrel. Remove the cap from the tube of vaginal cream and screw the tube into the barrel of the applicator. Squeeze the tube to fill the barrel to the prescribed amount. Disconnect the tube and replace its cap. Insert the applicator into the vaginal canal up and back and press the plunger to empty the barrel of medication. (The patient may do this herself if she wishes.) Remove the applicator, clean it with soap and water, and place it in a clean paper towel in the bedside stand. Remove gloves.

Make the patient comfortable. She should remain in bed for a minimum of 20 minutes. Dispose of gloves according to institutional procedure. Chart the medication.

SELF-TEST 1

Give the information requested for universal safeguards in administering medications. Answers may be found at the end of the chapter.

1. Universal safeguards should be applied when administering medications
   a. to all patients
   b. only to patients with HIV or hepatitis B virus

2. The type of safeguard to be used by the nurse depends upon _____

   _____

3. In administering medications, gloves must be worn when

   _____ and

   _____

4. After administering an injection, the syringe should be placed _____

   _____

5. Five safeguards stressed by the Centers for Disease Control inform the nurse when to use

   _____ ,   _____ , and

   _____ ,   _____

   _____ ,

6. In administering medications, hands must be washed

   a. _____

   b. _____

   c. _____

   d. _____

7. General safeguards in administering medications advise the nurse to use a clamp to _____

   _____

8. A gown should be worn to protect the nurse's uniform whenever _____

   _____

9. Goggles should be worn whenever _____

   _____

   _____

10. A mask should be worn when

   _____ or

   _____

SELF-TEST 2

Decide whether the following actions are correct or incorrect according to the safeguards in administering medications; explain your choice. Answers may be found at the end of the chapter.

1. A nurse wears gloves to remove an intravenous heparin lock from a patient's arm. This action is

    _____

    _____

2. A nurse who has just removed a gown and gloves puts them into the proper disposal container in the patient's room and leaves the room. This action is _____

    _____

3. In the medication room, a nurse puts on gloves to prepare an IV for administration. This action is

    _____

    _____

4. A nurse puts on a mask to administer an oral medication to a patient on respiratory isolation precautions. This action is _____

    _____

5. A nurse applies universal safeguards in caring for all patients on the unit. This action is _____

    _____

    _____

6. A nurse wears gloves to place a transdermal pad behind a patient's ear. This action is _____

    _____

    _____

7. A nurse puts on gloves and gown to administer 500 ml of a vaginal douche to a lethargic patient. This action is _____

    _____

8. A nurse whose finger has been stuck with a contaminated IV needle carefully washes his hands with soap and water and applies a Band-aid to the site. Because the patient's diagnosis is brain tumor, the nurse decides no further action is necessary. This action is _____

    _____

    _____

9. A nurse giving an injection to a patient makes the judgment *not* to wear gloves. This action is _____

    _____

    _____

10. A nurse puts on gloves to administer an oral tablet to an alert patient with a positive HIV blood count. This action is _____

    _____

11. After administering an injection, the nurse carefully caps the needle. This action is _____

_____

_____

SELF-TEST 3

Supply the following information. Answers will be found at the end of the chapter.

1. The primary reason patients should have individual eye medication is to _____

_____

2. Two methods of checking the positioning of a nasogastric tube are _____

_____ and

_____

3. For administration of a rectal suppository, the patient should lie _____

_____

4. How should each of the following be applied to a patient's skin?

   a. Powders _____

   b. Lotions _____

   c. Creams _____

   d. Ointments _____

5. How many SL nitroglycerin tablets may a patient take to relieve pain? _____

   At what time interval? _____

6. Identify these administration procedures as clean or sterile.

   a. SC injection _____   f. Nitroglycerin ointment _____

   b. SL tablet _____   g. Urethral suppository _____

   c. Vaginal suppository _____   h. Nasogastric route _____

   d. Nose drops _____   i. Intradermal _____

   e. IM injection _____   j. Rectal suppository _____

7. How should a vaginal applicator be inserted? _____

8. How should the skin be prepared for an injection? _____

_____

9. List three reasons for administering medication by injection. _____

_____

_____

10. What is the difference in administering ear drops to an adult and a 2-year-old child? _____

_____

_____

SELF-TEST 4

1. The purpose of the medication ticket in the ticket system is to identify the drug from the time the order is written until it is
   a. transferred to the Kardex
   b. poured
   c. administered
   d. charted

2. Which of the following is an appropriate action regarding medication tickets in the ticket system?
   a. All tickets are checked against the physician's order sheet.
   b. Tickets are made out only for standing orders.
   c. A new ticket is written each time a drug is given.
   d. The ticket is destroyed after charting a stat order.

3. Checking the Kardex before administering medication by ticket will enable the nurse to determine
   a. the name of the physician who ordered the medication
   b. if some tickets have been misplaced
   c. if a "stat" medication is to be administered
   d. whether the patient can have the next prn dose

4. When pouring an oral liquid medication, the nurse should
   a. place the cup on the tabletop and bend over to get the right level
   b. hold the cup in the hand and pour to the top of the meniscus
   c. hold the cup at eye level and pour to the center of the meniscus
   d. rest the cup on the medication shelf and pour to the mark at the side of the cup

5. Which statement is *false* regarding injections from powders?
   a. Read the label twice before drawing up and once after.
   b. Draw up one medication at a time.
   c. Always use sterile water as a diluent.
   d. Pull back on the plunger before injecting the medication.

6. Withdrawing medication from a vial is facilitated if a specific amount of air is injected into the vial before hand. Which of these statements explains this action?
   a. It creates a partial vacuum in the vial.
   b. It makes the pressure in the vial greater than atmospheric pressure.
   c. It makes the pressure in the vial the same as atmospheric pressure.
   d. It makes the pressure in the vial less than atmospheric pressure.

7. If a patient has difficulty swallowing medications, which oral form of drug may be crushed?
   a. Sugar-coated tablet
   b. Enteric-coated tablet
   c. Buccal tablet
   d. Capsule

8. A major advantage in the unit-dose system of drug administration is that
   a. the drug supply is always available
   b. no error is possible
   c. the drugs are less expensive than stock distribution
   d. the pharmacist provides a second professional check

9. When a drug is to be administered sublingually, the patient should be instructed to
   a. drink a full glass of water when swallowing
   b. rinse the mouth with water after taking the drug

    c. chew the tablet and allow the saliva to collect under the tongue

    d. hold the medication under the tongue until it dissolves

10. Ampules differ from vials in that ampules

    a. are glass containers

    b. contain only one dose

    c. contain solids as well as liquids

    d. are not used for injections

11. The Z-track technique for injections can be used to

    a. administer more than one drug at a single site

    b. inhibit hematoma formation by promoting drug absorption

    c. prevent skin discoloration by inhibiting drug seepage

    d. reduce allergic reactions at the injection site

12. Which action is *correct* in giving a Z-track injection?

    a. The skin is retracted and held to one side while the medication is given.

    b. The skin is massaged after the injection is given.

    c. The plunger is not pulled back when the needle has been inserted.

    d. Medication is injected quickly.

13. Which angle of injection is *correctly* matched with the route of administration?

    a. Intradermal—45° angle

    b. Intramuscular—90° angle

    c. Subcutaneous—90° angle

    d. Z-track—45° angle

14. A patient asks how he should put drops in his eye. The nurse instructs the patient to place the drops

    a. into the lower conjunctival sac

    b. under the upper lid

    c. directly on the cornea

    d. in the inner canthus

15. In administering a vaginal suppository, which statement is *false?*

    a. Universal safeguards should be used.

    b. The patient may insert the medication.

    c. The patient should be lying on her back.

    d. The applicator must be kept sterile.

16. In applying the next dose of a transdermal medication, the nurse should

    a. shave the new area and prepare with povidone-iodine

    b. cleanse the previous area and use a different site

    c. rotate the use of arms and legs as sites

    d. allow the previous patch to remain on the skin

17. Which is the muscle of choice to be used when an injection is irritating to the tissues?

    a. Deltoid—SC

    b. Dorsogluteal—Z-track

    c. Ventrogluteal—intradermal

    d. Vastus lateralis—IM

(continued)

SELF-TEST 4 (*Continued*)

18. Discomfort of an injection is reduced when the needle is inserted
   a. slowly into loose tissue
   b. slowly into firm tissue
   c. rapidly into loose tissue
   d. rapidly into firm tissue

19. After administering an injection, the nurse should
   a. immediately recap the needle
   b. break the needle off the syringe for safety
   c. place the used syringe in a nearby sharps container
   d. don gloves to carry the syringe to the utility room

20. Which statement is *incorrect* in the administration of drugs to mucous membranes?
   a. Eye medications must be labeled ophthalmic.
   b. Patients may insert their own urethral suppositories.
   c. Buccal medications are applied to the space between the teeth and cheek.
   d. Eye medications may be left in the client's bedside stand.

ANSWERS

SELF-TEST 1

1. To *all* patients. There is a risk of potential exposure to hepatitis B virus and human immunodeficiency virus that may not have been detected by standard laboratory methods.
2. The type of contact the nurse has with the patient.
3. When there is any direct "hands on" contact with patient's blood, bodily fluids, or secretions
   When handling materials or equipment contaminated with blood or body fluids
4. In a labeled puncture-proof container
5. Handwashing, gloves, gowns, masks, and goggles
6. a. Before preparing medications and after administering medicines to each patient
   b. After removing gloves, gowns, masks, and goggles, and before leaving each patient
   c. Immediately when soiled with the patient's blood or body fluids
   d. After handling equipment soiled with blood or body fluids
7. Hold contaminated IV needles being carried to a puncture-proof container
8. The nurse's clothing may become contaminated with a patient's blood or body fluids
9. A nurse is in extremely close contact with the patient and there is possibility of the patient's blood or blood-tinged fluids being splashed or sprayed into the nurse's eyes or mucous membranes
10. The patient is placed on *strict* or *respiratory* isolation precautions; carrying out a medication procedure may cause blood or body fluids to splash directly on the nurse's face

SELF-TEST 2

1. Correct. As the needle or catheter is removed there is a possibility of bleeding at the site. In addition, the nurse should use a clamp to carry the needle or catheter to a puncture-proof container.
2. Incorrect. The nurse must wash his or her hands before leaving the room.
3. Incorrect. It is not necessary to wear gloves to prepare an IV because there is no contact at this time with the patient's blood or body fluids.
4. Correct. Universal safeguards state that a mask must be worn when the patient is on strict or respiratory isolation precautions.
5. Correct. There is a potential risk of exposure to hepatitis B virus and human immunodeficiency virus. Laboratory testing may not show the presence of the virus or antibodies to the virus.
6. Incorrect. Transdermal pads are applied to intact skin. There is no danger of contact with the patient's blood or body fluids.
7. Correct. In carrying out the vaginal douche there is a possibility of exposure to vaginal secretions.
8. Incorrect. The nurse should squeeze the finger and, after washing his hands with soap and water, scrub the area with povidone-iodine (Betadine) or another accepted antiseptic. In addition, the needlestick should be reported to the proper authority and the protocol for exposure to blood carried out. Universal safeguards apply to all patients regardless of the diagnosis.
9. Correct. It is not necessary to wear gloves in giving an injection. Handwashing is adequate unless there is danger of exposure to blood or body secretions. In injection technique, the alcohol swab acts as a mechanical barrier.
10. Incorrect. Because the patient is alert and can take the medicine cup from the nurse, handwashing is adequate.
11. Incorrect. The CDC guidelines advise the nurse not to recap a needle but to place it immediately in a puncture-proof container.

SELF-TEST 3

1. Prevent cross-contamination
2. Aspirate stomach contents; place a stethescope on the stomach and insert 15 ml of air. A swishing sound indicates proper placement.
3. On the left side—left lateral recumbent position
4. a. Sprinkle on gloved hands and apply; use sparingly to prevent caking
   b. Pat on lightly with gloved hand or gauze pad

    c. Rub into skin while wearing gloves

    d. Use a gloved hand to apply an even coat and cover with a dressing

5. Three tablets; 5 minutes apart

6.
a.	Sterile	**f.**	Clean
b.	Clean	**g.**	Sterile
c.	Clean	**h.**	Clean
d.	Clean	**i.**	Sterile
e.	Sterile	**j.**	Clean

7. Back and up

8. Rub the skin with an alcohol pad in a circular motion from the center of the site out

9. The drug would be destroyed orally; a rapid effect is desired; the patient is unable to take the drug orally

10. In the adult, pull the ear back and up. In a 2-year-old child, pull the ear back and down.

SELF-TEST 4

1.	d	**11.**	c
2.	d	**12.**	a
3.	b	**13.**	b
4.	c	**14.**	a
5.	c	**15.**	d
6.	b	**16.**	b
7.	a	**17.**	b
8.	d	**18.**	d
9.	d	**19.**	c
10.	b	**20.**	b

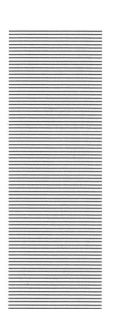

INDEX